Arterial Pollution

An Integrated View on Atherosclerosis

NATO Advanced Science Institutes Series

A series of edited volumes comprising multifaceted studies of contemporary scientific issues by some of the best scientific minds in the world, assembled in cooperation with NATO Scientific Affairs Division.

This series is published by an international board of publishers in conjunction with NATO Scientific Affairs Division

A	**Life Sciences**	Plenum Publishing Corporation
B	**Physics**	New York and London
C	**Mathematical and Physical Sciences**	D. Reidel Publishing Company Dordrecht, Boston, and London
D	**Behavioral and Social Sciences**	Martinus Nijhoff Publishers The Hague, Boston, and London
E	**Applied Sciences**	
F	**Computer and Systems Sciences**	Springer Verlag Heidelberg, Berlin, and New York
G	**Ecological Sciences**	

Recent Volumes in Series A: Life Sciences

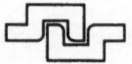

Arterial Pollution

An Integrated View on Atherosclerosis

Edited by

H. Peeters

Institute for Medical Biology
Brussels, Belgium

G. A. Gresham

The John Bonnett Clinical Labs
University of Cambridge
Cambridge, England

and

R. Paoletti

University of Milan
Milan, Italy

Plenum Press
New York and London
Published in cooperation with NATO Scientific Affairs Division

Proceedings of a NATO Advanced Study Institute on
Arterial Pollution: An Integrated view on Atherosclerosis,
held August 30–September 12, 1981,
in Maratea, Italy

Library of Congress Cataloging in Publication Data

NATO Advanced Study Institute on Arterial Pollution: an Integrated View on Atherosclerosis (1981: Maratea, Italy)
  Arterial pollution.

  (NATO advanced science institutes series. Series A, Life sciences; v. 58)
  "Proceedings of a NATO Advanced Study Institute on Arterial Pollution: an Integrated
View on Atherosclerosis, held August 30–September 12, 1981, in Maratea, Italy"—Ver-
so t.p.
  "Published in cooperation with NATO Scientific Affairs Division."
  Includes bibliographical references and index.
  1. Atherosclerosis—Congresses. I. Peeters, H. (Hubert), 1919–   . II. Gresham, G.
A. (Geoffrey Austin) III. Paoletti, Rodolfo. IV. North Atlantic Treaty Organization. Scientific
Affairs Division. V. Title. VI. Series.
RC692.N34 1981   616.1′36   82-24586
ISBN-13: 978-1-4684-4459-9   e-ISBN-13: 978-1-4684-4457-5
DOI: 10.1007/978-1-4684-4457-5

© 1983 Plénum Press, New York
Softcover reprint of the hardcover 1st edition 1983

A Division of Plenum Publishing Corporation
233 Spring Street, New York, N.Y. 10013

INTRODUCTION

This two week course on Arterial Pollution covered the field of atherosclerosis as a disease entity, and includes its anatomical, physiopathological, epidemiologic, preventive and therapeutic aspects.

With the cooperation of an outstanding group of international lecturers we have been able to present an overview of the disease and its accidents as it stands today. Such a scope differs greatly from the narrow workshops which only consider biochemical disorders, e.g., the lipoproteins or the risk factors.

We believe it was timely to study the entire physiopathological entity of arterial pollution and we included all aspects of the disease in one single sweep.

We are grateful to the Nato Advanced Institute Programs for accepting this topic on the list of their sponsored initiatives and especially Mr. di Lullo for his personal care.

Whether we succeeded was proved by the audience to the Nato Advanced Study Institute at Maratea in September 1981 and will become clearer through the audience these proceedings will gain in the medical community.

H. Peeters, editor
A. Gresham,
R. Paoletti, co-editors

CONTENTS

AN INTEGRATED VIEW ON ATHEROSCLEROSIS

Hubert Peeters

Institute for Medical Biology
Alsembergsesteenweg 196
B-1180   Brussels

It is the originality of the proceedings of the Nato Institute on Arterial Pollution held in Maratea (Italy) in September 1981 to give a balanced, integrated and comprehensive course on atherosclerosis not available at any teaching institution.

This Institute on 'ARTERIAL POLLUTION' was intended to describe the problem of atherosclerosis as a whole. The advances made over the last years in several domains - such as the physiology of lipoproteins, drug therapy - are usually documented in isolation but a general assessment of the interaction of these various domains has not been made.

The younger workers in the field are often not aware of the interactions between a host of problems that need to be solved in order to interpret the human atherosclerotic disease. They often specialize in one biochemical subtopic without sufficient reference to the thrombotic accident in man. The senior workers are better acquainted with general trends in food, diet, excercise patterns but less well with biochemical progress.

This means that a synthesis of our knowledge will cause interaction and correct or open perspectives between readers of several disciplines.

We aimed at a faculty with a BALANCED OUTLOOK on the many aspects of atherosclerosis in the presence of a student body eager to get a complete picture of the disease as a social and individual problem, as a biochemical entity, as a disease subjected to many unknown causes and predisposing factors.

1

A college of lecturers pertaining to several disciplines (pathology, epidemiology, pharmacology, biochemistry, internal medicine
etc...) was mustered for this occasion for a series of interactive
sessions.

Basically the Course was planned as follows.

1. Natural history of the disease :

This includes a description of the arterial lesion, the genesis of
the accident which can occlude a vital artery, the problem of
regression which is of great importance if therapy is to be efficient, a description of the incidence in modern times under so
called Western living conditions.
We assumed that the arterial lesion, the thrombotic accident, its
selective location e.g. coronary, cerebral or peripheral, the
recovery from an accident, the possibility of regression of lesions
and the epidemiology of these phenomena would all pertain to the
natural history of the disease.

2. Risk factors :

Risk factors can be subdivided into 5 subtopics.
  1. Inborn congenital disoders
  2. Environmental risk such as type of work, job stress, distur-
     bance due to circadian rhythm.
  3. Individual risk factors, such as hormone and sex-linked in-
     fluences, problems of diet including overweight, type of
     diet - lipids or carbohydrates - alcohol consumption, smo-
     king, sedentarity and lastly stress.
  4. Under the metabolic risk factors we considered arterial meta-
     bolism, the heart muscle itself and lipoproteins.
  5. Lastly platelets and coagulation play a pertinent role in the
     vascular accident.

3. Experimental approach :

Several animal models have been used extensively in connection with
the simulation of the metabolic disorders in man and the discovery
of drug therapy. Only a low percent of these experiments has lead
to the introduction of new drugs in man. In theory induction
procedures for the different model animals, the type, location and
regression of lesions and the extrapolation of such data to man
after experimental diet and therapy should be considered.

4. Prevention :

Recommended diets, their caloric and percent composition, the type
of protein, the type of lipid and the type of fiber would be

considered and next to that exercise programs, campaigns against
smoking etc. should be documented.

5. Therapy :

Drugs, derived from animal trials, have been only moderately
successful. Their aim is often to lower cholesterol. However
plasmalipids and lipoproteins require a more sophisticated
approach to evaluate drug effect.
After the accident, agents reducing the danger of further thrombotic accidents and some interventional measures, such as surgery,
become of importance.
It was considered that not only drugs with a cholesterol or triglyceride lowering effect but maybe also drugs improving on the
phospholipid quality of lipoproteins would be important and that
anti-coagulants would be described in their protective role against
thrombosis. Among the interventional measures surgery and plasma
exchange would be considered.

6. Prospective :

A balanced presentation of the problem of arterial pollution questions some a priori ideas about the disease. We should be induced
into fresh ways of discussing the problem and into new possibilities regarding the management of arterial pollution.
This last section would not only include an evaluation of
controversial issues but also describe new perspectives in
prevention and therapy.

     When these proceedings were prepared for publication we decided
on a slightly different outline partly because one can always
improve on a previous subdivision, and also the type and number
of papers available induced us to accept a new scheme. We decided
to start with NATURAL HISTORY,followed by ANIMAL MODELS. Next came
PHYSIOPATHOLOGY in which there are 4 subdivisions : the arterial
wall, the myocardium, the lipoproteins and the hemostatic mechanism.
EPIDEMIOLOGY AND RISK are followed by PREVENTION AND REGRESSION of
the disease and the last chapter is devoted to THERAPEUTIC MEASURES.

     At this point I would like to add a fresh idea that aroused
from the meetings discussions suggesting a specific role for apoprotein AII in HDL.
The AII polypeptide is a dimer in man and chimpanzee against
a monomer in rhesus and baboon. The small differences between
monomer and dimer are the presence of a cysteine bridge plus the
inversion of two amino acids. The HDL phospholipid distribution
on the contrary is different in the two groups of primates as can
be seen in table 1. Man and Chimpanzee have an HDL Lecithin to
Sphingomyelin ratio of about 6 against 14 in the Baboon and 20 in
the Rhesus.

Table 1 : Percent sphingomyelin and lecithin in HDL Phospholipids

		Sphingomyelin	Lecithin
Dimeric apo AII-	Man	13	75
	Chimpanzee	13	80
Monomeric Apo AII	Baboon	6	81
	Rhesus	4	88

This certainly stresses the importance of differences in polypeptide composition for the lipid distribution and the function of a lipoprotein. Let us also observe that the mutation of AII to a dimer in Man and Chimpanzee coincides with the appearance of spontaneous atherosclerosis in these species.

We would like to establish an analogy between this situation and this of the apo E mutants. An EII homozygote patient appears as being EIII deficient. The difference between EII and EIII lies in its primary structure and in the appearance of a second cystein-bridge in the EII mutant. This sequential modification leads to a different configuration of the polypeptide and influences the quality of HDL as a ligand towards the lipoprotein receptors on the cell surface. These facts are proposed to interpret dyslipoproteinemia of type III.

Let us now return to Apo AII. If the affinity of AII dimers for the LDL receptors was different from that of monomoners an HDL containing dimeric AII would compete differently for the protein receptor sites. The human primate could thus be in a phylogenetically inferior position to manipulate LDL with the consequences of increasing LDL circulation in the plasma to levels which are inexistent in baboon or rhesus and also causing intracellular lipid trouble ending up in arterial pollution.

Thus the dimeric AII mutant normally present in man could help to interpret why man is prone to become atherosclerotic, a disease which seems linked to his status in the animal kingdom.

The sequence and the steric structure of an AII dimer could influence the binding of HDL to the lipoprotein receptors at the cell surface and for this reason act as a general predisposing factor for atherosclerosis. In the light of this hypothesis the production of cystein free human monomeric AII by genetic manipulation could turn into a causal substitution therapy of atherosclerosis.

Looking for new relationships within a body of established facts excites our imagination to try out new ways of thinking about such a complex syndrome as arterial pollution.

After a few decennia of research the hardening of the arteries of man remains greatly unsolved. To make headway through the chalk of a hardened arterial wall seems to be a difficult task. We are still inside the tunnel. Hopefully the interaction between the papers of these proceedings will generate fresh knowledge about arterial pollution.

ATHEROSCLEROSIS: ITS ORIGINS
AND DEVELOPMENT IN MAN

G. A. Gresham

Professor of Morbid Anatomy

University of Cambridge

HISTORY

Arterial disease has been described in Egyptian mummies of the second century B.C.[1] However these lesions are not atherosclerotic but consisted of the medial calcification of Monckeberg's sclerosis which is well developed in the long arteries of the limbs. Anatomical descriptions of atherosclerosis were first made in the eighteenth and nineteenth centuries but the clinical features of coronary artery disease did not become manifest until the start of the twentieth century.

Sir William Osler did not mention heart attacks in the lectures that he gave in 1910 and the first clinical description of coronary artery thrombosis was given by Herrick in 1912. Since 1956 heart attacks have become increasingly frequent until ischaemic heart disease is now the principal killer in the Western World. There are strange variations in the incidence of ischaemic heart disease which are not entirely explicable in terms of the known, so called, risk factors. Only 50% of the incidence of the disease is, in fact, explicable in terms of exposure to risk factors such as diet, smoking and so on. For example France, Japan and China have a low incidence Sweden and Scotland have high rates. An extreme example is provided by the Masai of East Africa; a tribe of nomadic herdsmen living on a staple diet of milk supplemented by blood and meat.

Furthermore the milk of the Masai zebra cattle has
higher total lipids including cholesterol compared to
milk drunk in the United States of America. Despite this
their blood cholesterol and β lipoprotein levels are low
and clinical and autopsy evidence of coronary artery
disease is sparse. The explanation for this appears to
be a highly efficient negative feed back control mechanism
of endogenous synthesis of cholesterol which prevented
hypercholesterolaemia. This is a particularly important
observation because it shows that one cannot use isolated
parameters such as the dietary levels of cholesterol as
a pragmatic factor for the development of coronary
artery disease. Established notions of this sort have
seriously restricted advances in our understanding of the
process of atherogenesis. One needs to look at lipid
metabolism as a whole and the artery as a whole. It is
also important to keep a flexible approach to the potential ways in which arteries can react. They can, and do
behave like any other tissue responding by inflammation
repair, hypertrophy, hyperplasia and even neoplasia. It
is also important to look at atherosclerosis from the
comparative point of view for differences in incidence
and complications of the disease in different animal
species may point the way to factors involved in atherogenesis. In this respect severe atherosclerosis with its
complication of vasothrombosis is a disease of man. Minor
degrees of the disease occur in non human primates and in
other animals but only in man is it a prime cause of
morbidity and death. This anthropophilic tendency of
atherosclerosis should always be in the forefront of the
mind when trying to explain the occurence of the disease.

THE ATHEROSCLEROTIC SEQUENCE

There is no such thing as a typical artery and it is
unwise to extrapolate changes that can be induced in
one vessel, such as the aorta, to explain the occurrence
in another such as the coronary artery. Arteries vary
in structure and in their propensity to disease in
different parts of the human body. For example the
degree of atherosclerosis in the aorta correlates fairly
well with that in the coronary arteries. However there
is no such good correlation with atherosclerosis in the
cerebral vessels. Aortic, coronary and cerebral atherosclerosis only correlate well when hypertension is present.

    Human arteries also differ from animal arteries
especially in respect of their blood supply by the

vasa vasorum. Human arteries are the least well supplied
by vasa of all animal species. The wall of major vessels
is made up of stacks of lamellar units composed of
smooth muscle, elastin and collagen laid one upon the
other and yet only the outer half of the artery wall is
supplied by vasa vasorum. The inner part relies for
its nutriment on diffusion from the vessel lumen. It
follows that any process that leads to initial thickening
will imperil the inner part of the vessel wall.

Intimal changes start early in human life and vessel
wall changes have been described in stillborn babies.
De Sa[3] studied 286 stillbirths and infants and found
coronary artery lesions in 79 and myocardial necrosis in
111. The coronary artery lesions were associated with
conditions that might have caused severe hypoxia. It
is likely that the hypoxia caused inner medial damage to
the artery because of its impoverished blood supply
and that reparative intimal changes followed this. The
myocardial lesions are probably also a reflection of
damage to the inner myocardium which, like the artery,
is poorly supplied by its vasa vasorum which are the
coronary arteries.

Apart from the very early changes of this sort there
is a progressive thickening of the human arterial
intima that runs throughout life. It starts in childhood as a diffuse thickening composed of smooth muscle,
elastin and collagen and is followed in adolescence by
frank atherosclerotic disease. A detailed analysis
of these early changes and their possible relationship
to atherosclerosis is important because it now seems
clear that the foundations of atherosclerotic disease
are laid down in childhood. It is also clear that any
attempts to prevent atherosclerotic disease and
particularly that occuring in the coronary arteries
must be made in children and not in adults. Atherosclerosis is a paediatric problem.[4]

There is still considerable controversy about the
stages of development of atherosclerosis from birth to
old age. The arguments are concerned with the relationship of intimal thickening which Jores[5] considered to
be a normal age change to atherosclerosis and whether
the fatty streak or spot is the earliest visible
manifestation of the disease.

Intimal thickening appears in the first 3 or 4
decades of life and progresses during that period;

after that there is little further to see. In a recent
study in my laboratory we have examined serial block
sections of the coronary arteries from subjects in the
age groups 0 to 50. This has shown that the intimal
thickening is in two parts. The first to develop is a
musculo-elastic layer which is of fairly uniform thickness. Like Jores I think that this is a response to
progressive haemodynamic changes occurring with
increasing age. However, we have also shown a
subsequent development of a nodular intimal layer
internal to the first one. This is of irregular
thickness and can be regarded as focal proliferative
responses to arterial injury of one sort or another.
Movat et al [6] maintain that "atherosclerosis is most
severe in regions where the diffuse intimal thickening
is most marked". They also say that "the absence of
spontaneous arteriosclerosis in animals which show no
age changes in the intima strongly suggest that diffuse
intimal thickening predisposes to the development
of arteriosclerosis". However, animals do develop
intimal thickening. Stary and Strong [7] and several
subsequent authors have described diffuse and nodular
intimal thickenings in non-human primate coronary
arteries. The animals do not have visible atherosclerosis, nor do non-human primates develop it
subsequently.

Intimal thickenings have been studied from
different populations having different degrees of
atherosclerosis. There have been several reports and
they are contradictory. This is probably because of
failure to distinguish diffuse uniform thickening from
the later developing nodular variety. Other studies have
claimed that the intimal layer is thicker in newborn
male as compared to female infants. [8] This was said to
explain the greater tendency of the male to develop
atherosclerosis. Others however found that intimal
thickening began at birth but that there was no
difference between the sexes before the age of 20. [9] The
stimuli that cause diffuse intimal thickening in man are
still by no means clear. However, studies of hypertensive children indicate the important role of raised
blood pressure [10]. These workers found diffuse intimal
thickening of considerable degree twice as often as
atheromata in the children's coronary arteries.

Another important aspect of the early changes centres
upon studies of the internal elastic membrane of coronary
arteries at various stages of life. [11] These workers

examined arteries of 536 subjects up to the age of
40 years; about half of the number being males and half
females. They found changes in the internal elastic
lamella such as fragmentation and elastolysis. These
changes were less well developed in females from birth
to adolescence than they were in males. Furthermore the
intima was not so thick in females. Curiously enough the
sex differences were better seen in the left than in the
right coronary artery. The changes were conspicuous in
the left anterior descending and circumflex but not so
well seen in the right coronary artery. Furthermore
these intimal differences correlated well with the
incidence and distribution of atherosclerotic lesions in
men and women in later life. For example women tend to
develop plaques a decade later than men and the incidence
of atherosclerotic disease in three vessels in women was
about half of that in men.

     Another intimal change which increases steadily from
childhood to old age is the finding of small areas of
necrosis. These have been referred to already in the
study of still born and neonates. The change extends
centrifugally along the coronary vessels as age increases.
The histological features of the necrotic areas fall
broadly into three groups. These are mucoid, oedematous
or dissecting forms. The incidence of the change was
more frequent in males and was related[12] to the main
factors for coronary heart disease.

     The important question is whether this bewildering
array of intimal changes has any bearing on the
subsequent development of atherosclerosis. We have
already indicated that there is a correlation and it is
now possible to blend all of the observations into a
working hypothesis. Part of the intimal thickening may
be due to changing haemodynamic forces in arteries with
increasing age. The principal one being hypertension.
Other parts of the intimal thickening may be a reaction
to insudation of plasma constituents, such as lipoproteins, into the vessel wall because of altered endothelial permeability. Intimal necrosis is probably a
reflection of poor nutrition of the inner vessel wall
due to the lack of blood supply from the vasa vasorum.
This may be aggravated by spasm which is a factor that
has only recently been considered as a potential atherogenic agent. The subsequent development of clinical
atherosclerosis is superimposed on these intimal
processes which can all be regarded as an exudative and
proliferative response to vessel wall injury. The prime

injurious factor being ischaemia of the vessel walls.
It is reasonable to regard atherosclerosis as a proliferative response to vascular injury and all later changes
such as accumulation of lipid, fibrin, lipoprotein and
so on as a secondary event.

The cell that initiates and perpetuates this
response is the proliferating smooth muscle cell also
called a myointimal cell or myofibroblast.[13] It is the
same cell seen in healing wounds, reactive proliferations
of the connective tissues and so on. The myofibroblast
possesses much of the apparatus and functional properties
of fibroblasts and smooth muscle cells and is involved
in elastogenesis as well. Furthermore proliferation of
these cells is encouraged by a growth stimulating
factor derived from blood platelets. This links together
the thrombogenic and lipid insudation hypothesis of atherogenesis.

The next sequence of events in arteries is also
controversial, discussion having centred to a
large extent on the origin and subsequent fate of the
so-called fatty streak or spot. This a frequent lesion
in the arteries of adolescents appearing as a barely
raised streak or spot early in the carotid sinus region
of the internal carotid artery, above the aortic valve
cusps in the aorta and in the posterior thoracic aorta
in relation to the orifices of intercostal arteries.
They are particularly well seen after staining the whole
specimen with Sudan dyes. Even so more lesions are
invisible to the naked eye and are not demonstrable by
their sudanophilia. They can however be detected micro-
scopically.Velican and Velican[14] showed that coronary
atherosclerotic plaques were revealed only by microscopy
in 12% of adolescents and 28% of young adults. All the
plaques in adolescents and one third of them in young
adults escaped recognition on microscopic examination.
With increasing age the lesions extended centrifugally
down the coronary arterial tree. The initial site of
predilection in the main trunks of the coronary arteries
strongly suggests the operation of a local haemodynamic
factor affecting flow in that area. This could simply
be the kinking of the main trunks which can be shown
to occur angiographically at each heart beat.

Even at this early stage the plaques in adolescents
narrowed the lumen of undilated vessels by 55%; in young
adults the narrowing was 65%. Some of the plaques
contained no lipid but were of the gelatinous or mucoid

variety characterised by oedema, depolymerised mucopolysaccharide and collagen. The question arises
whether this is a potential fatty streak that has not
yet accumulated lipid or whether it is a different sort
of lesion. The partial answer to this might stem from the
observation that mucoid plaques were positively
associated with a history of cigarette smoking whereas
the lipid comtaining lesions were not.

The nature and fate of the fatty streak is of
considerable importance because lesions of this kind are
the ones most often found and produced experimentally in
other animals. If, as has been suggested, the fatty
streak is not the precursor of adult atheroma then much
of the research into atherogenesis in experimental
animals is invalid.

The major evidence for this controversy comes from
the International Atherosclerosis Project.[15] Aortas and
coronary arteries from 23,207 autopsies were examined and
the extent of fatty streaks, raised lesions and complicated lesions was estimated. The extent of aortic fatty
streaks did not predict the occurrence of raised lesions
in later life. In white populations there was a
relationship between fatty streaks in the coronary
arteries and raised lesions in later life. However, this
relationship did not hold for black people.

The clue to this problem is related to the factors
that may lead to progression, and more important
regression of fatty streaks and spots. There is a good
deal of human and experimental animal evidence for
regression.[16] It is thus not inconceivable that atherosclerotic lesions come and go in the young person
related to the growth and development of a vessel like
the aorta and the changing pressures within it. The
case for the fatty streak as a lesion independent of the
atherosclerotic sequence has not been convincingly made
as yet. As with other lesions in other tissues one must
be prepared to accept that lesions may heal and
disappear when the causative stimulus is removed.

Another probable explanation of the controversy of
the fate of the fatty streaks may lie in the fact that
not all fatty streaks are the same and that two lesions
may develop independently. The evidence comes from a
study of isoenzymes in the lesions. Black American
females who are heterozygous for glucose-6-phosphate
dehydrogenase show a mosaic of isoenzymes A and B in

most tissues including the arterial wall. However fibrous
plaques contain mostly one enzyme or the other. Fatty
streaks for the most part resemble normal arterial wall
in their isoenzyme pattern. However a minority of fatty
streaks show clonal characteristics intermediate between
normal artery and fibrous plaques. Intermediate clonal
streaks were found to be most frequent in middle age.
So it may well be that the more typical fatty streaks
have disappeared by this time and only those remain that
will evolve into fibrous plaques.[17]

    Observations on the fate of fatty streaks vary
according to the artery examined. In the carotid sinus
area of the internal carotid artery fatty streaks are
seen early in life and their conversion to fibrous
plaques and complicated lesions is progressive. Likewise coronary artery fatty streaks in youth are correlated with a tendency to form raised lesions later in
life. This observation comes from a geographical study
of the pathology of atherosclerosis which also showed
that aortic fatty streaks were less closely related to
the tendency to develop raised lesions.[18]

    Another interesting piece of evidence supports the
view that fatty streaks and dots and more advanced
lesions are related. This comes from two autopsy studies
ten years apart. The first study of material collected
between 1960 and 1968 showed that fatty streaks were
present in the youngest age group (10 - 14 years) and
were more extensive in blacks than whites. In the aorta
fatty streaks were replaced by fibrous plaques in later
life and by more advanced lesions subsequently. Raised
lesions in the aorta were most frequent and extensive
in white men. White women, black men and women had
fewer raised aortic lesions than white men. Raised
lesions in the coronary arteries were more extensive in
white men followed in order by black men, black women
and white women least of all. Sex differences were much
more conspicuous in the white race.[19]   The second study
for New Orleans was made on material collected between
1969 - 1972 when the mortality from coronary heart
disease was declining in the U.S.A. The area of coronary
intimal surface having raised atherosclerotic lesions
was considerably less in white men than in the previous
study. The extent in black men was little changed.[20]

    The next lesion to be considered in the athero-
sclerotic sequence is the fibrous plaque. When it is
heavily laden with lipid it can be called an atheroma.

It is important to recognise this entity which contributes a great deal to the occlusive effect of lesions
in the coronary arteries.

Fibrous plaques contain much collagen when examined histologically the fibrous tissue forming a cap
on the surface of the lesion with lipid in the deeper
parts. Chemical analysis confirms that 40 to 60% of
the dry mass of the lesion is collagen. The source of
the collagen in the lesions is a matter of debate. Some
say that it derives from transformed smooth muscle cells
consequent upon injury to the vessel wall. The
transformation of the smooth muscle cell to a collagen
secreting cell is mediated by the presence of intact
overlying endothelium. How this effect is produced is
not known.[21] Others argue that the presence of
cholesterol and its esters in the vessel wall stimulate
a granulomatous response which proceeds to the formation
of a fibrous plaque. Some esters of cholesterol have
been shown to be more fibrogenic than others. However
the effects of such fibrogenic esters may be modified
by the presence of phospholipid in the arterial wall.
This lipid opposes the fibrogenic action and may
explain the variable degree of fibrosis related to
deposits of arterial cholesterol.[22] There is yet
another view that the deposition of cholesterol in the
vessel wall is merely a deposition of lipid in dead
tissue. This is a universal pathological phenomenon
in many damaged tissues throughout the body.

Movat et al comment on the lack of reactive fibrosis
to early deposition of lipid in the arterial wall. They
consider that the production of collagen in the lesion
is due to the organisation of thrombi which are
progressively layered on to the fatty lesions.[24] This is
essentially reiterating the thrombogenic hypothesis of
atherogenesis which was first promulgated by Rokitansky.
This view is not now widely held and attention has
concentrated on the modified smooth muscle cell as a
producer of collagen and elastin. There are however
other cells including endothelial cells themselves
capable of subserving this function. The smooth muscle
cell is the particular favourite because it is
stimulated to proliferate by many factors associated
with enhanced atherosclerosis. For example β lipoproteins, a factor in the serum of diabetics and a
factor in the serum of patients with chronic renal
failure who are undergoing dialysis, all stimulate the
proliferation of smooth muscle cells. Patients with

hyperbetalipoproteinaemia, diabetes mellitus and chronic
renal failure are all liable to develop atherosclerosis
prematurely. There is also a factor derived from blood
platelets which will stimulate smooth muscle cell growth
so it may well be that some elements at least, of the
incrustation process are factors in atherogenesis.

The collagen content of arteries increases with age
and varied according to the vessel that was examined.
The collagen content of the normal intima varied from
16% in the young to 40% in the old. Fatty streaks
however contain about 26% of collagen and gelatinous
lesions have about 29%. Elastin on the other hand forms
about 20% of the intima in young people and 16% in the
elderly. Even less elastin (about 7 to 17%) is found
in the fibrous plaque.

The type of collagen present in the lesions is of
some interest. At the present time six basic types of
collagen are known (Table 1) and different sorts of cells
synthesise varied amounts of each type. For example, the
smooth muscle cell which plays such an important part in
the formation of the atherosclerotic lesion synthesises
Type I, III and IV. However, recent analyses of
collagen content of different parts of the artery have
revealed some provoking results. Examination of the
aortic media reveals 30% Type I collagen and 70% of Type
III whereas the pooled material from the intima showing
atherosclerosis shows 65% Type I and 35% Type III
collagen. This latter ratio of collagen types is much
more like that produced by fibroblasts. Furthermore,
electron microscopy reveals cells in the intima that
resemble fibroblasts rather than smooth muscle cells.
These results challenge the view held by some that the
proliferating smooth muscle cell is the basic process in
atherosclerosis. We are at present investigating the
distribution of different collagen types in the arterial
wall using fluorescent antisera to types of collagen
which may throw new light on the problems.

There is clearly a good deal of work yet to be done
in order to determine the precise histogenesis of the
fibrous lesion. Most of the evidence which has, so far,
been adduced supports the notion that atherosclerosis is
essentially a proliferative response to vascular injury.
A more difficult problem is to define the nature of such
injury or injuries which start to operate in childhood.
The further progression of the fibrous plaque is into the
more complicated lesion. These complications take the

form of calfication, medial degeneration and aneurysm
formation and superimposed thrombosis. The precise
trigger leading to thrombosis which may totally occlude
a coronary artery is not clear. Some consider that
stasis in the narrowed artery is the main factor, others
regard breaks of the plaque surface as essential.
Another view is related to the hypercoagulability of
blood in the vessel and another postulates haemorrhage
from capillaries within the plaque as the cause.

TABLE   1

COLLAGEN

TYPE   I   :-   BONE, TENDON, SKIN, VESSELS

TYPE   II   :-   CARTILAGE, EYE

TYPE III   :-   SKIN, VESSELS, SMOOTH MUSCLE ORGANS

TYPE   IV   :-   BASEMENT MEMBRANES

COLLAGEN A) BOTH RESEMBLE TYPE IV
)
)   ARE
)
COLLAGEN B) SYNTHESISED BY HUMAN
                SMOOTH MUSCLE CULTURE

Constantinides [25] studied thrombosed coronary
arteries and in every case where thrombi were present
he found cracks or fissures in the surface of the
atheromatous plaques. These cracks were overlain by the
older parts of the thrombi which suggested that it was
the fissure that initiated the thrombus formation and
this was followed by further extension of the thrombus.
The fissures tended to occur at the edges of atherosclerotic plaques but the reason for the fissuring has
not been fully explained.

Hellstrom[26] provides evidence in favour of a vasospastic
cause for coronary thrombosis. He explains that the
thrombus often contains extruded lipid debris from the
plaque. This could be caused by vascular spasm which
would also cause fracturing of the plaque surface.
Once the plaque surface is ruptured subendothelial
collagen is exposed, platelets adhere to it and
thrombosis results.

Aneurysms tend to form in the atherosclerotic
abdominal aorta but they may also occasionally be found
on the coronary arteries. They are the result of damage
to the arterial media probably largely due to ischaemia.
This is due to the great thickening of the intima which
impedes the diffusion of nutrients from the lumen of the
vessel wall. Spasm may also be a contributory factor
here because it also reduces wall diffusion leading to
hypoxia. Some have suggested that dissecting aneurysms
of the thoracic aorta which often occur in areas free of
atherosclerosis may also be caused by inner medial
ischaemia and subsequent necroses are due to aortic
spasm.

Calcification is a common accompaniment of the
atherosclerotic process. It is due to the deposition
of hydroxyapatite crystals on to elastic tissue coated
with mucopolysaccharide. It is seen more frequently in
the elderly and in hyperlipidaemic subjects. Precisely
why the hydroxyapatite is deposited on to elastic
tissue is not clear but it has been suggested that the
mechanism is ion binding by the mucopolysaccharide
coupled with the unmasking of polar amino acids of[27]
elastin with increasing age. The prevalence of
occlusions or of complicated lesions in the coronary
arteries is greater in ones with aortic calcification.
As might be expected if aortic calcification is also
an age change the significance of the presence of aortic
calcification in relation to coronary artery disease is
greater in the younger age groups.(ie. 30 to 50 rather
than 50 to 70).[28]

The effect of occlusive atheroma of the coronary
arteries upon the myocardium is greatly affected by the
extent of the coronary collateral circulation that may
develop. Widespread arterial anastomoses exist in the
normal heart especially in the epicardium. Anastomoses
can also be found between the coronary circulation and
the bronchial arteries. In a small proportion of cases
where all three main coronary arteries are blocked the

myocardium contrives to survive by means of these anastomoses with atrial and sino-atrial nodal vessels. A
variety of injection techniques have been used to
demonstrate the cardiac collateral circulation however
the mere demonstration of vessels does not necessarily
mean that they are functional. Opening up of these
collaterals after coronary occlusion depends upon a
variety of factors. These are the speed of development
of occlusion, the location of the occlusion, whether
it is proximal or distal in the artery and the presence
or absence of occlusions in other vessels in the heart.
A particularly important point affecting the opening of
collaterals is, of course, the level of pressure in the
local circulation.

After coronary occlusion the collateral arterioles
dilate the factors involved being chemical and haemo-
dynamic.With the passage of time the arterioles become
converted into arteries and become tortuous as well as
dilated.

This survey of the natural history of atherosclerosis reveals many points of controversy that still
require resolution. Further experimental work is
proceeding but is especially important in attempts to
demonstrate prevention and regression of the disease.

REFERENCES

1. M. A. Ruffer, On arterial lesions found in Egyptian
       mummies (1580 B.C. - 525 A.D.), J. Pathol.
       Bacteriol. 15:453 (1911).
2. Kang-Jey Ho, K. Biss, B. Mikkelson, L. A. Lewis
       and C. B. Taylor, The Masai of East Africa:
       some unique biological characteristics, Arch.
       Path. 91:387 (1971).
3. D. J. De Sa, Coronary arterial lesions and myo-
       cardial necrosis in stillbirths and infants,
       Arch. Dis. Child. 54:918 (1979).
4. M. J. Reisman, Atherosclerosis and pediatrics,
       J. Paediatrics 66:1 (1965).
5. L. Jores, Arterien, in "Handbuch der speziellen
       pathologischen Anatomie und histologie Band II
       Herz und Gefasse." F. Henke and O. Lubarsch, eds.,
       Publisher, Julius Springer Berlin (1924).

6. H. Z. Movat, R. H. More and M. D. Haust, The diffuse intimal thickening of the human aorta with ageing, Amer. J. Pathol. 34:1023 (1958).

7. H. C. Stary and J. P. Strong, Coronary artery fine structure in rhesus monkeys: non atherosclerotic intimal thickening, in: "Primates in Medicine", Publisher, Karger Basel (1976).

8. W. Dock, Predilection of atherosclerosis for coronary arteries, J. Amer. Med. Assoc. 131:875, (1946).

9. H. M. Neufeld, C. A. Wagenvoort and J. E. Edwards, Coronary arteries in fetuses, infants, juveniles and young adults, Lab. Invest. 11:837 (1962).

10. E. H. Oppenheimer and J. T. Esterly, Cardiac lesions in hypertensive infants and children, Arch. Pathol. 84:318 (1967).

11. D. Velican and C. Velican, Comparative study on age-related changes and atherosclerotic involvement of the coronary arteries of male and female subjects up to 40 years of age, 38:39 (1981).

12. C. Velican and D. Velican, Coronary intimal necrosis occurring as an early stage of atherosclerotic involvement, Atherosclerosis 39:479 (1981).

13. G. Gabiani, G. B. Ryan and G. Matno, Presence of modified fibroblasts in granulation tissue and their possible role in wound contraction, Experientia 27:549 (1971).

14. D. Velican and C. Velican, Atherosclerotic involvement of the coronary arteries of adolescents and young adults, Atherosclerosis 36:449 (1980).

15. H. C. McGill, Jr., in: "The Geographical Pathology of Atherosclerosis", H. C. McGill, ed., Publisher, Williams and Wilkins, Baltimore, Maryland (1968).

16. G. A. Gresham, Is atheroma a reversible lesion? Atherosclerosis 23:379 (1976).

17. T. A. Pearson, K. Solez, J. M. Dillman and R. H. Heptinstall, Evidence for two populations of fatty streaks with different roles in the atherogenic process, Lancet II:496 (1980).

18. H. C. McGill Jr. and J. P. Strong, The geographic pathology of atherosclerosis, Ann. New York Acad. of Sci. 149:2 (1968).

19. J. P. Strong, C. Restrepo and M. A. Guzman, Coronary and aortic atherosclerosis in New Orleans, Lab. Invest. 39:364 (1968).

20. J. P. Strong and M. A. Guzman, Decrease in coronary atherosclerosis in New Orleans, Lab. Invest. 43:279 (1980).

21. C. C. Chidi and R. G. DePalma, Collagen formation by transformed smooth muscle cells after arterial injury, Surg. Gynec. and Obstet. 152:8 (1981).

22. C. W. M. Adams, O. B. Bayliss, M. Z. M. Ibrahim, M. W. Webster Jr., Phospholipids in atherosclerosis the modification of the cholesterol granuloma by phospholipid, J. Pathol. Bacteriol. 86:431 (1963).

23. H. Kaunitz, Cholesterol and repair processes in arteriosclerosis, Lipids 13:373 (1978).

24. M. D. Haust, R. H. More and H. Z. Movat, The mechanism of fibrosis in arteriosclerosis Amer. J. Pathol. XXXV:265 (1959).

25. P. Constantinides, Plaque fissure in human coronary thrombosis, J. Atherosclerosis Res. 6:1 (1966).

26. H. R. Hellstrom, Evidence in favour of the vasospastic cause of coronary artery thrombosis, Amer. Heart J. 97:449 (1979).

27. M. B. Gardner and D. H. Blankenhorn, Aortic medial calcification, Arch. Pathol. 85:397 (1968).

28. D. A. Eggen, J. P. Strong and H. C. McGill, Calcification in the abdominal aorta, Arch. Pathol. 78:575 (1964).

FUNCTIONAL ASPECTS OF ATHEROGENESIS

Kenneth W. Walton

Department of Investigative Pathology
Medical School, University of Birmingham
Birmingham 15, England

1.0 INTRODUCTION

There is still a tendency to look upon arteries as impermeable tubes and upon 'arterial pollution' (atherosclerosis) as either arising from degeneration of intrinsic components of the arterial wall (1) or as due to the passive accumulation of a kind of 'sludge' on the inner surface (thrombi deposited on the intima) which subsequently undergoes breakdown and incorporation into the wall (2). However, modern physiological and pathological evidence suggests that, instead, arteries should be considered as composed of tubes of a living and reactive gel through which blood is pumped at a pressure such that there is <u>normally</u> an ultrafiltration or permeation of whole plasma through the wall with its removal or drainage from the outer coats by lymphatics (3).

It is proposed to survey the evidence for this last concept and its implications in relation to atherogenesis and the development of concomitant extravascular lesions.

2.0 COMPONENTS CONCERNED IN THE EVOLUTION OF ATHEROSCLEROSIS

It has already been stressed (4) that the atherosclerotic plaque, at almost all stages of its development and wherever it occurs in the arterial tree, contains lipid. Evidence that such lipid originates particularly from the 'family' of low-(LDL) intermediate-(IDL), and very low-density (VLDL) lipoproteins which share in common the same apolipoprotein B component (the LpB lipoproteins) is discussed below. The evidence suggesting that corresponding lipoproteins are concerned in experimental atherosclerosis in certain other species is discussed subsequently (see

Section 8.0). In addition to LpB, two other plasma proteins, fibrinogen and fibronectin, can be shown to be components of plaques.
These plasma components interact with the wall and evoke a cellular
response by certain cell types also discussed below.

2.1 The LpB lipoproteins

Indirect evidence relating the serum levels of LpB to the
prevalence of atherosclerosis in relation to age, sex, geographic
location, and in association with certain diseases has been reviewed
previously (3,5-7). More direct evidence for the implication of LpB
in atherosclerotic lesions has been obtained in the following ways:

2.1.1 Use of radioactivity-labelled lipoprotein. In occasional
instances in which autologous LpB (usually as low-density lipoprotein
or LDL), radioactively labelled in its protein portion, has been
administered intravenously for turnover studies in human subjects
and where subsequent autopsy examination has fortuitously been
possible, it was shown (8,9) that atherosclerotic arteries
accumulate radioactivity at a higher level per gram of tissue than
other organs. This suggested direct penetration of some of the
circulating labelled lipoprotein into the affected sites.

2.1.2 Examination of arterial extracts. Extracts of the arterial
wall prepared by homogenization, sonication, or by the use of a
tissue press have permitted the identification of lipids, by
chemical assays, and of lipoproteins, by immunochemical tests
(10-12). Using a technique involving electrophoresis of the proteins
of the interstitial fluid of arterial intima directly into anti-
serum-containing gels, it was shown (13-15) that the amount of LpB
recoverable from the intima is related to the levels of serum lipids
and lipoproteins in life.

The insudation of plasma into the arterial wall can be shown
convincingly by two-dimensional immuno-electrophoresis of the
interstitial fluid of the arterial intima. A pattern qualitatively
similar to that obtained with plasma from the same individual is
obtained (see Ref 17) even from 'normal' (lesion-free) intima.
This result is consistent with earlier immunohistological studies
(18-20).

2.1.3 Immunohistological techniques. In a study employing
fluorescein-labelled antisera to a range of plasma proteins of
varying molecular size it was shown (19) that: (a) A relatively
faint and diffuse but specific fluorescence is demonstrable in the
intima even of normal arteries to most of the plasma proteins
tested. This diffuse staining is most marked using antiserum to
plasma albumin, is less with antiserum to immunoglobulin G and is
least or is absent with antisera to macroglobulins (IgM,α_2M and
the low-density lipoprotein) in the vessels of children and young

adults. In the vessels of older subjects more marked reactivity, using the antisera to the macroglobulins, was observed and even areas of apparently uninvolved intima showed diffuse lipid infiltration (18,19). Quantitation of the LpB extractable with age showed a linear correlation for the earlier years but lack of correlation after the age of 40. These results suggest some selectivity of permeability into the arterial wall, on the basis of molecular size of the proteins concerned, in young subjects but a generalized increase of vascular permeability with age.

   (b) In contradistinction to the above results, in atherosclerotic plaques a close topographic relation is found between extracellular lipid, revealed by conventional lipid stains (such as Oil red O), and the intense specific fluorescence given with anti-LpB. This is seen even in the occasional plaque which is encountered as a rare finding in young children but is observed also at all stages of development of plaques in older subjects. Antibodies to lipoproteins are directed mainly or exclusively against the protein part of the molecule whereas dyes such as Oil red O are selectively soluble in lipids but unreactive with proteins. Where identity of distribution between lipid staining and the reaction for LpB is found, therefore, it can be inferred that the intact lipoprotein molecule is present. This has since been supported by the direct visualisation of lipoproteins in arterial lesions using the immunoperoxidase technique at the electron microscope level (see Refs 21 and 22).

   On the other hand, in relation to fat-filled cells within lesions, variable immunoreactivity for apo B was found (19). On a similar basis it was inferred that full immunoreactivity was compatible with the uptake of intact lipoprotein by phagocytic cells and relative lack or loss of immunoreactivity with progressive subsequent degradation of the lipoprotein by intracellular proteases. These, it was considered, first digest the apolipoprotein (site of antigenicity) leaving a lipid residue in the cell (possibly contributed to also by local synthesis of triglyceride and phospholipid) detectable by conventional lipid staining. The occurrence of fat-filled cells was thus suggested to indicate the activity of a cellular removal mechanism.

   2.1.4 Combined techniques. If intima bearing an atherosclerotic lesion is electrophoresed until no further plasma protein can be extracted and the same intimal sample is then examined by conventional histology and by immunofluorescence, it can be shown (15,17) that a 'firmly-bound' fraction is still demonstrable in the tissues. This fraction can only be removed from the tissues by enzymic digestion (23) or extraction of the tissues with a detergent (16). The 'bound' fraction was present in highest concentration in fibrous plaques, was less in fatty streaks and least in the apparently uninvolved intima and was thus considered to be of greater significance than the 'labile' fraction in relation to atherogenesis.

Possible mechanisms for the binding of this fraction in the arterial wall are considered later.

2.2 High-density Lipoproteins and Atherosclerosis

Case-control and propective observations in recent years have shown that serum levels of high-density lipoproteins (HDL) are negatively correlated with the incidence of coronary artery disease (24), ischaemic cerebro-vascular disease (25) and with peripheral vascular disease (26). Epidemiological observations on this negative association have been well reviewed by Heiss et al (29).

Two possible mechanisms have been suggested to account for the apparent anti-atherogenic effect of HDL (28). One hypothesis proposes that HDL transports cholesterol from peripheral tissues to the liver (the so-called 'reverse cholesterol transport mechanism') by a process involving the transformation of free cholesterol in HDL to cholesterol ester through the activity of the enzyme lecithin-cholesterol acyl transferase (LCAT). Additional free cholesterol could then be accepted by HDL from specifically located cells, such as those in the arterial wall.

An alternative. or additional, process by which HDL might exert a 'protective' effect may be by reducing arterial cellular uptake of cholesterol carried by LpB by interfering with LpB binding to cell surfaces. For the moment, neither hypothesis can be regarded as proven.

Direct studies on arterial extracts or by immunohistological methods have not clarified the matter. Electrophoretic extraction of both lesion free intima and intima bearing plaques, shows the presence of HDL (23) but this is almost entirely in the 'labile fraction' and is not bound to the tissue in the same way as LpB. Immunofluorescence on unextracted arterial tissue, using fluorescein-labelled anti-apo-lipoprotein A, shows reactive material to be present but diffusely distributed. The precise significance of the presence of HDL, at the arterial wall level, therefore still remains to be elucidated.

2.3 Other Blood-derived Components in Atherosclerosis

Thrombosis undoubtedly accounts for accretion upon, and thus to growth in size, of some established plaques. But it is difficult to accept whole blood thrombi or platelet aggregates adhering to the intima and subsequently becoming incorporated into the wall (29) as the universal mechanism of initial development of all plaques for general reasons which have been discussed previously (3). In

addition, the application of immunohistological techniques and of
immunochemical assays to arterial extracts has helped to clarify
the nature of the occurrence of various components of the coagulation system in the arterial wall.

    <u>2.3.1 Blood coagulation components</u>. Platelets are known to
adhere and to form aggregates at sites of slight damage to vascular
endothelium. Platelets have been shown to contain material antigenically closely related to plasma fibrinogen (30) and to fibronectin (31) and therefore possibly to be the vehicles transporting
these proteins into the wall. There are also intrinsic platelet
antigens in these cells which are unrelated to fibrinogen (32).
The LpB antigen is absent from platelets but lipid-rich membranes
and organelles are characteristic structural features making
platelets theoretical sources of, or contributors to, the lipid in
plaques.

    Immunohistological examination of <u>early</u> plaques has shown no
evidence of the presence of intrinsic platelet antigens (19, 33)
although such antigens are easily demonstrable in surface deposits
(thombi) in thrombosed vessels. It is therefore difficult to accept
platelets as the source of FRA or FN in uncomplicated plaques.

    In relation to lipids, comparison of the composition of the
lipids of platelets with that of the lipids in uncomplicated arterial
lesions (34) reveals such marked differences as to make platelets
a very unlikely source of plaque lipids. In any case, it has been
pointed out that the amount of lipid present in a given lesion is
often such as to require a very large mass of platelet material
(some twenty times greater than that of the lesion itself) to have
been deposited (35). Lastly, as previously stressed in Section 2.1
above, the available evidence overwhelming indicates that LpB
lipoproteins, permeating into the wall, serve as the primary and
major source of the lipid.

    With regard to other clotting components, a technical difficulty
arises from the fact that fibrin and fibrinogen are antigenically
so closely related as to be indistinguishable, using antisera to
intact fibrinogen. Nevertheless, it has been shown that FRA is
recoverable from arterial intima and that a proportion of such
material is clottable with thrombin (36). This establishes that
at least this fraction behaves functionally like native fibrinogen
and makes it likely that fibrinogen, like other plasma proteins,
enters the wall by an insudative process. On the other hand, other
haemostatic components of the coagulation system are demonstrable
in intima and the possibility cannot be excluded that these convert
some fibrinogen to fibrin <u>in situ</u> in the wall (37). The signifi
significance of the occurrence of degradation products of fibrinogen or fibrin in the wall is discussed in Section 5.0.

2.3.2 Fibronectin is an adhesive glycoprotein, synthesized by connective tissue cells, which serves to position and anchor cells to basement membranes, collagen and other substrata (38). FN is also present in plasma and binds to, and co-precipitates with, fibrinogen and fibrin in the cold, especially in the presence of heparin and other sulphated polysaccharides (39). For this reason it was originally designated as 'cold insoluble globulin' (40) but it has since been given other synonyms (41).

FRA and FN can be shown to be immunologically different and quite distinct (42). But in the artery wall (43) as in other sites (42) the two proteins are frequently co-distributed. The mechanism and possible significance of this is discussed later (see Section 4.0).

2.4 Cellular Components involved in Atherosclerosis

The intima, in which atherosclerotic lesions may form, consists normally of a network of fibro-elastic tissue supported in a gel of mucinous ground substance composed of tissue glycoproteins, proteoglycans and glycosaminoglycans. The intima is bounded on its inner surface by a single continuous layer of flattened endothelial cells and on its outer surface by the internal elastic lamina. It is devoid of capillaries or lymphatics so that its components are dependent for their nutrition upon diffusion or permeation of plasma from the lumen. The ground substance filling the spaces between the cells and fibres of the intima serves as a pathway by which nutrients and the plasma filtrate can pass through this layer and thence through the wall.

The connective tissues of the intima may alter in response to a variety of stimuli as the so-called intimal 'non-specific' mesenchymal reaction (44). Typically this is attended by oedema of the ground substance followed by cellular proliferation giving rise to the elaboration of new extracellular ground-substance, elastin and collagen. Where insoluble particulate material (and, in particular, material containing lipid or lipoproteins or their degradation products) is deposited in the ground substance, this may evoke a phagocytic cell response. The resulting fat-filled cells (foam cells) are of two types: 'myogenic foam cells' derived from smooth muscle cells (45); and lipid-filled macrophages, probably derived from circulating monocytes. These two populations of cells show distinctive and different cell marker charateritics (46).

3.0 MECHANISMS OF ENTRAPMENT OF PLASMA COMPONENTS IN THE ARTERIAL WALL

The mechanisms variously proposed have included:

3.0.1 Mechanical or functional 'barrier' effects due to: (i)
blockage of fenestrations in the internal elastic lamina (41); (ii)
intimal thickening and medial fibrosis (48); or (iii) enzymatic
medial defects due to anoxia (49).

However, firstly the mechanical 'damming-back' postulated by
these theories would be expected to cause accumulation of all the
proteins in plasma whereas the evidence discussed makes it clear
that selective entrainment as a 'firmly bound' fraction of only
certain proteins occurs. Secondly, the internal elastic lamina
is quite evidently not an effective barrier since involvement of
the media (especially in older subjects) is frequent even in areas
where only diffuse lipid infiltration of the overlying intima
(rather than discrete plaque formation) is demonstrable. Thirdly,
LpB, FRA and FN are demonstrable in early lesions (fatty streaks)
before changes can be found in the elastica or media (50,57).
Lastly, similar deposition occurs in heart valves in which no
muscular barrier exists (52).

3.0.2 A 'molecular sieve' effect of the ground substance (110).
But, as previously pointed out (3) it is not solely the macro-
globulin components of plasma which are demonstrable. For example,
alpha$_2$ macroglobulins (molecular weight 0.9×10^6) and immunoglobulin M (molecular weight 1.0×10^6) are not specifically
entrained in plaques whereas fibrinogen (molecular weight 300,000)
and fibronectin (molecular weight 450,000) are often present as
'firmly bound' components.

3.0.3 Interaction with the glycoaminoglycans or proteoglycans
of the ground substance (19,53). In relation to this proposal, it
seems of significance that: (i) the plasma components found in
plaques (LpB, FRA and FN) as part of the 'firmly bound' fraction
are precisely those which selectively form insoluble complexes
(co-a cervates) on the addition of charged polysaccharides to
plasma (39,54,55). Such reactions are given by strongly charged
sulphated polysaccharides, sulphated glycosaminoglycans
(S-GAG's) or proteoglycans (S-PG's), including materials isolated
from the arterial wall and other connective tissues (53,56, 57)
(ii) In the intact artery, histochemical methods and radiosulphate
uptake show a significant topographic correlation between the
distribution of S-GAG's or S-PG's and of LpB and FRA in plaques(58).
(iii) Very early intimal lesions, known as 'mucoid elevations',
are held by some authors (59,60) to be areas of localised oedema
(due to selective alteration of endothelial permeability)
preceding visible lipid accumulation (fatty spot or streak
formation) in the wall. These early lesions show localised
accumulation of S-GAG's (61). In this context it may be of
significance that many of the stimuli causing increased vascular
permeability also produce the 'non-specific mesenchymal reaction'
(44) in the subendothelial tissues of arteries, associated with

increased radiosulphate uptake due to increased local production of
S-GAG's. If the conditions giving rise to altered permeability
also promote synthesis of the arterial wall components which
precipitate or bind LpB, FRA and FN, it is possible to appreciate
how and why selective entrapment of these proteins may be initiated.

4.0 SIGNIFICANCE OF DISTRIBUTION OF BOUND PLASMA COMPONENTS

In the light microscope lipid is seen in the intima extracellularly: as lipid droplets apparently "peri-fibrous" (62) in
distribution on collagen and elastin; or disposed in relation to
the interstitial ground substance;or as 'lipid pools' underlying
a fibrous cap showing varying degrees of lipid deposition. Lipid
is also seen extracellularly as large aggregates and intracellularly
in fat-filled cells. By immunofluorescence, as previously
mentioned, the disposed extracellular lipid is identifiable as
LpB while the intracellular lipid and many of the large lipid
aggregates react variably or fail to react with antiserum to LpB.

4.1 Extracellular deposits of LpB

In the electron microscope, the use of the immunoperoxidase
technique has allowed direct visualisation of LpB molecules
in the ground substance, in lipid pools and on the outer surface
of bundles of micro-fibrils with the normal cross-striations of
mature collagen. This appearance conforms with the "perifibrous"
distribution seen by conventional microscopy. But LpB binding
to individual fibrils of collagen and elastin is also demonstrable
(22,63). It seems possible that LpB thus incorporated into the
matrix of fibrous tissue might correspond to the 'firmly-bound'
fraction of entrapped LpB (15,17).

In advanced plaques, LpB binding is also found in areas of
apparently new fibrous tissue formation at the periphery of
plaques. At these sites the lipoprotein may be found in relation
to an abnormal polymorphic form of collagen known as fibrous long-
spacing collagen (FLSC). In such instances LpB is bound at the
prominant transverse bands which occur at an 'abnormal' periodicity
of about 12 nm intervals along the fibrils (63).

The S-GAG's and S-PG's of connective tissues are intimately
involved in the structural organisation and assembly of collagen.
During fibrillogenesis they provide a framework allowing the
orientation and steric arrangement of micro-fibrils to allow their
cross-linking and aggregation. The insudation of LpB into the
environment of fully mature and assembled fibrils results in the
binding of the lipoprotein mainly on the outside of bundles of
fibrils as described above. There is no evidence to suggest that
this binding of lipoprotein to already-formed and mature collagen
is of any functional or structural significance in relation to
the integrity of the artery.

On the other hand, the finding of LpB binding to FLSC may be
of structural importance. This is because it has been reported
(64) that, when fibroblasts derived from arterial explants are
grown in tissue culture, the formation of FLSC by the cells occurs
in the presence of hyperlipidaemic but not of normolipidaemic
serum in the medium. In the FLSC found in intact arteries the
'abnormal' periodicity of binding of LpB is identical to the
periodicity with which interfibrillary binding and cross linking
of collagen molecules by S-GAG's is known to occur (65). Since
the tensile strength of FLSC is known to be much less than that of
'normal' collagen it is possible that the induction of FLSC by
LpB insudation into areas of new fibrous tissue formation in
arteries may underlie the hitherto unexplained tendency (in
biochemical terms) for atherosclerotic arteries to weaken, dilate
and even rupture.

4.2 Intra-cellular lipid

The entrainment of LpB in the intimal gel often evokes a local
cellular reaction with uptake of the lipoprotein. As previously
mentioned (see Section 2.4) the cells concerned are of two kinds,
probably originating from smooth muscle cells and macrophages
respectively. Cellular uptake and disposal of LpB by these cell-
types proceeds by different pathways. Smooth muscle-cells bind,
interiorise and degrade LpB by a 'receptor mediated' mechanism
which is critically dependent upon the initial step of interaction
of LpB, via its apolipoprotein B (apo B), with specific high
affinity surface receptors on the cell-membranes of these cells.
The binding of LpB to its receptors is considered to trigger a
feed-back mechanism which: (a) prevents overloading with LpB (and
hence with the cholesterol and other lipids carried by the
lipoprotein); and (b) controls intrinsic cholesterol synthesis
and esterfication within the cell (66). However, while the
'receptor-mediated' mechanism operates at and a little above
physiological concentrations of LpB in the environment, at higher
concentrations there is preliminary evidence that the mechanism
preventing overloading of the cell can be overcome. Lipoprotein
can then enter by a low-affinity (non-specific) uptake mechanism
which is probably a form of micropinocytosis but which gives an
end-result similar to that seen in actively phagocytic cells
such as macrophages.

In contrast to smooth muscle cells, macrophages have been
found to be capable of relatively little uptake of native LpB
but to show great avidity for denatured or chemically altered
LpB (67). There is current debate as to whether this 'scavenger
pathway' is non-specific or whether macrophages have a different
kind of specific cell-surface receptor for altered LpB (68).

5.0 THE FATE OF FIBRINOGEN AND FIBRONECTIN IN THE ARTERIAL WALL

In suitable material, FRA is identifiable as spots and streaks throughout the thickness of the arterial wall and in lymphatic vessels in the adventitia draining into venae vasorum (see Figs. 6A and B of Ref. 3). This presumably corresponds morphologically to the 'labile fraction' extracted by other techniques and shown to be thrombin-clottable (36). But in old fibrotic plaques, FRA is also seen by immunofluorescence lining or filling spaces resembling vascular or lymphatic channels between areas of fibrosis (see Fig.7 of Ref. 3). This material would seem more likely to correspond to the 'firmly bound' fraction only removable after enzymatic digestion (23). In fibro-fatty plaques containing fat-filled cells surrounded by areas of fibrosis, it is often assumed that the sclerosis arises from the fact that cholesterol, cholesterol esters and certain other lipids are released by fat-filled cells into their environment and promote a neighbouring cellular reaction in connective tissue cells, stimulating them to produce collagen and other products. It is perhaps of significance that FN and FRA are co-distributed in the immediate neighbourhood of fat-filled cells, in a mirror-image distribution from that of LpB. Since FN has been shown to bind strongly to newly-formed (immature) collagen in tissues (42) but not to older, mature collagen, it is possible that this accounts for the appearance found.

Both FN and FRA are sensitive to digestion and degradation by plasmin and by a number of proteolytic enzymes (including intracellular cathepsins) known to be present in the wall. Degradation products of fibrin or fibrinogen have been demonstrated in arterial extracts of intima subjected to electrophoresis (23) but whether digestion occurs in life, or is the result of the post-mortem autolysis to which all tissues removed from the body are subject, has not been resolved.

6.0 FACTORS INFLUENCING ARTERIAL "POLLUTION" AND THE FORMATION OF CONCOMITANT EXTRAVASCULAR LESIONS

The evidence discussed so far suggests that atherosclerotic lesions arise, in general, because certain macromolecular plasma proteins (LpB, FRA and FN) insude into the intima and interact with components of the connective tissues of the arterial wall. There is also evidence which points to this insudative mechanism as being a general one which also underlies the formation of lipid-containing deposits in connective tissues of certain extravascular sites. Consideration of these, along with true arterial lesions, is illuminating in relation to understanding the basic mechanisms involved.

If an insudative mechanism is provisionally accepted, then

the composition of the plasma in terms of LpB, FRA and FN will clearly be of importance. But it is also evident that the mere occurrence of these components in lesions does not explain their topographic distribution. This is made clear when one considers that lesions are restricted to certain sites only in arteries, and do not occur at all in veins, despite the fact that the composition of the blood in respect of LpB lipoproteins, fibrinogen and fibro- nectin is uniform throughout the vascular tree. It has also been objected that atherosclerosis may be encountered in individuals showing minimal or no elevations of serum lipid levels (69).

Moreover, for this or any other general theory of athero- sclerosis to be intellectually acceptable, and of any use in guiding either prophylaxis or treatment, it must take into account the fact that atherosclerosis is a multifactorial disease. In addition, it must help to explain why some of the major 'risk factors' identified by epidemiology (70) mutually re-inforce one another.

In seeking to answer these objections it is necessary to distinguish factors determining the <u>localisation</u> of lesions from those which <u>increase their severity</u> and also to understand how some factors may contribute both to the distribution of lesions <u>and</u> to their nature.

6.1 Factors determining localisation of lesions: Vascular Permeability

It seems likely that the prime factor determining the local- isation of lesions is increase of permeability of the vessel wall at the sites affected. The relative permeability of arterial endothelium by different plasma proteins, and thus the distribution of a given protein between the intravascular and extravascular compartments, is probably largely determined by the molecular size and shape of that protein. For example, in the case of a relatively small molecule like serum albumin, isotopic turnover studies have established that up to twice as much albumin is distributed in the extravascular fluid of the body as there is present in the circulation (71). By contrast, in the case of the LpB lipoproteins, similar methods have shown that, of the total body pool, about two-thirds is intravascular. Of the remaining one-third, much is accounted for by pools in the liver and intestine (sites of synthesis of LpB lipoproteins) so that approximately 5 per cent only of the total pool is in extra- vascular fluid (72). In addition, labelled LpB molecules introduced into the circulation have been found to reach full equilibrium very slowly with the extravascular pool (73).

These observations lead to the conclusion that LpB lipoproteins are normally largely confined to the circulation. The corollary

to this is that if they can be shown to have gained access at some
point to the arterial wall (which, by definition, is <u>outside</u> the
circulation) then there must be some abnormal influence at that
point allowing the 'escape' of these proteins from their normal
intravascular habitat.

The ultrastructural basis of altered endothelial permeability
is difficult to study in humans but in experimental animals the
nature of the structural changes, occurring in response to a
variety of stimuli have been studied by Constantinides and
Robinson (74). These investigations suggest that plasma proteins
probably enter the arterial wall by two pathways. One is a
pathway <u>through</u> the cell by a process of transcellular passage by
micropinocytotic vesicles which is probably relatively slow and
not capable of great augmentation. The other pathway, which is
rapid, involves the formation of gaps <u>between</u> endothelial cells
allowing direct access to the subendothelial spaces.

The various factors capable of inducing localised or diffuse
alteration of endothelial permeability have been discussed
previously (3).

6.2 Other Factors in Localisation of Lesions:obstructed outflow

Apart from factors causing increased <u>ingress</u> of plasma
infiltrate (trauma, allergic injury to arteries etc.) it can also
be envisaged that obstructed <u>outflow</u> into the lymphatics draining
the outer coat of the vessel might also be of importance. There
is a well-documented tendency for atherosclerosis to be more severe
when it supervenes in arteries affected by various forms of granulomatous arteries such as temporal arteritis , Takayasu's disease
or syphilitic arteritis (75,76). A chronic inflammatory process
affecting arteries can be envisaged as giving rise to a segmental
increase of permeability in the affected areas but also influencing
outflow from the wall because of involvement of the adventitial
coat with the obstruction of lymphatic drainage which is
characteristic of these granulomatous arteritides.

6.3 Factors affecting the Severity of Lesions

6.3.1 Serum lipids and atherosclerosis. Once increased
permeability is established at a particular point in an artery,
it can be envisaged that an increased <u>volume</u> of plasma permeates
through the affected segment in unit time, <u>as well as</u> there being
initiated ingress of the large molecules normally largely
excluded. This might explain why atherosclerosis is encountered
in <u>normolipidaemic</u> individuals. However, clearly the process
envisaged would be further accelerated with concomitant hyperlipidaemia (hyperlipoproteinaemia).

6.3.2 Mechanisms involved in the control of plasma lipids and
lipoproteins. The serum levels of lipoproteins depend upon the
balance between their synthesis and catabolism. There is evidence
that the apolipoproteins of HDL and of LDL are synthesized, and
the intact lipoproteins assembled, in both the liver and the
intestinal wall (77). Little is yet known about: the respective
contributions made by each site of synthesis to the total body
pools of these lipoproteins; whether the contributions made by
each synthetic site vary relative to one another or are constant;
nor how control of the rate of synthesis at each site is exerted.
It might be expected that dietary variation, hormonal effects and
diseases affecting the liver or intestinal tract might exert effect
at one or other or both sites.

Metabolic studies have established that VLDL are sequentially
degraded (by lipoprotein lipases) to LDL before final catabolic
disposal occurs. It has been shown that the catabolism of LDL
takes place not only in the liver, as was once believed, but also
in other tissues widely dispersed throughout the body (78). It
has been estimated that the specific LDL receptor-mediated pathway
(see Section 4.2) accounts for between one-third (79) and one-
half (80) of overall LDL catabolism in health but for a reduced
proportion in certain familial hyperlipidaemias (see below,
Section 6.3.4).

6.3.3 Moderate hyperlipidaemia. The effects of age, sex,
ethnic origin, cultural conventions etc. upon serum lipid levels
and the incidence of atherosclerosis have been discussed previously
(6). Most surveys have shown a positive association of LpB
lipoproteins, and a negative association of HDL, with cardiovascular disease morbidity and mortality (27,89,95,96).

6.3.4 Severe hyperlipidaemia. Marked elevation of serum
lipids and lipoproteins occurs (a) Secondarily in association with
certain disease processes (see Table I) or (b) Primarily as
familial hyperlipidaemia (Table II). (a) The secondary hyperlipidaemias, although otherwise pathogenetically diverse, and showing
various patterns of derangement (Types) of hyperlipidaemia,
nevertheless share in common an overall increase of LpB
lipoproteins and a high incidence of atherosclerosis (For
references see Refs 5 and 6). (b) Primary hyperlipidaemias
classified by the system proposed by the World Health Organisation
(81) show varying risks of cardiovascular disease (see Table III).

Studies of the turnover and distribution of LDL in both the
primary and the secondary hyperlipidaemias which are associated
with a high incidence of atherosclerosis have established that
although the mechanisms underlying the elevation of LpB lipoproteins may differ, the common factor is a marked increase in
total body pool, reflected in increases of both intra- and extra-

Table   I   Conditions associated with an increased incidence of
            atherosclerotic cardiovascular disease and with
            hyperlipidaemia (serum lipids: N + 2 to 3 S.D)

Condition	Usual Type of hyperlipidaemia
Hypothyroidism Nephrotic syndrome with non- selective proteinuria	Type IIA or IIB
Recurrent pancreatitis Chronic alcoholism Diabetes mellitus Occasional cases of myelomatosis (esp. IgA) Occasional cases of macroglobulinaemia Lipoid nephrosis of childhood Some cases of gout	Type IV or V
Obstructive biliary disease	Distinctive pattern with abnormal Lp(LpX)

Table II   Patterns of alterations of LpB lipoproteins in primary
            (familial) hyperlipidaemias and risk of cardiovascular
            disease (CVD)

Type*	Pattern in serum	Risk of CVD
I	Gross chylomicronaemia; all other LpB lipoproteins diminished; deficient lipoprotein lipases	not increased
IIA	Marked increase of LDL	very high
IIB	Increased LDL & moderate increase of VLDL	high
III	Increase of LDL & abnormal IDL (floating betalipoprotein)	high
IV	Marked increase of VLDL	increased
V	As for IV but with chylomicronaemia also	increased

* Based on W.H.O. classification of Beaumont et al (81)

vascular pools of LpB (82). It seems possible that, in particular,
the increase in extravascular pool is given expression not only in
the development of lipoprotein deposits in arteries but also in the
precocious development of the corneal arcus (83) and the frequent
occurrence of xanthomata (98), which are characteristic
associated features of such cases.

  6.3.5 Atherogenic potential of lipoproteins. Consideration of
the reported incidence of overt cardiovascular disease in
association with the primary hyperlipidaemias (as shown in Table II)
allows certain broad inferences to be drawn regarding the relative
atherogenic potential of lipoproteins of different molecular sizes.
For example, the rare Type I pattern, characterised by gross
chylomicronaemia, reduced levels of lipoproteins of smaller molecular
size (VLDL, IDL and LDL) and reduced or absent lipoprotein lipases,
is not associated with the accelerated development of atherosclerosis.
This suggests that chylomicra are either too large to enter the
arterial wall unchanged or, if they do enter, are disposed of
rapidly.

    The former of these possibilities is favoured by Zilversmit
(84) who suggests that the lack of endothelial lipase in Type I
hyperlipidaemia patients prevents degradation of chylomicra to a
size permitting their permeation through endothelium. It is
striking that correction (by a low fat diet) of the defect in these
cases, greatly reduces the level of chylomicra and increases that
of LDL. It would be of interest to know whether the 'correction'
is associated with an increased risk of cardiovascular disease in
treated case of Type I hyperlipidaemia.

    On the other hand, at the other end of the scale, it might
be expected that the smallest lipoprotein molecules of the LpB
'family' (the LDL class) might penetrate most easily through the
endothelial barrier. This accords with the data of Slack (85)
who found that men with the Type IIA or IIB abnormality
(preponderant increase of LDL) have an earlier onset of
ischaemic heart disease than do men with Types III-V abnormalities.
Nevertheless, the incidence rate is high even in persons with a
predominant increase of VLDL (Types IV & V abnormalities). A
possible reason for this association is disscussed below.

  6.3.6 Immunohistological and electron microscopic observations.
Inferences regarding the molecular sizes of the lipoproteins
involved in atherogenesis have also been made from work done using
immunohistological techniques. It was shown that not only
apolipoprotein B (apo B) which is common to VLDL, IDL and LDL, but
also apolipoprotein C (apo C) found in lipoproteins larger in size
than LDL, can be detected in lesions (86). In some individuals
the antigen (apo-Lpa) characteristic of Lp(a) lipoprotein, which
is denser but larger than LDL, was additionally demonstrated (87).

The topographic distribution of apo C or of apo Lpa was found to be closely similar to that of apo B in plaques from both hyper-lipidaemic and normolipidaemic subjects. This suggested that both antigens were closely associated spatially in the tissue, as might be expected if molecules carrying apo B plus apo C (intact IDL or VLDL) or apo B plus Lpa (intact Lp(a) lipoprotein) were present in the lesion along with LDL (characterised solely by apo B). These observations were taken to be suggestive evidence that lipoproteins even larger than LDL gain entry to the intimal gel.

More direct visual evidence relating to this question has been obtained using the immunoperoxidase technique and electron microscopy (21,22,65). This technique when applied directly to isolated LDL preparations shows an appearance of spherical particles (molecules) uniformly covered by electron-dense material (see Fig. 1 of Ref. 63). When applied to plaques containing 'pools' of lipid, large numbers of spherical particles of varying size are seen (see Fig. 5 of Ref. 22). Some of these are similarly covered by electron-dense material (the osmicated reaction product of diaminobenzidine reacting with the peroxidase coupled to anti apo B binding to the particle). In other instances the plane of section transects the particles. The great majority of the particles thus identified as apo B-containing lipoproteins have diameters of a range corresponding to LDL. But a minority of particles are of larger diameter thus appearing to offer con-firmation that lipoproteins bigger than LDL can participate in atherogenesis. This at first-sight accords with the clinical observation (alluded to above) that types IV & V hyperlipidaemia (with preponderant increases of VLDL without, or with chylomicron-aemia) show an augmented incidence of atherosclerotic cardio-vascular disease.

However, it has long been known that the VLDL and IDL fractions, even from healthy individuals, as isolated ultracentrifugally, are heterogeneous in moelcular size when examined by negative staining techniques in the electron microscope (88). In a recent study (89) it has been noted that the IDL fraction from Types IV & V shows an even greater heterogeneity of size, with a larger proportion of molecules of below average diameter, than normal. This abnormality appears to be associated with an abnormal composition of the 'core' components of these lipoproteins. The occurrence of an abnormally high proportion of 'small' molecules in the fractions preponderating in the serum of Types IV & V thus might explain the apparently paradoxical predilection to the development of atherosclerosis in such cases.

6.4 Interaction of Hyperlipidaemia and altered Vascular Permeability

6.4.1 Age and sex effects. Alterations in serum lipids with

age and sex show a broad parallelism with the incidence of atherosclerosis with age and between the sexes, especially in the
developed countries. The increase in serum lipids seen with age
and sex is invariably given expression in the LpB lipoproteins
and not in HDL levels which differ significantly between the sexes
(being higher in women) but show relatively little change with age.
Serum triglycerides show an association with VLDL levels, total
serum cholesterol with LDL levels (90).

There is also evidence that vascular permeability increases
with age and, in the later decades, this is the case for both sexes.
The effect of this, acting in conjunction with the moderate hyperlipidaemia characteristic even of healthy subjects of advanced
years, is seen in the aortas of these elderly individuals as a
diffuse lipid (LpB) infiltration of the intima even in areas not
directly involved by plaque formation (7,51).

In many populations, the incidence of the corneal arcus
(arcus senilis) and of atherosclerosis increase with age in parallel
with increase of LpB proteins (for References, see Ref. No 91). It
has been shown that the arcus itself is a process of lipid
deposition in the region of the superficial and deep limbal vascular
processes and that the lipid, as in arteries elsewhere, is in the
form of LpB lipoproteins (91).

6.4.2 Effects of trauma. The direct effect of injuries to
arteries internally or externally applied in localising and
accelerating atherosclerosis has been studied in experimental
animals (92) but is not possible in man. On the other hand, the
localising effect of trauma is demonstrable in relation to the
pathogenesis of human xanthomata. These occur in man in
association with both primary and secondary hyperlipidaemias and
are typically distributed at sites subjected to minor traumata.
For example, they occur at sites of pressure (elbows, knees
buttocks); in skin subjected to constant creasing or folding
(palmar creases); in tendons subjected to frictional stress over
joints (finger tendons) or postural tensional stress (tendo
Achillis). It has been shown (93) that when autologous radioactive
LDL is injected into hyperlipidaemic subjects with actively
progressive xanthomata symmetrically disposed on both elbows,
greater localisation of radioactivity occurs into a lesion
subjected to slight but repeated trauma than into the contralateral
lesion if the latter is protected and the limb bearing it is
immobilised.

6.5 Hypertension

Increase of blood pressure occurs with age in developed
countries (94) and has been clearly established as a factor
increasing the severity, or ace lerating the rate of development,

of arterial disease in man. It can be envisaged that, once selective
alteration of permeability has been established in a given artery,
with the onset of hypertension an even greater <u>volume</u> of plasma
would transude through the affected segment in unit time. In this
way the total amount of potentially reactive plasma proteins (LpB,
FRA and FN) available for interaction with components of the wall
at that site would increase, even if their plasma levels were
normal. But clearly the effect would be magnified with increase
of their concentration (for example, by hyperlipidaemia). This
mechanism may explain the clinical observation that hypertension
increases the risk of development of cardiovascular disease but
that the risk is magnified in hyperlipidaemic individuals.

Examples of how the effect if hypertension in both localising
and increasing the severity of atherosclerotic lesions at particular
sites in the vascular tree have been cited previously (95).

7.0 SYNERGISM BETWEEN RISK FACTORS

Epidemiological studies have shown not only that atherosclerosis
is multifactorial in origin but also that the identifiable adverse
(or 'risk') factors mutually re-inforce one another. For example,
it was shown in one study (96) that if (say) three adverse factors
(e.g., serum cholesterol, blood pressure and smoking habit) were
identifiable in a given group, the nett effect was to increase the
'standard' risk of development of ischaemic heart disease not
merely 3 times, but between 9 and 10 times. This geometric rather
than arithmetic summation of effect has been given mathematical
expression for certain populations (97). Calculations based on
one of these formulas give rise to predictions of summation of
effects of a kind which have been illustrated previously (3).

Possible ways in which adverse factors might operate and
summate <u>at the level of the arterial wall</u> have been discussed in
the foregoing sections and are summarised in Table III.

8.0 EXPERIMENTAL VALIDATION OF THE INSUDATIVE HYPOTHESIS

In certain species (including the dog, the rat and the
hamster) the principal lipid-carrying protein in the plasma is
a high-density lipoprotein. These species are highly resistant
to the development of atherosclerosis both naturally and experimentally. In other species in which the principal lipid-carrying
proteins are low-density lipoproteins, as in man, dietary
manipulation can be shown to increase the plasma levels of these
lipoproteins and this is accompanied by the development of
lipid-filled arterial lesions. Among this latter group of
animals is the rabbit.

Table   III   Possible mechanisms of summation of effect of adverse
              factors at the level of the arterial wall

Adverse Factors	Possible mechanism
1. Age, smoking (hypoxia) extrinsic or intrinsic vaso-active agents,trauma.	Increased vascular permeability (increased inflow) & generation of entrapping agents (S.GAG's) due to 'mesenchymal response'
2. Age, sex (maleness) high fat intake	Moderate hyperlipidaemia increased input of LpB even with unchanged inflow)
3. Primary or secondary hyperlipidaemias	Grossly increased input of LpB (effect as in 2 but more pronounced).
4. Hypertension	Further increase of inflow (effect especially marked with hyperlipidaemia)
5. External injury to artery or co-existent arteritis	Inflammation of wall increasing permeability; obliterated lymphatics impeding outflow.

8.1 Plasma Lipids and Lipoproteins in the Lipid-fed Rabbit

Whether rabbits are maintained on cholesterol-supplemented
diets, or on a diet containing beef lard without added cholesterol,
the animals develop a hyperlipidaemia and also a hyperlipoproteinaemia. In the cholesterol-fed animal there is a marked increase
of a lipoprotein with VLDL-like density characteristics but containing a much higher proportion of cholesterol than normal (98).
The protein portion of this abnormal' lipoprotein also contains
a high proportion of a peptide probably analogous with human
apolipoprotein E (99) and is unusually large in molecular size
as visualised by electron microscopy (100). Cholesterol-fed
animals often show a reciprocal reduction in HDL (98).

On the other hand, beef-fat fed rabbits show a more moderate
hyperlipidaemia with an increase of the total low-density lipoproteins (TLDL) and of HDL. The TLDL show a distribution of
subclasses which approximate more closely to normal than is the
case in the cholesterol fed animal (98).

8.2 Metabolic effects of Lipid-feeding in Rabbits

At the height of the hyperlipidaemia induced by cholesterol
feeding there is evidence that the synthesis of lipids and
lipoproteins by the liver in rabbits is greatly reduced (101). It
has therefore been inferred that, under these circumstances, the
great bulk of the circulating lipoproteins must be of intestinal
origin (95).

Using immunofluorescence the presence of the major lipoprotein
apoproteins have been demonstrated in human intestinal epithelial
cells (102) and employing the immunoperoxidase technique it has
been shown that in these cells, the smooth endoplasmic reticulum
Golgi apparatus and secretory vesicles form a pathway for the
assembly, transport and secretion of lipoprotein particles
(molecules) into intestinal lymph (102) in a similar to that
seen in the liver (103). The same techniques have shown that
analogous assembly of LpB lipoproteins occurs in rabbit intestinal
cells (Walton, Morris and Poonia, unpublished) in cholesterol-fed
rabbits, suggesting that the inference that the bulk of circulating
lipoprotein in the lipid-fed rabbit are of intestinal origin is
probably correct.

8.3 Experimental atherosclerosis

Irrespective of the nature of the dietary lipid supplement,
rabbits developing hyperlipoproteinaemia are found to develop
atherosclerotic lesions and also to show the presence of a
corneal arcus and spontaneous xanthomata (98,104,105). Differences
in the rate and severity of development of arterial lesions between
groups of animals on the two different dietary supplements
reflect differences in the duration and intensity of hyperlipoproteinaemia between the groups (105).

Arterial lesions in cholesterol fed animals are more
extensive and contain larger numbers of fat-filled cells than
lesions in beef-fat fed animals. In rabbit arterial lesions, as in
humans, precise agreement is found between the distribution of
lipid reacting with Oil red O and specific fluorescence for LpB
in endothelial cells and in extracellular deposits in the
intimal ground substance or on collagen in the intima. But fat-
filled cells, again as in humans, show variable immuno-reactivity
(105). On the other hand, in the medial coat, cells which are
indisputably smooth muscle cells are seen to contain lipid and to
give strong immunofluorescent reactivity. The distinction is
seen particularly clearly in material fixed in cold ethanol and
wax embedded. In such sections the lipid solvents used during
the embedding process remove lipids from the tissue, converting
the intimal cells to foam cells but cells in the medial coat still
retain immuno-reactivity for apo B (see Fig. 13 of Ref. 105).

These observations suggest that initial foam-cells even if of myogenic origin, differ from lipid-filled fully differentiated myocytes in the media, the latter degrading the LpB molecule less readily.

Lipid (as LpB lipoproteins) is also demonstrable in lipid-fed rabbits in heart-valves, in large muscular arteries (carotids, coronaries) and, in severely hyperlipidaemic animals, even in the pulmonary artery and small visceral arteries and arterioles (105). In addition as previously mentioned, the animals develop a corneal arcus and lipid (lipoprotein) infiltration of other intra-ocular structures (10A), and spontaneous xanthomata (98). All these lesions show evidence of regression and resolution with discontinuance of lipid-feeding and diminution of LpB serum levels.

8.4 Experimental Induction of Ocular Lesions in Lipid-fed Rabbits

The eye-lesions in lipid fed rabbits are broadly similar to those accompanying corneal arcus formation in man but in the rabbit,deposits in the cornea itself are less prominent in the earlier stages of the process, while lipid deposition is more severe in the iris and in the ureal tract. These differences from the human are due to anatomical dissimilarities in the vascular supply to the affected areas. As in arterial lesions, FRA is also identifiable in the lesions and deposition is mainly perivascular and is maximal in areas showing an increase of S-GAG's of the ground substance of the tissues involved. Subsequent uptake and degradation of LpB-S-GAG complexes by macrophages may give rise to the release of cholesterol and other lipids into the tissues, provoking a later sclerotic reaction. In these respects the pathogenesis of the process is similar to that occurring in arteries and may serve as a model for the study of atherogenesis (106).

8.5 Xanthomatosis in Lipid fed Rabbits

'Spontaneous' xanthomata occur in lipid-fed animals on the foot pads and around the carpal joints as Anitschkow (107) observed originally. Some authors have also recorded xanthomata in the nuchal skin. The reason for this localisation was unknown although Anitschkow suggested that altered vascular permeability at the affected sites might be a factor.

This was supported by the observations that: (i) xanthoma formation on the foot pads of lipid-fed animals is prevented or delayed in animals kept in cages with a solid floor padded with straw whereas lesions develop quickly in animals maintained in cages with a wire-mesh floor. This suggests that trauma to the feet localise the lesions - perhaps by inducing increased

permeability of the vessels in the damaged tissue and thus allowing
lipoprotein-rich plasma to 'leak' into these areas; (ii) nuchal
xanthomata are observed to occur only in animals lifted by grasping
the skin of the scruff of the neck and not in animals otherwise
handled. This again suggests trauma (pinching or grasping the
skin) is a localising factor.

The suggestion was further supported by the effects resulting
from giving daily intracutaneous injections of histamine to lipid-
fed and control rabbits. In the former, nodules were induced at the
elective site which, when biopsied, showed the histological
appearance of typical xanthomata whereas no lesions occurred in
the controls. The vehicle transporting lipid into the lesions in
the lipid fed animals was identified as LpB by the use of isologous
rabbit LpB labelled with radioactive iodine which localised in the
injected site; and by immunofluorescence (98,106).

8.5 General Conclusions concerning Experimental Atherosclerosis in the Rabbit

No single animal model is universally accepted as reproducing
all aspects of human atherosclerosis (for reviews see Refs 108,109).
There are certain aspects of the rabbit's response to lipid-
feeding which produce features unlike those seen in humans. For
example, on high and continuous cholesterol feeding, rabbits
develop a 'cholesterol storage disease' which is characterised
by large deposits of cholesterol in the reticulo-enothelial
system and in interstitial cells in the heart, kidneys, lungs and
elsewhere.

Nevertheless, from the restricted view-point of view of view
of examining, under experimental conditions, whether an insudative
mechanism operates in atherogenesis in species other than man, the
lipid-fed rabbit is indeed a useful model since, as indicated above,
it is possible not only to induce arterial disease but also some of
the extravascular accompaniments of human atherosclerosis (corneal
arcus, xanthomas etc.) and even to induce certain of these at
elective sites so that all stages of the insudative process can be
studied.

9.0 SUMMARY

It is submitted that the evidence surveyed overwhelmingly
favours the view that both human and experimental atherosclerosis
arise in general because certain reactive macromolecular components
of the plasma insude in increased amounts into the arterial wall
at sites of increased vascular permeability. The latter sites
may be determined by a variety of causes but show certain areas of
predilection in the arterial tree. The plasma components which
are of significance are LpB lipoproteins, fibrinogen and fibro-

nectin which share in common the physio-chemical characteristic of forming insoluble complexes with charged polysaccharides. These are macromolecules closely associated with the evolution of the fibrous structural proteins of the connective tissue.

Morphologically, LpB lipoproteins, fibrinogen and fibronectin are seen to be entrained in arterial intima, extracellularly, in the interstitial ground substance or bound to elastin and collagen; or intracellularly in fat-filled cells. The latter may be either myogenic in origin or arise from monocytes/macrophages. Cellular uptake occurs by both 'receptor mediated' (in smooth muscle cells) and by 'scavenger' (in macrophages) pathways and is a removal mechanism which may be reinforced by the activity of high-density lipoproteins.

Critical examination of the existing evidence available suggests that while thrombosis certainly augments the size of existing atherosclerotic plaques it is probably not an initiating mechanism of atherogenesis. Blood platelets probably do not serve as the vehicles carrying fibrinogen or fibronectin into plaques since, where these proteins are detectable in established plaques, intrinsic platelet antigens are not detected. Platelets are also a very unlikely source of plaque-lipids which other evidence indicates largely to arise from LpB lipoproteins.

The evidence surveyed further suggests that the insudative mechanism proposed is a general one which also operates to explain lipid (lipoprotein) deposition in certain extravascular lesions (corneal arcus formation, xanthomatosis) which are broadly associated with atherosclerosis and hyperlipidaemia. Epidemiological studies have stressed the multifactorial nature of atherosclerosis and the way in which the identifiable adverse ('risk') factors mutually re-inforce one another. Consideration of the patho-physiological mechanisms underlying the formation both of athero-sclerosis itself, and of associated conditions referred to above, allows understanding of how adverse factors inter-relate and re-inforce another also at the level of the arterial wall.

While cellular uptake and degradation of the plasma proteins bound in arterial intima normally serves as a clearance and disposal mechanism, in some circumstances the degradation products (and in particular those deriving from the LpB lipoproteins) may give rise to the release of cholesterol and other components which stimulate normal or abnormal fibrosis, or result in the accumulation of 'atheromatous gruel' in the plaque. These changes may, in turn, initiate any of the later complications of atherosclerosis (necrosis of the plaque, haemorrhage, ulceration, calcification, medial involvement and degeneration, aneurysmal dilatation or arterial rupture. To prevent or alleviate such effects all the identifiable factors in any given individual, rather than a single factor (say hyperlipidaemia) should be clinically controlled.

10.0 REFERENCES

1. R. Thoma, Über die Abhängigkeit der Hindegewebsneubildung in
    der Arterienintima von den mechanischen Bendingungen dis
    Blutumlaufes, Virch. Arch. Path. Anat. 93: 443 (1883).
2. C. von Rokitansky, A Manual of Pathological Anatomy, Vol.4,
    p. 261. Translated by G.E. Day, Sydenham Society, London
    (1852).
3. K.W. Walton, Pathogenetic Mechanisms in Atherosclerosis, Amer.
    J. Cardiol. 35: 542 (1975).
4. G.A. Gresham, - this volume.
5. K.W. Walton, The Biology of Atherosclerosis, in "The Biological
    Basis of Medicine", E.E. Bittar and N. Bittar, eds. Vol. 6,
    pp. 193-233, Academic Press, New York (1969).
6. K.W. Walton. Atherosclerosis and Aging, in "Textbook of
    Geriatric Medicine and Gerontology", pp. 77-112,
    J.C. Brocklehurst, ed. Churchill Livingstone, Edinburgh
    (1973).
7. K.W. Walton, Hyperlipidaemia and the Pathogenesis of Athero-
    sclerosis, in "Perspectives in Ischaemic Heart Disease",
    A.B. Simmonds, ed. pp. 55-67, Advances in Drug Research,
    Vol. 9, Academic Press, New York (1974).
8. K.W. Walton, P.J. Scott, J. Verrier-Jones, R.F. Fletcher and
    T.P. Whitehead, Studies on low-density lipoprotein turnover
    in relation to Atromid therapy, J. Atheroscler. Res., 3:396
    (1963).
9. P.J. Scott and P.J. Hurley, The distribution of radioiodinated
    serum albumin and low-density lipoprotein in tissues and the
    arterial wall, Atherosclerosis, 11: 77 (1970).
10. H. Ott F. Lohss and J Gergely, Der Nachweis von Serumlipoprotein
    in der Aortenintima, Klin. Wschr., 36: 383 (1958).
11. R.E. Tracey, E.B. Merchant and V.C. Kao, On the antigenic
    identity of human serum beta and alpha-2 lipoproteins and
    their identification in the aortic intima, Circ. Res. 9:472
    (1961).
12. A.N. Klimov, A.D.Denishenko and E.Y. Magracheva, Preparation of
    tissue fluid of the vessel wall and determination of its
    lipoproteins, Atherosclerosis, 19:243 (1974).
13. E.B. Smith and R.S. Slater, Relationship between low density
    lipoprotein in aortic intima and serum lipid levels, Lancet
    1:463 (1972).
14. H.F. Hoff, C.L. Heideman, J.W. Gaubatz, A.M. Gotto, E.E.Erikson
    and R.L. Jackson, Quantification of apolipoprotein B in
    grossly normal human aorta, Circ. Res., 40:56 (1977).
15. K.W. Walton and G.V.H. Bradby. The significance of 'bound' and
    'labile' fractions of low-density lipoprotein and fibrinogen
    in the arterial wall, in "Atherosclerosis - Metabolic,
    Morphologic and Clinical Aspects", pp.888-893, G.M. Manning
    and M.D. Haust, eds., Plenum Press, New York (1975).

16. H.F. Hoff, C.L. Heideman, J.W. Gaubatz and A.M. Gotto, Quantitation of apoB in human aortic fatty streaks - A comparison with grossly normal intima and fibrous plaques, Atherosclerosis, 30:263 (1978).

17. G.V.H. Bradby, K.W. Walton and R. Watts, The binding of total low-density lipoproteins in human arterial intima affected and unaffected by atherosclerosis, Atherosclerosis, 32:403 (1979).

18. V.C.Y. Kao and R.W. Wissler, A study of the immunohistochemical localization of serum lipoproteins and other plasma proteins in human atherosclerotic lesions, Exp. Mol. Pathol., 4:465 (1965).

19. K.W. Walton and N. Williamson, Histological and immunofluorescent studies on the evolution of the human atheromatous plaque, J. Atheroscler. Res. 8:599 (1968).

20. H.F. Hoff, J.T. Lie, R.L. Jackson, M.E. DeBakey, R.J. Bayards and A.M. Gotto, Localization of apo-low-density lipoproteins (apo-LDL) in atherosclerotic lesions of human normo- and hyperlipemics, Arch. Path., 99:253 (1975).

21. H.F. Hoff and J.W. Gaubatz, Ultrastructural localization of apolipoprotein B in human aortic and coronary atherosclerotic plaques, Exp. Mol. Pathol. 26:214 (1977).

22. K.W. Walton and C.J. Morris, Studies on the passage of plasma proteins across arterial endothelium in relation to athero-genesis, Progr. Biochem. Pharmacol., 13:138 (1977).

23. E.B. Smith, I.B. Massie and K.M. Alexander, The release of an immobilised lipoprotein fraction from atherosclerotic lesions by incubation with plasmin, Atherosclerosis, 25:71 (1976).

24. G.J. Miller and N.E. Miller, Plasma high density lipoprotein concentration and development of ischaemic heart disease, Lancet, 1:16 (1975).

25. S. Rössner, K.G. Kjellin, K.L Mettinger, A. Siden and S.E. Söderström. Dislipoproteinemia in patients with ischaemic cerebrovascular disease, Atherosclerosis, 30:199 (1978).

26. G.V.H. Bradby, A.J. Valente and K.W. Walton, Serum high density lipoproteins in peripheral vascular disease, Lancet, 2:1271 (1978).

27. G. Heiss, N.J. Johnson, S. Reiland, C.E. Davis and H.A. Tyroler, The epidemiology of plasma high-density lipoprotein cholesterol levels, Circulation 62 (suppl IV:116 (1980).

28. R.I. Levy and B.M. Rifkind. The structure, function and metabolism of high-density lipoproteins: A status report, Circulation 62 (Suppl. IV): 4 (1980).

29. J.B. Duguid, The thrombogenic hypothesis and its implications, Postgrad. Med. J. 36:226 (1969)

30. M. Seligmann, B. Goudemaud, A. Janin, B. Bernard and P. Grabar, Etudes immunochimiques sur la présence de fibrinogène dans des extraits de plaquettes humaines lavées et dans certains extraits leucocytaires, Rév. hémat., 12:302 (1957).

48 K. W. WALTON

31. E.F. Plow, C. Birdwell and M.H. Ginsberg, Identification and quantitation of platelet-associated fibronectin antigen, J. Clin. Invest., 63:540 (1979).
32. P. Wolf, The nature and significance of platelet products in human plasma, Brit. J. Haematol., 13:269 (1967).
33. K.C. Carstairs, The identification of platelets and platelet antigens in histological sections, J. Pathol. Bact. 90:225 (1965).
34. E.B. Smith, in "Atherosclerosis: Proceedings of the Second International Symposium", R.J. Jones, ed., p.106, Springer Verlag, Berlin.
35. E.B. Smith, Quantitative and qualitative comparison of the lipids in platelets, aortic intima and mural thrombi, Cardiovasc. Res., 1:111 (1967).
36. E.B. Smith, R.S. Slater and J.A. Hunter, Quantitative studies on fibrinogen and low-density lipoprotein in human aortic intima, Atherosclerosis, 18:479 (1973).
37. E.B. Smith, Haemostatic factors in human aortic intima, Lancet, I:1171 (1981).
38. S. Stenman and A. Vaheri, Distribution of a major connective tissue protein, fibronectin, in normal human tissues, J. Exp. Med., 147:1054 (1978).
39. M.W Mosesson, Structure of human plasma cold-insoluble globulin and the mechanism of its precipitation in the cold with heparin or fibrin-fibrinogen complexes, Ann. N.Y. Acad.Sci. 312:11 (1978).
40. J.T. Edsall, G.A. Gilbert and H.A. Scheraga, The non-clotting component of the human plasma fraction I-1 ('cold insoluble globulin'), J. Amer. Chem. Soc. 77:157 (1955).
41. K.M. Yamada and K.Olden, Fibronectins - adhesive glycoproteins of cell surface and blood, Nature 275:179 (1978).
42. D.L. Scott, A.C. Wainwright, K.W. Walton and N. Williamson, Significance of fibronectin in rheumatoid arthritis and osteoarthritis, Ann. Rheum. Dis., 40:142 (1981).
43 K.W. Walton and D.L. Scott, The role of fibronectin in the progression of human atherosclerotic plaques, - in preparation.
44. W.H. Hauss, U. Gerlach, G. Junge-Hülsing, H. Themann and W. Wirth, Studies on the 'non-specific mesenchymal reaction' and the 'transit zone' in myocardial lesions and athero-sclerosis, Ann. N.Y. Acad. Sci., 156:207 (1969).
45. M.D. Haust, R.H. More and H.Z. Movat, The mechanism of fibrosis in arteriosclerosis, Amer. J. Pathol., 35:265 (1959)
46. T. Schaffner, K. Taylor, E.J. Bartucci, K. Fischer-Dzoga, J.H. Beeson, S. Glagov and R.W. Wissler, Arterial foam cells with distinctive immunomorphologic and histochemical features of macrophages, Amer. J. Pathol., 100:57 (1980).

47. J.W. Gofman and W. Young, The filtration concept of athero-
    sclerosis and serum lipids in the diagnosis of athero-
    sclerosis, in "Atherosclerosis and its origin" pp. 197-229,
    M. Sandler and G.H. Bourne, eds. Academic Press, New York
    (1963).
48. S.L. Wilens and R.T. McCluskey, The permeability of excised
    arteries and other tissues to serum lipid, Circ. Res.,
    2:175 (1954).
49. C.W.M. Adams, O.B. Bayliss and M.Z.M. Ibrahim, A hypothesis to
    explain the accumulation of cholesterol in atherosclerosis,
    Lancet, 1:890 (1962).
50. N. Woolf and T. Crawford, Fatty streaks in the aortic intima
    studied by an immunohistochemical technique, J. Pathol. Bact.,
    80:405 (1960).
51. K.W. Walton, The role of serum lipoproteins in very early and
    late atherosclerotic lesions, in "Connective Tissue and
    Ageing", H. Vogel, ed., pp. 34-37, Excerpta Medica,
    Amsterdam (1973).
52. K.W. Walton, N.Williamson and A.G. Johnson, The pathogenesis
    of atherosclerosis of the mitral and aortic valves,
    J. Pathol., 101:205 (1970).
53. S. Gerö, J. Gergely, T. Devenyi, L. Jakab, J. Szekely and
    S. Virag. Role of mucoid substances of the aorta in the
    deposition of lipids, Nature, 187:152 (1960).
54. K.W. Walton, The biological properties of a new anticoagulant
    possessing heparin-like properties, Brit. J. Pharmacol.
    7:370 (1952).
55. K.W. Walton and P.J. Scott, Estimation of the low-density (β,
    lipoproteins of serum in health and disease using large
    molecular weight dextran sulphate, J. Clin. Path., 17:627
    (1964).
56. A.J.Anderson, The formation of chondromucoprotein - fibrinogen
    and chondromucoprotein - β - lipoprotein complexes.
    Biochem. J., 88:460 (1963).
57. J.S. Amenta and L.L. Waters, The precipitation of serum lipo-
    proteins by mucopolysaccharides extracted from aortic tissue,
    Yale J. Biol. Med. 33:112 (1960).
58. R.C. Curran and W.A.J. Crane, Mucopolysaccharides in the
    atheromatous aorta, J. Pathol. Bact., 84:405 (1962).
59. H.D. Moon and J.F. Rinehart, Histogenesis of coronary arterio-
    sclerosis, Circulation, 6:481 (1952).
60. M.D. Haust, The morphogenesis and fate of potential and early
    atherosclerotic lesions in man, Human Pathol., 2:1 (1971).
61. W.H. Hauss, G. Junge-Hülsing and H.J. Hollander, Changes in
    the metabolism of connective tissue associated with ageing
    and arterio - or atherosclerosis, J. Atheroscler. Res.,
    2:50 (1962).
62. E.B. Smith, P.H. Evans and M.D. Downham, Lipid in the aortic
    intima: the correlation of morphological and chemical
    characteristics, J. Atheroscler. Rec., 7:171 (1967).

63. C.J. Morris, G.V.H. Bradby and K.W. Walton, Fibrous long-
    spacing collagen in human atherosclerosis, 31:345 (1978).
64. J. Larrue, D. Daret, J. Demond and H. Bricaud. Fibrous long
    spacing collagen in aortic explants of normal rabbit
    cultured in hypercholesterolaemic serum. Atherosclerosis,
    28:53 (1977).
65. B.B. Doyle, D.W.L. Hukins, D.J.S. Hulme, A. Miller and
    J. Woohead-Galloway, Collagen polymorphism - Its origin in
    the amino-acid sequence, J. Molec. Biol., 91:79 (1975).
66. J.L. Goldstein and M.S. Brown, The LDL pathway in human fibro-
    blasts: a receptor-mediated mechanism for the regulation of
    cholesterol metabolism, in "Current Topics in Cellular
    Regulation", B.L Horecker and E.R. Stadtman, eds. pp. 147-
    181, Academic Press, New York.
67. R.W. Mahley, T.L. Innerarity, K.H. Weisgraber and S.K. Oh,
    Altered metabolism (In vivo and in vitro) of plasma lipo-
    proteins after selective chemical modification of lysine
    residues of the apoproteins, J. Clin. Invest., 64:743
    (1979).
68. Goldstein, Y.K. Ho, M.S. Brown, T.L. Innerarity and R.W. Mahley,
    Cholesteryl ester accumulation in macrophages resulting from
    receptor-mediated uptake and degradation of hypercholesterol-
    emic canine β-very low density lipoproteins, J. Biol. Chem.,
    255:1839 (1980).
69. G.W. Pickering, Pathogenesis of myocardial and cerebral
    infarction: nodular arteriosclerosis, Brit. Med. J., 1:517
    (1964).
70. G. de Backer - this volume.
71. S. Cohen, T. Freeman and A.S. McFarlane, Metabolism of
    ^{131}I-labelled human albumin. Clin. Sci., 20:161 (1961).
72. P.J. Scott, P.W. Dykes, J. Davis and K.W. Walton, Turnover
    studies of ^{131}I-labelled β-lipoprotein in health and in
    thyroid disease in "Biochemical Problems of Lipids",
    A.C. Fraser. ed., pp. 318-324, Elsevier, Amsterdam, (1963).
73. P.J. Hurley abd P.J. Scott, Plasma turnover of S O-9 low-
    density lipoprotein in normal men and women. Atherosclerosis,
    11:51 (1970).
74. P. Constantinides and M. Robinson, Ultra-structural injury of
    arterial endothelium, Arch. Pathol., 88:99;106;113 (1969).
75. H.M. Turnbull, Alterations in arterial structure and their
    relation to syphilis, Q. J. Med., 8:201 (1915).
76. R.S. Ross and V.A. McKusick, Aortic arch syndromes, Arch. Intern.
    Med., 92:701 (1953).
77. D. Steinberg, Lipoprotein structure and metabolism: Inhomo-
    geneity, variability and species specificity, in "Athero-
    sclerosis V", A.M. Gotto, L.C. Smith and B. Allen, eds.
    pp. 616-623, Springer Verlag, New York (1979).
78. D. Steinberg,R.C. Pittman, A.D. Attie, T.E. Carew, S. Pangbourn
    and D. Weinstein, The role of the liver in LDL catabolism in
    "Atherosclerosis V" A.M. Gotto, L.C. Smith and B. Allen, eds.
    pp. 800-803, Springer Verlag, New York (1979).

79. C.J. Packard, S. Bicker, H.G. Morgan, T.D.V. Lawrie and
    J. Shepherd, Receptor dependent low density lipoprotein
    catabolism in normal and familial hypercholesterolemic
    subjects, in "Proceedings of Vth International Symposium
    on Atherosclerosis", Houston, Texas, November 1979,
    Abstract No. 202.
80. R.W. Mahley, Dietary fat, cholesterol and accelerated athero-
    sclerosis, in "Atherosclerosis Reviews", R. Paoletti and
    A.M. Gotto, eds. Vol. 5, pp. 1-34, Raven Press, New York
    (1979).
81. J.L. Beaumont, L.A. Carlson, G.R. Cooper, Z. Fejfar,
    D.S. Fredrickson and T. Strasser, Classification of hyper-
    lipidaemias and hyperlipoproteinaemias, Bull, Wld. Hlth. Org.
    43:891 (1970).
82. K.W. Walton, The metabolism of low-density (β) lipoproteins in
    health and disease, in "Physiology and pathophysiology of
    Protein Metabolism", G. Birke, R. Norburg and L.O. Plantin,
    pp. 145-148, Pergamon Press, Oxford (1969).
83. A.K. Khachadurian, The inheritence of essential familial
    hypercholesterolaemia, Amer. J. Med., 37:402 (1964).
84. D.B. Zilversmit, A proposal linking atherogenesis to the inter-
    action of endothelial lipoprotein lipase with triglyceride-
    rich lipoproteins, Circ. Res. 33:633 (1973).
85. J. Slack, Risks of ischaemic heart disease in familial hyper-
    lipoproteinaemic states, Lancet, 2:1380 (1969).
86. K.W. Walton, Identification of lipoproteins involved in human
    atherosclerosis, in Atherosclerosis III, G. Shettler and
    A Weizel, eds. pp. 93-95, Springer Verlag, Berlin, (1974).
87. K.W. Walton, J. Hitchens, H.N. Magnani and M. Khan, A study of
    methods of identification of Lp (a) lipoprotein and of its
    significance in health, hyperlipidaemia and atherosclerosis,
    Atherosclerosis, 20:323 (1974).
88. E. Grosjek and S.M. Grundy, Electron microscopic evidence for
    particles smaller than 250 A° in very low density lipo-
    proteins of human plasma, Atherosclerosis, 31:241 (1978).
89. C.J. Morris, H.N. Magnani, K.W. Walton and A.J. Valente,
    Variation in particle size of human and intermediate
    density lipoproteins in health and in hyperlipidaemias:
    An electron microscope study, in preparation.
90. B. Lewis, A Chait, I.D.P. Wootton, C.M. Oakley, D.M. Krikler,
    G. Sigurdsson, A. February, B, Maurer and J. Birkhead,
    Frequency of risk factors for ischaemic heart disease in a
    healthy British population, Lancet, 1:141 (1974).
91. K.W. Walton, Studies on the pathogenesis of corneal arcus
    formation. I. Corneal arcus formation in the human and its
    relation to atherosclerosis as studied by immunofluorescence.
    J. Pathol. 111:263 (1973).
92. P. Constantinides, Lipid deposition in injured arteries, Arch.
    Pathol. 85:280 (1968).

93. P.J. Scott and C.C. Winterbourn, Low density lipoprotein
    accumulation in actively growing xanthomas. J. Atheroscler.
    Res., 7:207 (1967).
94. W.E. Miall and S. Chinn, Blood pressure and ageing: results of
    a 15-17 year follow-up study in South Wales, Clin. Sci. Mol.
    Med., 45:suppl 1, 23S (1973).
95. K.W. Walton, Models for the study of tissue deposition and
    synthesis of lipoproteins, in "The Lipoprotein Molecule ",
    H. Peeters, ed. pp. 255-260, Plenum Press, New York (1978).
96. T.R. Dawber, W.B. Kannel, N. Revotskie and A. Kagan, The
    epidemiology of coronary heart disease - the Framingham
    enquiry, Proc. R. Soc. Med. 55:265 (1962).
97. A. Keys, C. Aravanis, H. Blackburn, F.S.P. van Buchem,
    R. Buzina, B.S. Djordevic, F. Fidanza, M.J. Karvonen,
    A. Menotti, V. Puddu and H.L. Taylor, Probability of middle-
    aged men developing coronary heart disease in five years,
    Circulation, 45:815 (1972).
98. K.W. Walton, C. Thomas and D.J. Dunkerley, The pathogenesis of
    cutaneous xanthomata, J. Pathol. 109:271 (1973).
99. G. Camejo, V. Bosch. C. Arreaza and H.C. Mendis, Early changes
    in lipoprotein structure and biosynthesis in cholesterol-
    fed rabbits. J. Lipid Res. 14:61 (1973).
100. G. Camejo, V. Bosch and A Lopez, The very low density lipo-
    proteins of cholesterol-fed rabbits - A study of their
    structure and in vivo changes in plasma, Atherosclerosis,
    19:139 (1974).
101. B. Shore and V. Shore, Rabbits as a model for the study of
    hyperlipoproteinaemia and atherosclerosis, Adv. Exp. Biol.
    Med., 67:123 (1976).
102. K.W. Walton, G.V.H. Bradby and C.J. Morris, Intestinal bio-
    synthesis of human serum lipoproteins, in "International
    Conference on Atherosclerosis, L.A. Carlson, R. Paoletti,
    C.R. Sirtori and G. Weber, eds. pp. 303-310, Raven Press,
    New York (1978).
103. R. H Hamilton, Synthesis and secretion of plasma lipoproteins,
    Adv. Exp. Biol. Med., 26:7 (1972).
104. K. W. Walton and D.J. Dunkerley, Studies on the pathogenesis
    of corneal arcus formation, II, Immunofluorescent studies
    on lipid deposition in the eye of the lipid-fed rabbit,
    J. Pathol., 114:217 (1974).
105. K.W. Walton, D.J. Dunkerley, A.G. Johnson, M.K. Khan,
    C. Morris and R.B. Watts, Investigation by immunofluorescence
    of arterial lesions in rabbits on two different lipid
    supplements and treated with pyridinol carbamate, Athero-
    sclerosis, 23:117 (1976).
106. K.W. Walton, Atherosclerosis of heart valves and the formation
    of the corneal arcus as models for the study of athero-
    sclerosis, Nutr. Metab., 15:37 (1973).

107. N. Anitschkow, Experimental arteriosclerosis in animals, in
     "Arteriosclerosis", E.V. Cowdry, ed, pp. 271-322, Macmillan,
     New York (1933).
108. R.F. Scott, A.S. Daoud and R.A. Florentin, Animal models in
     Atherosclerosis, in "The Pathogenesis of Atherosclerosis",
     R.W. Wissler and J.C. Gear, pp. 120-146, Williams and
     Wilkins Co., Baltimore, (1972).
109. D. Vesselinovitch, Animal models of atherosclerosis, their
     contributions and pitfalls, Artery, 5:193 (1979).
110. E.B. Smith, Molecular interactions in human atherosclerotic
     plaques, Amer. J. Path., 86:665 (1979).

ANIMAL MODELS OF ATHEROSCLEROSIS

G. A. Gresham

Professor of Morbid Anatomy

University of Cambridge

A vast amount of experimental work has been done in producing atherosclerotic disease in many kinds of animals. In more recent years attention has been directed to work on prevention and regression of lesions using diet, drugs, ileal diversion and so on. In this chapter we shall attempt to provide an overview of past work up to the present day. A few key references are appended to enable the reader to gain access to the precise details of the experiments that have been done.

The choice of a suitable animal model which best represents the human situation has always been a hotly debated problem for experimentalists. Starting with the rabbit a series of experiments involving other mammals and birds have been done. The choice of a suitable model depends to some extent on the nature of the investigation. For example, genetic factors are best exemplified by bird models such as the White Carneau pigeon. Lipid accumulation is best and most easily achieved in the rabbit and so on. However if it is accepted that atherosclerosis is a proliferative response to injury then most animals are suitable. It also follows, if this thesis is accepted, that any stimulus that causes arterial damage will initiate the response. Further events such as lipid accumulation, calcification, and thrombosis are regarded as secondary to the initial injury.

Broadly speaking there have been two basic methods of approach. One involves the use of established risk factors such as hyperlipidaemia, hypertension, smoking

and so on. The other methods use unnatural stimuli such
as freezing arteries, scraping off endothelium and the
like. These are designed to study the role of certain
wall components such as endothelium or smooth muscle
cells in the atherogenic process. Chemical studies of
lipoproteins, apoproteins and glycosaminoglycans often
are involved in either experimental approach.

Experimental work has often attempted to explain
a number of important questions that arise from the
study of atherosclerosis in man. It is an exclusively
human disease in its most severe form of thrombo-
atherosclerosis. Its changing incidence, differences
in severity in various human races require explanation
and animal experiments may help. They also help to
elucidate the precise mode of action of the various
postulated risk factors though some of them still defy
experimental confirmation. For example there is strong
epidemiological evidence in favour of the role of
cigarette smoking in atherogenesis but the precise
mode of action of the smoke has not been revealed by
experiment. Cigarette smoke may act via hypoxia, allergy
to tobacco glycoproteins, nicotine or smoking may only
be an indication of a particular type of
atherosclerosis-prone personality.

It is often said that atherosclerosis is a
multifactorial disease but there are many who seek for
a single causative stimulus taking the view that the
other factors involved merely complicate the initial
event. Champions of the "single insult" theory have
turned their attentions to endothelial injury possibly
mediated by platelet aggregation, adherence and
release of vasoactive components as a possible cause of
atherosclerotic disease. A final important question
which relates to the interpretation of experimental
work is the fate of the fatty streak. This is the
lesion most often produced experimentally but some
maintain that it does not progress to the more complex
stages of atherosclerosis. Studies in birds have
shown that such a progression does exist.

The precise mode of action of the various
postulated risk factors has been the concern of many
in the experimental field. For example hyperlipidaemia
may produce effects in several ways. It may result in
death of endothelial cells, it may encourage platelet
aggregation and lipoproteins do stimulate the
proliferation of smooth muscle cells. Certain
cholesterol esters are more histotoxic than others and

and this is another way that lipids can damage the arterial wall.

Hypertension produces atherogenic effects in a variety of ways. The endothelial sheet is subjected to stretching and shear forces and foci of endothelial cell death have been shown using Evans blue staining. Various vasoactive amines such Angiotensin II which may be associated with hypertension lead to increased endothelial permeability and more easy access of lipoproteins and other plasma constituents into the inner vessel wall.

The effects of hormones on atherogenesis are in opposite directions. They cause cell proliferation in the intima of rats and are associated with a tendency to vasothrombosis. On the other hand they are associated with higher levels of high density lipoproteins and oestrogen blocks the growth stimulation effect of low density lipoproteins on smooth muscle cells. Both of these factors are thought to be antiatherogenic.

Cigarette smoking has a strong epidemiological association with ischaemic heart disease but experimental support for its role in atherogenesis is weak.

Smoking may act in a variety of ways. These may be a hypoxic effect, or one due to nicotine. Even sensitivity to tobacco glycoprotein has been postulated Hypoxia increases endothelial permeability and also predisposes to the development of fatty change in the arterial wall.

RABBIT EXPERIMENTS

Rabbits have been used for the study of experimental atherosclerosis since the first decade of this century. Lipid laden lesions are easily and rapidly produced by feeding cholesterol though it was not appreciated for some time that individual animals within a breed responded more rapidly than others. Complications of atherosclerosis such as haemorrhage into the plaque, thrombosis and ulceration do not occur unless other stimuli such as vitamin D and epinephrine are added to the experimental regime.[1] Only early lesions in rabbits have been seen to regress when the experimental regime is stopped. Later, more fibrotic plaques are not altered. Those using rabbits and also rats have always appreciated that cholesterol feeding induces a

generalised lipidosis in many organs. This has led to
speculation about the significance of such experiments
in relation to atherogenesis in man.[2]

RAT EXPERIMENTS

Rats do not usually develop spontaneous
atherosclerosis and for this reason many advocate their
use in this field of research. In order to produce
lesions in the heart and aorta it is necessary to feed
40% of the diet as fat with 5% cholesterol and other
agents such as thiouracil and cholic acid. This results
in extensive lipidosis of the liver, spleen and other
organs. However an interesting result emerged relating
to the type of fat that was fed. If it was 40% butter
the animals developed massive intracardiac thrombosis
and myocardial infarction but no atherosclerosis was
found. Feeding 40% of peanut oil resulted in lipid-
laden atherosclerotic plaques in the aorta and
proximal coronary arteries.[3] This raised the
interesting question of the mechanisms of action of
the saturated and unsaturated fats: whether both
affected platelet aggregation leading to thrombosis
on the one hand and smooth muscle stimulation and
atherosclerosis on the other. To clarify this issue
attempts were made using radioactive phosphorus in
small doses to deplete the platelet stores. However
this proved to be too toxic.

More recently strains of rats with naturally
occurring hypo[4] and hypercholesterolaemia have
been described[4] as well as spontaneously hypertensive
strains that we have already described. These may
provide more suitable models.

BIRD EXPERIMENTS

Much early work was done in chickens. We have
already referred to spontaneous disease in these
animals. Feeding cholesterol to cockerels produces
aortic lesions and lesions in the small branches of
the coronary arteries. This model has been valuable
in showing that oestrogens ameliorate the coronary
lesions but have no effect on the aortic disease.[5]
Some of the earliest work on possible regression of
atherosclerosis was done by the same team.[6] They
observed regression of cholesterol induced

atherosclerosis when a diet containing cholesterol was withdrawn.

Experiments with chickens have made the important point that aortic and coronary atherosclerotic lesions do not always behave in the same way. This reinforces the view that the results of experimentally induced aortic disease cannot always be extrapolated to interpret factors which may affect coronary atherosclerosis.

The observations that turkeys often develop dissecting aneurysms of the posterior aorta in the interrenal area led to experimental studies with this animal.[7] This point of weakness was marked by a fibro-muscular intimal plaque which contained some lipid and occasional fragments of calcification. Such lesions had been produced in other animals by dietary fat and it was postulated that the highly artificial diets of these domestic animals might be responsible for the lesions. Various dietary modifications were made none of which affected the disease. The occurrence of similar lesions in wild Texan Turkeys also made the dietary hypothesis less tenable. However the extent of the aortic disease can be aggravated by feeding cholesterol. An important feature of these birds was the presence of hypertension and that the level of blood pressure and the extent of lesions increased with age. The use of hypotensive agents lowered the incidence of rupture. In the turkey hypertension is probably the most potent atherogenic factor.

The White Carneau pigeon is probably one of the most useful birds for experiment. They have naturally occurring atherosclerosis which closely resembles the disease in man.[8] Feeding small amounts of cholesterol to these animals leads to conspicuous enlargement of lesions and obstructive lesions of the coronary arteries lead to myocardial infarction. At the same time serum lipids become elevated. The pigeon is unique in that short-term cholesterol feeding leads rapidly to the appearance of lesions in predictable sites. This makes the model especially valuable for the study of early metabolic changes in atherosclerotic vessels. The patterns of spontaneous disease vary in different strains of pigeon so that cross breeding experiments can be done to study the role of genetic factors in atherogenesis.

PIG EXPERIMENTS

Atherosclerosis occurs naturally in the pig and
young animals are often affected. Large domestic
and razor-backed mini-pigs have been used. They
respond readily to cholesterol enriched diets :
blood lipids rise and atherosclerosis increases.
Blood clotting factors have also been studied in
these animals and patterns of platelet deposition
in artificial arteriovenous shunts interpolated into
the circulation produce deposits at sites when
atherosclerosis might be expected to develop in normal
blood vessels. They readily develop cerebrovascular
disease when fed on waste foods. This work has been
extensively reported from Philadelphia.[9]

Lesions have also been produced by scraping the
aortic surface and the sequence of development of
atherosclerosis has been studied in this way.
Irradiation of the thorax of the pig coupled with
cholesterol feeding leads to the rapid production of
coronary disease in a few months. This emphasizes the
role of arterial injury in atherogenesis and provides a
model for speedy induction of disease.[10] It is also
a useful experimental method for the study of
pathophysiological mechanisms in sudden death.

EXPERIMENTS IN OTHER ANIMALS

We shall discuss non-human primates shortly
particularly in relation to studies of regression. Here
we shall briefly discuss other species that have only
occasionally been used for atherosclerosis research.
Mice have not often been used. Studies have been done
on diet and irradiation. Irradiation, wheather acute
or repeated shortens survival times in mice. When
this is combined with cholesterol feeding lipid
accumulates in intimal and smooth muscle cells of the
aorta, coronary, renal and pulmonary arteries.[11] By
using inbred strains it is possible to obtain consistent
results.

Dogs have been little used because they need to be
made hypothyroid before cholesterol feeding will produce
any atherogenic effect. Cats respond more readily and
develop hypercholesterolaemia and coronary artery
lesions when the diet contains 2% cholesterol. Little
has been done with domestic farm animals other than

pigs. Naturally occuring disease has been described
in cows and sheep will develop atherosclerosis if fed
1% cholesterol and 10% lard.

In general feeding cholesterol induces
hypercholesterolaemia in most animals. More interesting
are those creatures such as chinchillas and mongolian
gerbils which are naturally hypercholesterolaemic but
have no arterial disease. We have already suggested
that the explanation for this fact in other animals
such as mink, is due to the fact that the bulk of their
plasma cholesterol is associated with high density
lipoprotein.

NON-HUMAN PRIMATE EXPERIMENTS

Non-human primates are the subjects of much
research into the causes of atherosclerosis. The
subject has been extensively reviewed recently.[12] They
are attractive because they have morphological and
biochemical features that are similar to those in man
and may develop atherosclerosis similar to the human
disease.

Within the primate order both Simidae and Pongidae
have been studied. The latter are expensive animals and
most work has therefore been done with the baboon,
rhesus, cebus, vervet and squirrel monkeys. Early
experiments involving feeding cholesterol and
thyroidectomy did not give promising results. Experiments
which purported to show that methionine deficiency or
pyridoxine deficiency were factors could not be
confirmed. However subsequent workers were able to
produce severe coronary atheroma by feeding cholesterol
and experimentally induced hypertension in monkeys was
also shown to be atherogenic.[13]

Feeding butter with 2% cholesterol to young
baboons produced a rise in serum lipids after three
months. In particular the low density lipoproteins
were elevated after feeding fat. At the end of
eighteen months abundant fatty streaks were found
in the thoracic aorta and occasional lesions in the
coronary arteries.[14]

More recently species of the genus Macacca have
been shown to be highly susceptible to dietary
induced atherosclerosis of the proximal main coronary
arteries and myocardial infarction has been reported.

GENERAL CONSIDERATIONS

Clarkson[2] has summarised the various indications
that have emerged from the vast amount of experimental
work that has been done in this field. In most
species atherosclerosis is aggravated by feeding
cholesterol. Some species of animal are more
susceptible to it than others. For example rabbits
and pigeons have exacerbation of their vascular
disease with only minor additions of cholesterol to the
diet. Furthermore cholesterol feeding will also induce
lesions in animals like the rat in which they do not
naturally occur.

However the elevation of blood cholesterol may not
always be associated with the appearance of
atherosclerotic lesions. This is because the
cholesterol is associated with lipoproteins other than
those of low density. Even within a strain of animals
such as rabbits or squirrel monkeys there is also a
variation in the response to cholesterol feeding.
Furthermore different arteries also respond differently
in the same subject. The question of the subsequent
fate of the fatty streak is a topic that permeates the
whole field of experimental atherosclerosis. The
answer to the question depends on the particular artery
studied and the particular species of animal that is
used.

Finally we come to the question of regression.
In 1970 only 2% of the projects supported by the
National Heart Institute of N.I.H. were related to
studies of regression. Since that time much has been
done.

In the early 1970's Armstrong and his team showed
that by withdrawing an atherogenic stimulus lipid could
be mobilised from lesions and that some types of
collagen would break down.[15] The morphological changes
during the regression phase were studied in detail by
Stary.[16] He saw death of macrophages loaded with lipid
and determined a decline in the proliferative activity
of endothelial cells, smooth muscle cells and foam cells
during the regression phase. At the end of thirty two
weeks practically all of the foam cells had
disappeared.

A number of drugs have been used to promote
regression. The experimental evidence available so
far suggests that cholestyramine is probably the most

practical agent in this regard. Other studies have
indicated the value of lowering blood pressure.
In a study by Hollander et al[17] blood pressure levels
of 180/120 were produced by coarctation of the aorta
and blood cholesterol levels of 510 mgm/dl were
produced by feeding 2% cholesterol and 10% butter in
the diet. In one group cholesterol was withdrawn
after six months and in another cholesterol was
withdrawn and hypotensive therapy was given. The latter
regime proved to be the most effective in reducing the
extent of coronary artery narrowing.

One of the principal problems in all of this work
is that of assessing the degree of disease in the
living animal. Invasive techniques only complicate
the issue by generating more arterial damage and hence
further lesions. For the future we look to non-
invasive ultrasound and other techniques that will
construct images of arterial lesions in man and
experimental animals.[18]

REFERENCES

1. P. Constantinides, Experimental atherosclerosis in
    the rabbit, in "Comparative Atherosclerosis",
    J. C. Roberts and R. Straus, eds., Publisher,
    Harper (Hoeber) New York, 276, (1965).
2. T. B. Clarkson, Animal models of atherosclerosis,
    Adv. in vet. science and comp. med. 16:151
    (1972).
3. G. A. Gresham and A. N. Howard, The independent
    production of thrombosis and atherosclerosis
    in the rat, Br. J. exp. pathol. 41:393 (1960).
4. H. N. Adel, Q. B. Deming and L. Brun, Genetic
    hypercholesterolaemia in rats, Circulation 39
    Supp. 3:1 (1969).
5. R. Pick, J. Stamler and L. Katz, The inhibition
    of coronary atherosclerosis by oestrogens in
    cholesterol-fed chicks, Circulation 6:276
    (1952).
6. L. Horlick and L. N. Katz, Regression of athero-
    sclerotic lesions on cessation of cholesterol
    feeding in the chicken, J. lab. clin. med.
    34:1427 (1949).
7. G. A. Gresham and A. N. Howard, Aortic rupture in
    the turkey, J. atheroscler. res. 1:75 (1961).
8. T. B. Clarkson, R. W. Prichard, M. G. Netsky and
    H. B. Lofland, Atherosclerosis in pigeons. Its
    spontaneous occurrence and resemblance to

human atherosclerosis, A.M.A. Arch. pathol.
68:143 (1959).

9.   H. L. Ratcliffe and H. Luginbuhl, The domestic
     pig: a model for experimental atherosclerosis,
     Atherosclerosis 13:133 (1971).

10. K. T. Lee, D. M. Kim and W. A. Thomas, Method for
     rapid production in swine of advanced coronary
     occlusive disease with myocardial infarction
     and sudden death, Circulation 41 Supp.3:III:9
     (1970).

11. D. Vesselinovitch and R. W. Wissler, Experimental
     production of atherosclerosis in mice. Part
     II Effects of atherogenic and high fat diets
     on vascular changes in chronically and acutely
     irradiated mice, J. Atheroscler. res. 8:497
     (1968).

12. G. A. Gresham, Primate atherosclerosis, in
     Monographs on atherosclerosis 7
     Publisher, S. Karger Basel (1976).

13. G. A. Gresham and A. N. Howard, Comparative
     pathology of spontaneously occurring and
     experimentally induced atherosclerotic lesions,
     Meth. Achievm. exp. Path. 1:314 (1966).

14. G. A. Gresham, Vascular lesions in primates,
     Conference on comparative cardiology,
     N.Y. Acad. Sci. 127:694 (1965).

15. M. L. Armstrong and M. B. Megan, Arterial fibrous
     proteins in cynomolgous monkeys after
     atherogenic and regression diets, Circ. Res.
     36:256 (1975).

16. H. C. Stary, Regression of atherosclerosis in
     primates, Virchows Arch. A. Path. Anat. and
     Histol. 383:117 (1979).

17. W. Hollander, I. Madoff, J. Paddock and
     B. Kirkpatrick, Aggravation of atherosclerosis
     by hypertension in a subhuman primate model
     with coarctation of the aorta, Circ. Res.
     38: (Supp. II) 63 (1976).

18. G. A. Gresham, Reversing atherosclerosis in
     "America Lecture Series", Charles C. Thomas,
     Ed., Publisher Springfield, Illinois (1980).

ATHEROSCLEROSIS IN ANIMALS:

COMPARATIVE ASPECTS

G. A. Gresham

Professor of Morbid Anatomy

University of Cambridge

Of all animals man is most seriously affected by
atherosclerosis and its complications. In an attempt
to explain this fact extensive surveys of many different
kinds of animals have been made ranging from fish to
elephants and eagles. This was done primarily to try to
identify factors in the life style of man and by
comparison with other animals which may promote or
prevent the development of atherosclerosis.

Many animals such as old pigs and many sorts of
birds develop atherosclerosis similar to that seen in man.
The lesions are both proliferative and degenerative
containing myofibroblasts lipids and so on. If the term
arteriosclerosis is used to encompass arterial thickenings
of all sorts, of which atherosclerosis is but one,
arteriosclerosis is a common feature of many animal
arteries. For example intimal sclerosis of the kind
seen in young people is often found in the arteries of
aged horses, ruminants and carnivores. It shows a
predilection for the abdominal aorta occurring near to
branches and often involving the peripheral arteries as
well. These are basically uncomplicated lesions
containing smooth muscle cells, glycosaminoglycans and
multiple elastic layers. They do not usually advance
to form complicated lesions as seen in advanced human
atherosclerosis. Other varieties of arteriosclerosis
occur in animals such things as amyloid deposition in the
coronary arteries of dogs and calcification of the media
of large vessels occur in many species including the
elephant. The ultimate aim of these comparative studies

is to find an animal model which develops arterio-
sclerotic lesions similar to human atherosclerosis. We
shall now review a series of animal groups with this
in mind. All sorts of animals including mammals
develop intimal thickenings and medial changes as well.
The occurrence of such lesions occasionally provide
some clues to the aetiology of the disease.

FISH AND REPTILES

The coronary arteries of cartilaginous and teleost
fish often show intimal lesions and these are found
both in freshwater and marine mammals. Mostly the lesions
consist of foci of intimal thickening but occasionally
lipid-laden lesions have been reported as for example in
the tuna fish.[1] Moore et al[2] have related the number,
severity and location of coronary artery lesions in
Pacific salmon and later in Steelhead trout to stages of
their spawning migration and to sexual maturity. The
number of intimal lesions increased steadily as the
time of spawning approached. The lesions were found
mainly in the large coronary arteries and increased in
size with sexual maturity. The lesions consisted of
focal proliferations of smooth muscle cells which
projected through gaps in the internal elastic lamella
into the intima. The newly formed cells were often
orientated at right angles to the existing smooth muscle
cells of the media. Occasional medial changes occurred
as well. They consisted of medial thinning, loss of
elastic fibres and degeneration of smooth muscle cells.

The earliest change that has been described in
these fish months before spawning consists of
endothelial cell swelling and vacuolation with
separation of endothelial cells from the internal
elastic lamella. This is then followed by proliferation
of smooth muscle cells into the intima. Various attempts
have been made to relate these changes to the activities
of the fish. However they are not due to adaptation to
freshwater as they are frequent in ocean fish. Nor have
they been linked with starvation, prolonged stress,
distance of migration and the sex of the fish.
Administration of cortisol likewise had no influence
on the occurrence of the lesions. The lesions were
exacerbated by sexual maturation which points to some
relation to hormonal activity.[3]

Lesions in the Steelhead trout were more severe than
in the Pacific salmon and were found in all animals.[4]

Other workers found that 95% of prespawning trout had
lesions when in fresh water but only 7% of the animals
had lesions when returning to spawn from the ocean.[5]
So the intimal lesions of the trout regress after they
return to the ocean. This is a most interesting
observation in relation to the potential regression of
atherosclerosis. The ease of regression was probably
due to the fact that lesions in the trout were purely
intimal and there was no lipid present. Other workers
have reported regression of these lesions as the size
of the gonads falls after spawning. Another factor that
might be associated is the level of hormones in the
blood. Injections of testosterone, oestradiol and human
chorionic gonadotrophic induce such lesions in juvenile
trout.[6] Studies in other animals such as the rat
indicate that the hormones oestradiol and testosterone
produce effects in arteries. High levels of oestradiol
cause degradation of the elastic tissue and testosterone
stimulates collagen synthesis.[7]

Few examples of coronary artery disease have been
recorded in reptiles. Intimal proliferations have been
reported in an anaconda and in crocodiles. Fatty streaks
and plaques have been recorded in a 20 year old two
banded monitor.

BIRDS

Many birds develop atherosclerosis of one sort or
another and diffuse intimal thickening is a common
finding. Vastesaeger[1] observed it in 20% of over 500
birds that he examined. Coronary atherosclerosis was
not frequent (about 1.3%) much less so than aortic
atherosclerosis which is common in birds of various
species. Some birds are more affected than others:
for example rheas, ostriches and some galliforms.
Closely related birds often show a discrepant incidence
of the disease. The captive congolese peacock has much
more intimal sclerosis than its domestic counterpart.

Ratcliffe and his team have made extensive studies
on the effects of captivity upon the arteries of various
animals including birds. He described three changes in
the nature and distribution of cardiovascular disease
in animals in the Philadelphia Zoo over a period of
30 years.[8] Between 1936 and 1955 the incidence of
aortic atheroma had increased from 4% to 20%. Then
followed a period when lesions became less frequent

in the brachio-cephalic arteries and aortic arch of
larger psittacines. This was associated with a change
in the diet. In the 60's a new development was the
appearance of fibrosis in the myocardial branches of the
coronary arteries which was accompanied by fibrosis and
infarction of the myocardium. This accompanied attempts
to assemble and maintain stocks of breeding mammals and
birds. That is an increased frequency of small coronary
artery disease was associated with a change in the
social environment. The precise factor which causes this
rise in incidence of small vessel disease is not clear.
However the increased incidence was associated with
increased adrenal weights suggesting a possible role of
hypertension generated by social interaction. It is
recorded that the blood pressure rises less in isolated
laboratory animals than in those that are crowded
together.[9]

Atheroma of the large vessels was greater in birds
than in mammals. Two cranes had such severe aortic
atheroma that they developed aortic thrombosis with
gangrene. Atheroma in the psittacines (parrots, macaws
and cockatoos) was often due to feeding a diet rich in
sunflower seeds which contain 30% of fat. Within six
months of changing to a mixed low-fat ration the lesions
were greatly reduced in size. The lesions of the small
coronary arteries, which were thought to be the result
of social interaction, consisted of proliferations of
smooth muscle and fibrous tissue in the intima. There
was often accompanying medial fibrosis.

Some birds which develop spontaneous atherosclerosis
have been used as experimental animals to study factors
affecting the disease. They are principally chickens,
pigeons and turkeys. An early study by Dauber in 1944[10]
of adult chickens obtained from a Chicago market showed
visible aortic lesions of the aorta in about 50% of
roosters and hens. However the lesions were rather
different. In the abdominal aorta of the rooster they
were linear and fibrous; in the hen they contained
more lipid. In addition the hens had fatty streaks
in the proximal aorta. This difference could be
associated with enormous fluctuation of plasma
cholesterol levels which occur in the egg laying hen.

Another study of white leghorns showed a progressive
increase in cholesterole content and severity of the
atherosclerotic lesion in both males and females with
age. However the lesions were seen most often in the
abdominal aorta in contrast to cholesterol induced

lesions which tended to favour the thoracic part of the
vessel. This observation makes interpretation of
cholesterol feeding experiments difficult in relation
to the pathogenesis of human atherosclerosis. Other
workers showed that hypertension and atherosclerosis
both increased with age in chickens but that a close
relationship between the two processes was not clearly
established.[10] The coronary arteries are rarely affected:
intimal fibrosis occurs in the coronary arteries of
cockerels but lipid-containing lesions have not been
reported in natural conditions.

The pigeon has been extensively used as a model
in atherosclerosis research. Several sorts of pigeon
develop atherosclerosis but the White Carneau has been
studied more extensively than the rest. In these birds
lipid begins to accumulate in the intima during the
first few weeks of life. By the age of four years
100% of the birds have grossly visible aortic lesions
particularly at the origin of the coeliac artery.
Coronary atherosclerosis develops more slowly but
by the age of 8 years lipid laden lesions are present
in 70% of the birds. Neither aortic not coronary
lesions showed any sex predilection.

Aortic atherosclerosis in the White Carneau is
histologically very similar to the human disease.[11]
The lesions in mature birds are yellow or yellow and
white with depressed centres and rather ovoid in shape.
They are larger in the older animals. Up to the age
of five years about 8% of the aortic surface was
involved and about 10% in birds aged 6 to 12. Not
only did the lesions increase in size but also in
extent with age. This is strictly comparable to the
human situation.

The pigeon plaques also resemble many human
atheromas in that they contain about 40% lipid grouped
in the centre of the plaque and covered by a fibrous
cap. Lipid is initially contained in cells which are
either macrophages or smooth muscle cells and is also
found extracellularly. As the amount of lipid increases
with age cholesterol clefts and foci of calcification
develop. Once again these histological features are
strikingly similar to the human disease. In addition
the pigeon disease tends to develop the complications of
vascularisation, haemorrhage, ulceration and thrombosis.
In these respects it differs from disease in the
chicken and the turkey. About 20% of the lesions have

become ulcerated and develop superimposed thrombosis.

Atherosclerosis of the coronary arteries occurs in about 70% of adult White Carneau pigeons and they increase in number with age. During the first two years of life there is no association between the development of coronary and aortic disease. Thereafter a weak relationship exists. The coronary lesions often calcify but other complications are infrequent as compared to the aortic lesions. Coronary vessels of all sizes are affected and there is no difference between the sexes. The degree of luminal narrowing caused by the lesions is usually slight and of the order of not more than 8%. Myocardial infarcts have been the cause of death in a few birds but these are due to atheromatous emboli derived from the aortic root.

The White Carneau pigeon provides a good example of genetic influences in atherogenesis which is a rare phenomenon in the animal kingdom. When compared with other pigeons such as the Show Racer 30% of the White Carneau squabs have intimal lipid lesions after one week of life. Only 10% of Show Racer squabs show such lesions histologically. At four years 100% of White Carneaux have disease whereas only 15% of Show Racers show disease at 7 years of age.

Studies of the sterol and sterylesters in the two sorts of pigeon have shown differences. A greater amount of sterol and degree of sterylesterification in the abdominal aorta of the White Carneau was found. In addition the cholesterol content was increased. This is interesting because this sterol has been isolated from human lesions and feeding it to rabbits can induce atherosclerosis.[12]

Lesions in pigeons, in particular the White Carneau are consistently found at the coeliac bifurcation in the same way that atherosclerotic lesions are consistently found in the carotid bifurcation in man. Similarly the lesions are lateral to the orifice and progress up-stream suggesting low shear rates in the areas. Furthermore the fatty streaks at these locations in pigeon and human arteries show steady progression into fibrous plaques.[13]

The turkey has also been the subject of research in atherogenesis since a report in 1952 that a significant number of the Broad Breasted Bronze variety

died before reaching market age (5 - 6 months).
Subsequently it was reported that extensive linear
atherosclerosis occurred in the abdominal aorta of birds
with aortic rupture in those that survived.[14] The aortic
lesions were of two kinds. Fatty streaks were seen and
these increased in extent with age. Another lesion was
a linear fibromuscular plaque containing a little lipid
in the interrenal part of the aorta. This was the
usual site of aortic rupture. The reason for rupture was
partly explained by a high systolic blood pressure
(about 280 mm Hg) found in these animals. Coronary
artery atherosclerosis was also seen in poults at
twelve weeks of age. They were histologically similar
to the lesions in the aorta and were occasionally
associated with deposits of lipid in the media.

Much work has been done to determine the cause of
spontaneous atherosclerosis in the turkey. Some of it
deals with the influence of rapid growth which might
lead to defective formation of elastin in the aorta
which predisposes to migration of smooth muscle cells
from the media into the intima. The linear raised
muscular lesions occur in the abdominal aorta just
distal to the origin of the coeliac artery and it is at
this point that the normal structure of the aorta
changes. The proximal aorta and its brachiocephalic
vessels are thick elastic tubes composed of closely
packed elastic lamellae separated by collagen and
mucopolysaccharide. The distal aorta is by contrast
thin, composed of smooth muscle cells separated by
thin irregular strands of elastic tissue. During the
early period of growth fragmentation of internal and
external elastic membranes is a feature of the
abdominal but not of the thoracic aorta in the turkey.
This is related to the presence of polar amino acid
residues and chemically unstable dehydrolysinoleucine
which is a cross linking substance for elastic tissue.[15]
When the animal becomes mature the elastin stabilises.

Growth in domestic turkeys is rapid and is promoted
by intensive feeding. It might be expected that the
rapid growth is related to the production of plaques in
the aorta and if growth could be suppressed then plaques
would not develop. This experiment was done inadvertantly
by feeding Triparanol to reduce cholesterol levels in
order to see what effect this had on the incidence of
aortic rupture in turkeys fed β aminopropionitrile. It
had no effect. However the drug did inhibit growth
which likewise had no effect on the incidence of aortic
diseases.[16] It has also been found that feeding

diethylstilboestrol to turkeys increases the incidence
of rupture but this drug has no effect after 16 weeks
of age. This suggests that something occurring in the
growing aorta is the principal reason for the
appearance of lesions.[17]

MAMMALS

     Of all the mammals man is unique in having a high
incidence of extramural coronary atherosclerosis,
coronary thrombosis and myocardial infarction, whereas
stenotic lesions of the intramural vessels are common
in other animals and cause foci of myocardial necrosis
and fibrosis.[18] However disease of large and small
coronary arteries has been described in a wide variety
of captive and wild animals. Carnivores and strict
herbivores tend to develop less disease than
omniverous species and reports tend to be more
numerous in those animals that have been used to study
atherogenesis. Thus there are several accounts of
naturally occurring disease in rabbits, rats, pigs
and non-human primates. However it is more useful to
study those animals which do not develop atherosclerosis
spontaneously because they might provide a clue to
mechanisms of atherogenesis. We have already discussed
this point in relation to the Masai tribe in Africa.

     There is repeated reference throughout the
literature to medial calcification in the arteries of
several animals. This pathological process has nothing
to do with atherosclerosis but has often been confused
with it by several authors. This change which is
similar to Monckeberg's sclerosis in man has been
described in rabbits, pigs, old female breeder rats and
in dogs and cats. It can occur alone or together with
intimal disease.

     We have already referred to periodic hyperlipidaemia
in the laying hen chicken and suggested it is an
explanation for the occurrence of fatty streaks in the
proximal aorta. The advantages of comparative studies
reveal that such simplistic views are not tenable. This
is well illustrated by the seasonal hyperlipidaemia
and hypercholesterolaemia in particular, in the European
badger. The hyperlipidaemia occurs during the cold
months of the year and yet the animal has not been
shown to develop atherosclerosis.[19]

We have also suggested previously that the intimal changes in the arteries of infants and young children might be the basis for the subsequent development of atherosclerosis. This may well be true in man but there are other animals such as cattle where intimal changes are frequent but developed atherosclerosis is rare. Cattle provide a good example of this. Extensive calcified plaques occur in the aorta of cattle with Johne's disease but these are more akin to the non-atherosclerotic medial calcification. Lesions of a different sort were found in the coronary arteries of cows (3 to 10 years old). They consisted of swollen intimal elastic fibres which were often duplicated, fragmented and stained unevenly. Similar changes were seen in the media and were associated with an increased level of sulphated acid mucopolysaccharides.[20] The microscopic appearances occurred even though lesions were not macroscopically evident. Here then is an example of an animal showing early changes similar to those seen in man which do not proceed to the development of more complicated atherosclerotic disease.

The African elephant provides an interesting example of the effects of changing habitat on the incidence of atherosclerosis.[21] A survey was made of arterial disease in elephants living in an undisturbed habitat in the indigenous forests compared with those in scrubland with no shade; ill suited for the elephant (a so called disturbed habitat).

Uncomplicated intimal sudanophilia occurred in the aorta and large arteries of all elephants being particularly common in suckling calves and lactating and pregnant females. However in animals culled from the 'disturbed' habitat, especially in scrubland, lesions resembling human atheroma were found. They consisted of intimal hyperplasia, fragmentation of the internal elastic lamella, hyaline degeneration and calcification. Another feature was medial sclerosis. Such intimal and medial changes were not found in animals from the "natural" montane habitat. The suggestion that arose from these observations was that population pressure was a factor in atherogenesis. A view which was also proposed by Ratcliffe. Other workers have described sudden death from coronary artery disease in captive elephants, others have studied the arteries of captive and wild elephants and have found no difference in the degree of atherosclerosis in either group.[22] The arterial disease was only related to the age of the

animal and the medial fibrosis and calcification was
subsequently correlated also with the serum calcium
levels.[23]

Pigs, rabbits and rats have been extensively used
in studies of experimentally induced atherosclerosis.
It is therefore appropriate at this point to discuss
naturally occurring disease in these animals. Pigs are
large expensive animals and are costly to feed. However
they do develop atherosclerosis spontaneously and
because the lesions are large provide an excellent source
of material for chemical as well as morphological studies
of atherosclerosis.

An excellent account of intimal changes in the
arteries of ageing swine was given by French et al.[24]
They examined animals from 4 to 10 years of age and
found intimal thickenings in the coronary arteries
similar in structure and distribution to those seen in
man. There was elastic tissue fragmentation followed
by proliferation of intimal smooth muscle cells. In
later lesions lipid was found. These changes are almost
identical with those which we have described in infants
and children. Other workers have described atherosclerotic plaques in the aorta and at the coronary
orifices in a number of pigs over the age of one year.[25]

Of all animals the rabbit has received most
attention in the field of atherosclerosis research. It
readily develops atherosclerosis after cholesterol
feeding and then initially lipid-rich lesions turn
into fibrofatty plaques as the regime is continued.
The occurrence of spontaneous lesions varies with the
breed of rabbit as does the response to cholesterol
feeding. Some breeds are hyperresponders and develop
high cholesterol levels in a few weeks of cholesterol
feeding, other breeds take longer to develop the same
blood cholesterol levels as the hyperresponders. A
survey of 1089 rabbits of different breeds showed the
differences in incidence of aortic disease.[26] 46%
of Flemish giants showed disease as opposed to 13% of the
Dutch breed. In addition considerable variation in
incidence was found between strains of New Zealand white
rabbits from three separate sources in the U.S.A. For
example in New Jersey rabbits taken from suppliers only
70 miles apart there were differences in incidence
ranging from 70 to 36%. These differences have not been
explained by external influences such as diet, climate
and so on and must therefore be considered when selecting
rabbits for experimental work.

Concomitant with the intimal lesions in rabbits were medial areas of sclerosis and calcification. Both types of lesion had however been recorded separately and as in pigs, cattle and elephants there was no clear causative relationship between intimal and medial changes.[27]

Similar strain differences exist in rats though in general rats are much more resistant than rabbits to develop experimentally induced atherosclerosis. We have used hooded rats which in general have responded well to feeding experiments. The Wistar strain however proved much more resistant. Certain strains of rat have been bred which are especially susceptible to atherosclerosis. Such an animal is the spontaneously hypertensive, obese and hyperlipidaemic rat produced by crossing a Kyoto Wistar strain with a normotensive Sprague - Dawley rat. The stable strain was isolated after selective inbreeding of hypertensive offspring. The animals were hyperphagic and showed a hyperlipidaemia similar to that of type IV in man: namely hypertriglyceridaemia with moderate hypercholesterolaemia. The blood pressures were 180 mm of Hg or more rising progressively with increasing age.[28]

Examination of the cardiovascular system in these animals showed a thick firm left ventricle with small foci of necroses. No lesions were found in the coronary arteries apart from slight intimal smooth muscle cell proliferation. However the splanchnic vessels showed aneurysms and thromboses with extensive proliferative intimal lesions composed of smooth muscle cells in a myxoid stroma. Occasionally polyarteritis developed and death was often due to renal failure.

The vascular lesions were aggravated by feeding a 1% saline solution and this particularly affected the cerebral vessels[29] this is very similar to the situation in the Japanese male where a high salt intake is related to hypertension and stroke.

In more recent times a number of non-human primates have been used to study atherosclerosis. Animals such as the baboon have many morphological and biochemical similarities to man and this has proved an attractive feature for experimental studies. 20 species studied showed diffuse intimal thickenings similar to those seen in man[30] McGill et al found fatty streaks in the aortas of three quarters of the Kenya baboons that he examined and others have described aortic plaques in a large proportion of squirrel monkeys.[31]

Primates vary considerably in the occurrence of lesions. They are rare in the marmoset and in Macaca nigra for example. However the development of spontaneous diabetes mellitus in the latter[32] aggravates the development of atherosclerotic disease.

This account of spontaneously occurring atherosclerosis in a variety of animals provides a spectrum of the disease and a range of possible atherogenic stimuli that is a challenge to the investigator. Each species has some light to throw on the process of atherogenesis which is essentially no more than a proliferative response of the arterial wall to injury.

REFERENCES

1. M. M. Vastesaeger, Coronary arterial lesions in exotic vertebrates, Ann. N. Y. Acad. Sci. 127:709 (1965).
2. J. F. Moore, W. Mayr and C. Hougie, Number, location and severity of coronary arterial changes in spawning pacific salmon, J. Comp. Pathol. 86:37 (1976).
3. J. E. McKenzie, E. W. House, J. Mcwilliam and D. W. Johnson, Coronary degeneration in sexually mature rainbow and steelhead trout, Salmo gairdneri, Atherosclerosis 29:431 (1978).
4. J. F. Moore, W. Mayr and C. Hougie, Number, location and severity of coronary arterial changes in steelhead trout, Atherosclerosis 24:381 (1976).
5. R. L. Van Citters and N. W. Watson, Coronary disease in spawning steelhead trout, Science 159:105 (1968).
6. S. P. Schmidt and E. W. House, Time study of coronary myointimal hyperplasia in precocious male steelhead trout, Atherosclerosis 34:375 (1979).
7. G. M. Fisher and M. L. Swain, Effect of sex hormones in blood pressure and vascular connective tissue in castrated and non-castrated male rats, Amer. J. Physiol. 232:4671 (1977).
8. H. L. Ratcliffe, Age and environment as factors in the nature and frequency of cardiovascular lesions in mammals and birds in the Philadephia Zoological Garden, Ann. N. Y. Acad. Sci. 127:715 (1965).
9. M. Hallback, Consequences of social isolation in blood pressure, cardiovascular reactivity and design in spontaneously hypertensive rats, Acta Physiol. Scand. 93:455 (1975).

10. A. Grollman, C. Ashworth and W. Suki, Atherosclerosis in the chicken - correlation of the arterial blood pressure and arterial changes in the chicken, Arch. Pathol. 75:618 (1963).

11. R. W. Pritchard, T. B. Clarkson, H. O. Goodman and H. B. Lofland, Aortic atherosclerosis in pigeons and its complications, Arch. Pathol. 77:244 (1964).

12. M. T. R. Subbiah, B. A. Kotke and I. A. Carlo, Studies in spontaneous atherosclerosis - susceptible and resistant pigeons, Int. J. Biochem. 5:63 (1974).

13. R. F. Santerre, T. N. Wight, S. C. Smith and D. Brannigan, Spontaneous atherosclerosis in pigeons. A model system for studying metabolic parameters associated with atherogenesis, Amer. J. Pathol. 67:1 (1972).

14. G. A. Gresham and A. N. Howard, Aortic rupture in the turkey, J. Atheroscler. Res. 1:75 (1961).

15. R. J. Bouce, N. L. Noble, Z. Gunta-Smith and C. F. Simpson, Consideration of aortic elastin chemistry in the genesis of the intimal plaques (broad-breasted white turkey), Exp. and Molec. Pathol. 31:400 (1979).

16. P. E. Waibel, R. E. Burger, R. A. Ball, J. H. Sautter I. E. Liener and B. S. Pomerot, Effect of triparanol on β - aminopropionitrile-induced dissecting aneurysm and blood lipid levels in the turkey, Proc. Soc. Exp. Biol. and Med. 104:673 (1960).

17. C. F. Simpson, R. H. Harms and F. C. Neal, Influence of high dietary sodium chloride on aortic ruptures in turkeys induced by diethylstilboestrol, Proc. Soc. Exp. Biol. and Med. 116:334 (1964).

18. D. K. Detweiler, H. L. Ratcliffe and H. Luginbuhl, The significance of naturally occurring coronary and cerebral arterial disease in animals, Ann. N. Y. acad. sci. 149:868 (1968).

19. P. M. Lapland, L. Beaubatie and D. Maurel, A spontaneously seasonal hypercholesterolaemic animal: plasma lipids and lipoproteins in the European badger, (Meles meles L.), J. Lipid Res. 21:724 (1980).

20. I. N. Likar, L. J. Likar and R. W. Robinson, Bovine arterial disease Part 3 elastic tissue and acid mucopolysaccharides in bovine coronary arteries without gross lesions, J. athero sclerosis res. 8:643 (1968).

21. S. K. Sikes, The disturbed habitat and its effect
    on the health of animal populations with special
    reference to cardiovascular disease in elephants,
    Proc. Roy. Soc. Med. 61:160 (1968).
22. K. McCullagh and M. G. Lewis, Spontaneous
    arteriosclerosis in the wild African elephant.
    Its relation to the disease in man, Lancet
    II:492 (1967).
23. K. G. McCullagh, Arteriosclerosis in the African
    elephant, Part 2 medial sclerosis,
    Atherosclerosis 21:37 (1975).
24. J. E. French, M. A. Jennings, J. C. F. Poole,
    D. S. Robinson and Sir Howard Florey, Intimal
    changes in the arteries of ageing swine
    Proc. Roy. Soc. B 158:24 (1963).
25. B. H. Skold, R. Getty and F. K. Ramsey,
    Spontaneous arteriosclerosis in the arterial
    system of ageing swine, Amer. J. Vet. research
    27:257 (1966).
26. E. M. Gaman, A. S. Feigenbaum and E. A. Schenk,
    Spontaneous aortic lesions in rabbits Part 3
    Incidence and genetic factors, J. Atherosclerosis
    7:131 (1967).
27. E. A. Schenk, E. Gaman and A. S. Feigenbaum,
    Spontaneous aortic lesions in rabbits II
    Relation to experimental atherosclerosis,
    Circulation Res. XIX:89 (1966).
28. S. Koletsky, Pathological findings and laboratory
    data in a new strain of obese hypertensive rats,
    Amer. J. Pathol. 80:129 (1975).
29. F. Hazama, A. Ooshima, T. Tanake, K. Tomimoto and
    K. Okamoto, Vascular lesions in the various
    substrains of spontaneously hypertensive rats
    and the effects of chronic salt ingestion,
    Jap. Circ. J. 39:7 (1975).
30. L. C. Stout and L. W. Thorpe, Histology of normal
    aortas in non-human primates with emphasis
    on diffuse intimal thickening, Atherosclerosis
    35:165 (1980).
31. G. A. Gresham and A. N. Howard,"Comparative
    pathology of spontaneously occurring and
    experimentally induced atherosclerotic lesions,"
    Meth. achievm. exp. path. ed. E. Bajusz Mass
    and G. Jasmin, Publishers, Montreal, 1:314
    (1966).
32. C. F. Howard, Aortic atherosclerosis in normal
    and spontaneously diabetic Macaca nigra,
    Atherosclerosis 33:479 (1979).

ATHEROSCLEROSIS:

SOME COMPONENTS OF THE LESION

G. A. Gresham

Professor of Morbid Anatomy

University of Cambridge

We have already indicated the need to regard the
arterial wall as any other tissue capable of basic
pathological processes such as inflammation and repair
and have postulated the view that atherosclerosis is a
proliferative response to injury by the arterial wall.

In this chapter we shall examine some of the
cellular and intercellular components of the vessel
wall in normal and in diseased arteries. The
proliferative atherosclerotic response is probably
generated at first by injury to the endothelium which
leads to a change in permeability allowing the entry of
materials such as lipoproteins into the intima. The
nature of the initial injury is uncertain but hypertension and hyperlipidaemia are two likely contenders
in this respect.

ENDOTHELIAL INJURY

In recent years a great deal has been learned about
endothelial cells. They have been studied in a variety
of ways. Hautchen preparations strip off a sheet of
endothelial cells and enable the flat sheet to be viewed
"en face", a new technique of vascular casting using
a modified Batson No. 17 injection technique and then
peeling the arterial tissue off the cast.[1] Other methods
involve labelling with tritiated thymidine in order to
study mitoses in different parts of the endothelial

79

sheet. Tissue culture has also been used to study the
growth and by-products of endothelial cells. Finally
much work has been done by means of scanning and
transmission electron microscopy.

As a result of all this work endothelial cells
have been shown to grow in a single sheet unlike
arterial smooth muscle cells which grow as little
hillocks in tissue culture. The endothelial cellular
sheet consists of closely opposed cells with well
defined intercellular junctions that control the
width of the intercellular space.[2] The intercellular
junctions are covered over on the luminal side of
the cells by a flap-like extension of the cytoplasm
acting as a microvalve controlling entry into the
intercellular space.[3] Not only can this microvalve act
to prevent entry of substances into the vessel wall
it can also exert a trap door effect preventing egress
of substances that have entered the intima. We shall
discuss this "trap-door effect" later.

Studies using tritiated thymidine indicate that
the "turn over" of cells is greatest at branchings and
divisions of arteries and also in areas of increased
Evan's blue uptake which are thought to be areas of
increased permeability to albumen. This is important
in relation to the vulnerability of such sites to
atherosclerosis in man and in the experimental animal.
These studies have also shown that the mean generation
time of endothelial cells increases with advancing age
of the animal.[4] However the turnover even in young
animals is slow only about 0.2% of all cells enter
mitosis each day so that the whole endothelial sheet
turns over in 500 days.

The rate of regeneration of endothelial cells
speeds up considerably if the endothelium is abraded
for example by a balloon catheter. In addition collagen
and smooth muscle cells increase in the area of the
damaged endothelium. Endothelial injury leads to
proliferation and the extent of this depends on the
degree and depth of vessel wall damage. Severe injury
induces lesions that clearly resemble those of atherosclerosis.[5]

Synthesis of new collagen is achieved by proliferating smooth muscle cells. However recent work has
shown that endothelial cells are also capable of
producing a basement membrane type of collagen. This

synthesis of collagen after arterial injury by balloon catheterisation proceeds most rapidly after the damaged area has been recovered by endothelial cells. It appears that smooth muscle cells in the intima require the interaction with overlying endothelium before they can be transformed into cells capable of secreting collagen. The precise nature of this interaction is not known at present.[6] Other workers do not agree with these observations and conclude that injured intimal areas which are rapidly covered by endothelium are protected from the development of a fibrocellular intimal lesion.[7]

Endothelial cells are also metabolically active. They are capable not only of synthesising collagen but they can also produce glycosaminoglycans and lipids including cholesterol. They secrete prostaglandins including prostacyclin and this is important in relation to the interaction between platelets and endothelial cells. In relation to the coagulation process they secrete von Willebrand factor and the factor VIII antigen. We shall shortly be discussing the inter-action of endothelial cells with vasoactive amines in the blood and in this respect the production of angiotensin converting enzyme is important.

Atherosclerosis and athero-thrombosis is largely a disease of man and it is interesting to speculate why this should be. Searching about for characteristics that differentiate man from other animals we light upon hypertension and stress. A few other animals such as rats and some birds are hypertensive but most of the primate order, excluding Homo sapiens is not.

Hypertension produces effects upon vessels and cardiac chambers in both systemic and pulmonary circuits. Atheromatous changes may for example develop rapidly in the pulmonary arteries of children with chronic heart failure or ventricular septal defects. It is also a profound cause of atheroma in the systemic circulation particularly affecting the cerebral arteries which may also develop tiny aneurysms that rupture to produce haemorrhage into the brain. Severe cerebral atheroma rarely appears in the absence of hypertension[8] and hypertension must be considered as one of the most important contributory factors in causing atherosclerosis.

Hypertension may act upon the vessel wall in several ways. It may act purely mechanically or by

means of chemical mediators which are found in the blood
of some hypertensive patients. Evidence of mechanical
stretching of the endothelial sheet causing the cells
to separate has been obtained by electron microscopy
using tracers such as ferritin, horseradish peroxidase
and colloidal carbon.[9] Vasoactive amines may also exert
an effect. One of these found in some hypertensives
is angiotensin II. This and other vasoactive amines
have been shown to increase endothelial permeability
in a variety of ways.[10] Four main changes were
described in endothelial cells exposed to vasoactive
amines perfused into the limb vessels of experimental
animals. Tyramine caused rupture of the plasmalemma
and extravasation of the contents of the cytoplasm.
Angiotensin acted mainly by opening the endothelial
junctions; this was caused by contraction of the
endothelial cells. Dopamine and epinephrine caused
oedema both inside and outside the cells. Intracellular oedema was also caused by serotonin and
bradykinin; these substances also led to opening of
junctions between the endothelial cells.

It has also been demonstrated that patchy death
of endothelial cells occurs in hypertension. Dead
cells stain with nigrosin or Evans blue. In rats
and rabbits such dead cells have been shown at divisions
and branches in the artery points where haemodynamic
strain is excessive.[11] These are also sites of predilection for atherosclerosis.

Evidence of increased permeability at these sites
in the vascular tree has also been obtained by immunohistological methods for Ig G and fibrinogen. They
show accumulation of globulin and fibrinogen in the
intima at sites of hypertensive injury. Microthrombi
have also been shown at these sites and these in turn
may lead to platelet aggregation on the intimal surface.

PLATELET AGGREGATION

Though platelets are strictly speaking not
components of the vessel wall their close relationship
to vessels, particularly those that are injured in one
way or another, merits some discussion here. It is also
important to realise the possibility that platelets
themselves may act to injure the vessel and trigger the
whole process of fibrocellular intimal thickening that
leads to more advanced atherosclerosis. Platelets
contain vasoactive amines such as 5 hydroxytryptamine,

the amount that is present varies in different animals. Whilst it has not yet been shown that platelets may adhere to intact endothelium and injure it, it is possible that the constant flux of endothelial cells which are normally being replaced by slow regeneration may leave gaps in the endothelial sheet to which platelets may adhere.

Extreme examples of intimal adherence of platelets leading to occlusive atherosclerosis are seen in the coronary arteries in transplanted hearts and in patients or experimental animals with homocysteinaemia. Homo-transplantation of hearts or segments of aorta leads to accelerated atherosclerosis. Severe occlusive disease of coronary arteries in such cases has been reported within 18 months of transplantation of the heart of a young subject into a severe diabetic patient.[12] Sheets of endothelial cells are lost in patients with homocystein-aemia and in animals with induced homocysteinaemia. In these cases considerable smooth muscle cell proliferation occurs. If experimental animals are fed cholesterol as well lesions that closely resemble atherosclerosis are produced.[13] A similar result is obtained after denuding endothelium with a balloon catheter followed by feeding of cholesterol.[14]

It has been shown recently that platelets contain a mutagenic factor which causes the proliferation of smooth muscle cells and fibroblasts.[15] It is a protein of low molecular weight which acts in minute amounts to increase the synthesis of D.N.A. by smooth muscle cells or embryonic mouse fibroblasts in tissue culture. Evidence is steadily accumulating to implicate the platelet as an atherogenic agent. In human subjects with severe arterial disease which has been shown angiographically, platelet survival is often reduced by as much as 80% and levels of platelet factor 4 were raised suggesting platelet break-down. All of this may be explained by the formation of multiple thrombi in the diseased vessels. However there is experimental evidence from homocysteinaemia in the baboon which shows that atherosclerosis can be reduced in these animals if platelet aggregation is inhibited by the administration of dipyridamole or sulphinpyrazone.[16]

ARTERIAL SPASM

Little attention has been paid to this physiological component of the vessel wall in relation to the possi-bility that it might also have a pathogenic role in the production of arterial disease. Sustained spasm of

arteries is clearly undesirable for the tissue supplied
by the vessel but is also deleterious to the vessel
itself. As we have already indicated the inner arterial
media is poorly supplied by vasa vasorum and relies for
its nutriment from diffusion from the lumen of the vessel.
Spasm is likely to impair this diffusion and damage the
inner artery wall by hypoxia.

Arterial spasm, hypertension, release of catecholamines and other events are a feature of stress. Stress
is a factor which has often been linked with atherogenesis
but it is difficult to define and consequently difficult
to produce in the experimental situation. Whether or not
vascular spasm is a feature of stress is debatable.
However spasm is a feature in ischaemic heart disease
and it has been shown angiographically in patients with
variant angina and with single coronary artery disease[17]
that spasm occurs at sites of atherosclerotic plaques
Boyd[18] discusses the reasons for spasm at these sites. It
may be due to the presence of the lesion. On the other
hand spasm may induce plaque formation in the way that we
have already discussed namely by causing hypotoxic damage.
This is then followed by reactive proliferation to
produce a plaque. Vascular spasm can be produced by
hypothalmic stimulation in the rabbit and this
association lends support to the notion that stress and
vascular spasm are related and that stress might play[19]
a role in atherogenesis.

Not only may it play an atherogenic role, it may also
contribute to the formation of lesions in other vessels.
Dissecting aneurysm of the aorta has been an enigma for
many years. It occurs in the arch where atherosclerosis
is often absent and where overt medionecrosis is often
sparse. Spasm in this region of the aorta could weaken
the inner wall and predispose to it. At the other
extreme arteriolar hyaline change could be explained
again in terms of spastic injury to the vessel wall
leading to insudation of lipid,fibrinogen and other
plasma constituents.

GLYCOSAMINOGLYCANS

The role of glycosaminoglycans in the normal and
diseased artery wall has been the subject of much debate.
In recent times the important action of heparan sulphate
at the endothelial surface has been recognised in the
sequence of lipid metabolism. Heparan sulphate forms
an important anchor for lipoprotein lipase fixing it

to endothelial cell proteins. This enzyme at the
vascular surface acts upon circulating chylomicra
leading to the progressive breakdown to lipoproteins
and to triglyceride release. Abnormalities in this
surface system might be expected to affect lipid disposal
from the blood and hence the process of atherogenesis.
Studies have shown, using fat tolerance tests that there
is a delay in the removal of ingested fat from the blood
in atherosclerotic subjects.[20] Heparan sulphate is
closely related to heparin which is present in blood.
Hypertriglyceridaemic and hypercholesterolaemic subjects
have a low level of circulating heparin. Heparin like
heparan sulphate localises on the endothelial surface and
can be shown as a metachromatic layer on the vascular
intimal surfaces in animals and in man. We have already
discussed the role of heparan sulphate at the intimal
surface. Heparin also acts at that level in a variety
of ways. It reduces the positive electrical charge that
appears at the surface when the endothelium is injured.
Thus it restores the normal electronegativity. In
addition heparin binds and inactivates many agents that
can react with and damage the vessel surface. Amongst
these are many of the vasoactive enzymes that we have
discussed already, lysozyme, components of complement
some viruses and many toxins. Viral infectious
immunological injury coupled with hypercholesterolaemia
and platelet adhesion have all been shown to be
atherogenic and these factors are antagonised by heparin.
In addition human platelets contain a factor capable of
degrading heparin and this degradation is opposed by
heparin. This leaves intact the lipoprotein lipase
attachment which is central to the clearance of
postprandial hyperlipidaemia. Glycosaminoglycans of
various sorts occur in vessel walls. The principle one
in the artery is chondroitin sulphate B. The presence
of this and other polysaccharide materials has been
reviewed and investigated by a number of workers notably
Bertelson in Denmark.[21] He showed a progressive increase
in acid and neutral mucopolysaccharides with increasing
age in the media of human arteries and in these areas
granules of calcium salts begin to appear after the
second decade.

     Acid mucopolysaccharides appear first in the intima
in the first two decades. Later on neutral mucopolysaccharides appear and the amount of acid substance gets
less. The precise role of these substances in relation
to ageing and atherosclerosis is not clear. The
mucopolysaccharides appear to be related to the formation
of collagen fibres and dermatan sulphate

binds both the low density and very low density lipoproteins.   These properties may indicate a role in
atherogenesis.

    Comparative studies of glycosaminoglycans in the
aortic wall of a variety of animals has cast more light
on their significance.[22]   Dermatan sulphate was the main
constituent of the adventitia in all of the 15 sorts of
animals examined.   Chondroitin 6-sulphate was proportionately higher in the intima and media of atherosclerosis
susceptible animals.   In atherosclerosis resistant
mammals dermatan sulphate and heparan sulphate pre-
ponderated.   This is an interesting observation in
relation to the role of heparan sulphate in lipoprotein
lipase degradation of blood lipids which we have already
discussed.

ARTERIAL CELLS

    Cells appear and disappear from the arterial wall
under a variety of circumstances.   We have already
discussed factors that affect the numbers and positions
of smooth muscle cells or myofibroblasts.   We shall now
consider other cell types in relation to their possible
role in the atherogenic process.   The cells to be
considered are mast cells, lymphocytes and plasma cells
which have received scanty consideration in past years.

    Mast cells are present in the adventitia of
arteries and in the myocardium of young animals.   Their
numbers tend to decrease with increasing age.   A
relationship was found between the number of mast cells
and the grade of coronary atherosclerosis.   High counts
were related to lesser degrees of coronary artery
disease and also to a lower incidence of myocardial
infarction.[23]   It is interesting to speculate on these
observations because mast cells produce both histamine
and heparin in man both of which have potential parts to
play in the atherogenetic process.

    The question is whether the decrease in mast cells
precedes the development of atherosclerosis or is a
consequence of the ischaemia induced by vascular
narrowing.   In favour of the former view is a higher
mast cell count in African negroes as compared to white
people.   Africans have a low incidence of angina
pectoris and myocardial infarction.   Another point is
the observation of a low serum cholesterol level in
patients with idiopathic mastocytosis.   Once again this

may support the fact that heparin is acting to prevent
the atherosclerotic process via its link with heparan
sulphate and lipoprotein lipase.

Another possible way in which heparin might act
is as an inhibitor of smooth muscle cell proliferation.
Guyton et al.[24] Using non-anticoagulant heparinoid
compounds they showed an inhibitory effect on smooth
muscle cell proliferation in the rat. They denuded the
endothelium of the exposed carotid artery by air drying
and then observed the subsequent proliferation of smooth
muscle. Heparan sulphate which is a by product of the
production of heparin from ox lung inhibits smooth muscle
cell proliferation in these circumstances.

It would be dubious to propose the use of non-
anticoagulant heparin for the treatment of atherosclerosis but it might prove useful in circumstances
where smooth muscle cell proliferation might occur more
rapidly than in atherosclerosis. Examples being in
saphenous vein coronary artery by-pass grafting and
after arterial embolectomy using a Fogarty balloon
catheter.

There are other cells to be found in atherosclerotic
vessels that have received little attention in times
past. These include lymphocytes and plasma cells. It
is particularly important to consider them in the light
of the notion that allergy may be an important part of
the process of atherogenesis. It was suggested in 1962
that adventitial lymphocytic infiltrates might be
correlated with the degree of early atherosclerosis.[25]
The more the plaque was raised the greater the degree of
cellular infiltration. It did not relate to the site
of the lesion in the arterial tree nor was it correlated
with age. A number of authors have suggested that the
cellular infiltrates may reflect an allergic event in the
vessel wall.[26] Sometimes the inflammatory component is so
intense that it may resemble a giant celled arteritis
and giant cells also occur sometimes which are not
always related to lipid in the vessel wall. In support
of the allergic hypothesis are the reports of auto-
antibodies in atherosclerotic arterial walls and the
suggestions that elastin, glycoprotein or lipoprotein
might be the antigenic stimuli. Also supporting an
allergic basis for atherosclerosis is the proposal that
activated serum complement is a key factor involved in
endothelial injury.[27] The complement system activates
the inflammatory response and it can be brought into
action by immune complexes, infective agents and even

non specifically by circulating macromolecular
aggregates. Circulating immune complexes have been
found in a substantial proportion of patients with
vascular disease.[28] In general the cellular response
in the arterial wall becomes more intense with increasing
severity of the lesion. So that even though allergy may
not play an initial role in atherogenesis it may cause
the lesions to progress as more and more antigenic
material accumulates in the atherosclerotic lesion.

REFERENCES

1. M. J. Levesque, J. F. Cornhill and R. M. Nerem,
    Vascular casting, Atherosclerosis 34:457 (1979).
2. T. Shimamoto, Y. Yamashita and T. Sunaga, Scanning
    electron microscopic observation of endothelial
    surface of heart and blood vessels, Proc. Jap.
    Acad. 45:508 (1969).
3. S. Bjorkerud, H. A. Hansson and G. Bondjers,
    Subcellular valves and canaliculi in arterial
    endothelium and their equivalence to so-called
    stigmata, Virchows Arch. - Abt. B. Zellpath
    II:19 (1972).
4. J. Kunz and U. Keim, On the regeneration of aortic
    endothelium at different ages, Mechs. of Ageing
    and Development 4:361 (1975).
5. B. C. Christensen, J. Chemnitz, I, Tkocz and
    C. M. Kim, Repair in arterial tissue, Acta. path
    microbiol. scand. sect. A 87:265 (1979).
6. C. C. Chidi, Klein, LeRoy, R. G. DePalma, Effect of
    regenerated endothelium on collagen content in
    the injured artery, Surg. Gynec. Obstet. 148:839
    (1979).
7. C. C. Haudenschild and S. M. Schwartz, Endothelial
    regeneration restitution of endothelial
    continuity, Lab. Invest. 41:407 (1979).
    S. Sadoshima, T. Kurozumi, K. Tabaki, K. Ueda,
    K. Takeshita, Y. Hirota, T. Omae, H. Uzawa
    and S. Katsuki, Cerebral and aortic athero-
    sclerosis in Hishayama, Japan, Atherosclerosis
    36:117 (1980).
9. I. Huttner, R. H. More and G. Rona, Fine structural
    evidence of specific mechanisms for increased
    endothelial permeability in experimental
    hypertension, Amer. J. Pathol. 61:395 (1970).
10. P. Constantinides and M. Robinson, Ultrastructural
    injury of arterial endothelium. I effect of pH
    osmolarity, anoxia and temperature. II effects
    of vasoactive amines, Arch. Pathol. 88:99 (1969).

11. A. L. Robertson and P. A. Khairallah, Arterial endothelial permeability and vascular disease, the trap-door effect, Exp. and Molec. Pathol. 18:241 (1973).

12. J. G. Thomson, Production of severe atheroma in a transplanted human heart, Lancet ii:1088 (1969).

13. L. Harker, R. Ross, S. Slichter and C. Scott, Homocystine induced arteriosclerosis. The role of endothelial cell injury and platelet response in its genesis, J. Clin. Invest.58:731 (1976).

14. H. R. Baumgartner, Eine neue methode zur erseugung von thromben durch gizielte Uberdehnung der Gefasswand, z. Ges. Exp. Med.137:227 (1963).

15. R. Ross and J. A. Glomset, The pathogenesis of atherosclerosis, N. Engl. J. Med. 295:369 and 420 (1976).

16. L. A. Harker, R. Ross, R. J. Wall and J. M. Harlan, Pharmacological prevention of endothelial cell injury and homocysteine induced arteriosclerosis, J. Clin. Invest. (to be published) (1979).

17. A. Maseri, A. Pesola, M. Marzilli, S. Severi, O. Parodi, A. L'Abbate, A. M. Ballestra, F. Maltinti, D. De Nes and A. Biagini, Coronary vasospasm in angina pectoris, Lancet i:713 (1977).

18. G. W. Boyd, Stress and disease: The missing link. A vasospastic theory. II The nature of degenerative arterial disease, Med. Hypoth. 4:420 (1978).

19. N. Weckman, Local constriction and spasm of large arteries elicited by hypothalmic stimulation, Experimentia 16:34 (1960).

20. H. Engelberg, Heparin and Atherosclerosis. A review of old and recent findings, Amer. Heart J. 99:359 (1980).

21. Bertelsen, Sr., Problems concerning the definition and grading of the aortic atherosclerosis, Acta. path. microbiol. scandinav. 61:249 (1964).

22. O. M. S. Toledo, P. A. S. Mourao, Sulfated glycosaminoglycans in normal aortic wall of different mammals, Artery 6:341 (1980).

23. M. Fernex and N. H. Sternby, Mast cells and coronary heart disease, Acta. path et microbiol. scandinav. 62:525 (1964).

24. J. R. Guyton, R. S. Rosenberg, A. W. Clowes and M. J. Karnovsky, Inhibition of rat arterial smooth muscle cell proleferation by heparin, Circulation Res. 46:625 (1980).

25. J. R. A. Mitchell, C. J. Schwartz, "Arterial disease" Publisher, Blackwell Scientific Publications, Oxford (1965).

26.   R. N. Poston and D. F. Davies, Immunity and
        inflammation in the pathogenesis of athero-
        sclerosis, <u>Atherosclerosis</u> 19:353 (1974).
27.   P. Geertinger and H. Sorensen, Complement and
        arteriosclerosis, <u>Atherosclerosis</u> 18:65 (1973).
28.   G. Fust, E. Szocudy, J. Szekely, I. Nanii and
        S. Gero, Studies on the occurence of
        circulating immune complexes in vascular
        disease, <u>Atherosclerosis</u> 29:181 (1978).

CHARACTERISATION OF THE ARTERIAL WALL USING ULTRASOUND

P.C. Clifford

Department of Surgery
Southampton General Hospital
Southampton, Hants, England

INTRODUCTION

Much of the present day arterial surgery is concerned with athero-sclerotic occlusive disease of the lower limb. 'Non-invasive' diagnostic ultrasound techniques are now available to help the vascular surgeon apply his operative skills successfully. Using these methods it is possible to characterise the anatomy, position and dimensions of blood vessels; and their physiological properties including the perfusion pressure, blood velocity, arterial wall elasticity and haemodynamic responses to environmental changes.

Clinical application of Doppler systolic pressure has led to new methods of identifying and localising arterial stenosis. The functional assessment of aorto-iliac stenosis using femoral artery Doppler signals is an example and three methods, Pulsatility Index (PI), Laplace Transform (LT) and principal component analysis are currently available.

The recent development of ultrasonic imaging systems suitable for clinical use now permit objective diagnostic studies which were previously impossible. The multi-channel pulsed Doppler scanner allows rapid visualisation of the moving flow stream, and has been used to image arterial grafts and to study the ischaemic lower limb. "Duplex" scanners combine high-resolution B mode real-time scanning with sampling of Doppler waveforms. The combination of these two techniques provides a comprehensive assessment of arterial morphology.

ULTRASOUND ASSESSMENT TECHNIQUES

The simple continuous-wave Doppler instrument can be used to
monitor blood velocity signals from most of the major blood vessels
(1). Its clinical value lies in its ability to display the waveform
which allows a subjective assessment of the artery to be made.
Also objective measurements such as the blood pressure at the
ankle, calf, thigh and arm can be taken (4,5,6).

Doppler Systolic Pressures

The ratio of systolic pressure at a site in the lower limb
divided by systolic pressure at the comparable site in the upper
limb is termed the Pressure Index (7).

In health this is greater than 1.0, whereas in lower limb
ischaemia it falls below unity. To measure systolic pressure the
ultrasonic flowmeter is placed over the artery distal to an
occluding cuff. Ankle systolic pressure (mmHg) is recorded at the
level at which audible flow signals return during deflation of the
cuff. The ankle/brachial systolic pressure index (ASPI) is able
to separate normal subjects from patients with intermittent claudication or ischaemic rest pain. Accuracy of diagnosis and localisation of disease is improved by increasing the number of arterial
segments studied. Several authors report good correlation of
segmental pressures with angiography (9-12) others have used
segmental pressures for indicating healing after below knee
amputation (13-15).

The usefulness of ASPI alone in diagnosis is limited since
either proximal or distal occlusion results in the same pressure
reduction. Nonetheless measurement of ASPI has become a valuable
and widely used screening test.

Doppler Waveform Analysis

Since atherosclerosis converts a smooth internal lining into
one which is roughened, later narrowed and finally occluded, it
is reasonable to assume that the velocity patterns are changed in
a predictable manner. Damage by atheroma to the media and internal
elastic lamina may also contribute to these alterations in waveform
shape by a fall in arterial compliance. Doppler shifted signal
detect the presence or absence of a flow and alterations in pitch
secondary to changes in acceleration or velocity. Directional
Doppler devices produce a composite waveform of the forward and
reverse flow velocities. In 1969 Gosling and King described
Pulsatility index (PI), which provides a numerical estimate of the
waveform shape (2). Recently Skidmore and Woodcock introduced a
new more sophisticated method termed Laplace Transform analysis

(LT) (3). These numerical methods describe the <u>shape</u>, rather than the amplitude of the waveform and therefore, are independent of beam/vessel angle.

In 1975 PI was defined as the ratio of the maximum vertical excursions (i.e. peak forward velocity and peak reverse velocity) divided by the mean value (20). Arterial occlusion produces vasodilating metabolites which cause a fall in peripheral resistance. PI has previously been shown to be sensitive to changes in peripheral resistance, and femoral artery PI falls with lower limb vasodilatation. This effect is also demonstrable in the upper limb. PI is also affected by changes in arterial wall elasticity: increased blood pressure increases the static elastic modulus of the arterial wall and induces reflex vasoconstriction, both tending to increase PI.

Recently a more sensitive method of waveform analysis using a Fourier transform has been described (21,22). Preliminary clinical results have suggested that LT Damping is a sensitive indicator of proximal stenosis (24) and that LT stiffness may be used to measure changes with age, smoking and vasectomy (25).

Ultrasonic Imaging

Ultrasonic imaging is now of improved resolution such that it is proving to be a very informative technique with the advantage that it can be repeated without risk (26,27). The commonest use of B mode ultrasound scanning is in obstetrics but the next most popular use is in the field of organ and tissue pathology, including the study of aneurysms and arterial stenosis (Figure 1). Real time imaging is a recent innovation where scans are produced so rapidly that movement is easily seen. Duplex scanners are real time (B mode) scanners with integral pulsed Doppler flowmeter attachments.

Doppler Imaging

Pulsed Doppler imaging systems detect blood flow and interpret it as a dot on a storage oscilloscope screen. Probe movement enables a composite image of the flow patterns to be built up. Multichannel devices have a fast scanning speed and a three dimensional imaging capability (28).

One pulsed Doppler scanner, MAVIS*, uses thirty-channels and

---

* Multichannel Artery and Vein Imaging System (MAVIS)
  GEC Medical Equipment Ltd., PO Box 2, East Lane, Wembley,
  Middlesex. HA9 7PP, UK.

AORTIC ANEURYSM

COMMON FEMORAL ARTERY STENOSIS

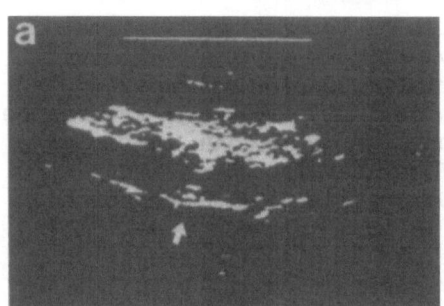
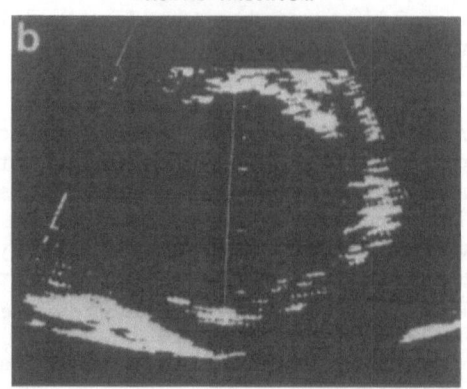

Fig. 1

Real time B mode scanning of a common
femoral artery atheromatous plaque
causing stenosis (a) and aortic
aneurysm in cross section (b).

Fig. 2

Neointimal hyperplasia in a
prosthetic graft.

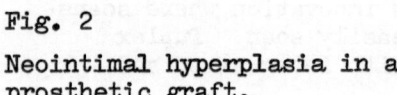
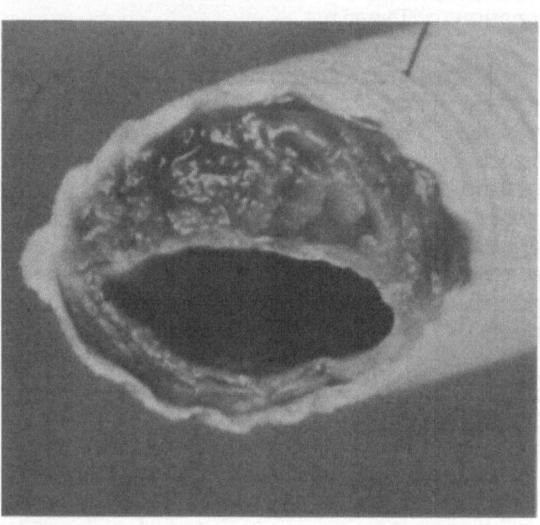

the 5MHz transducer is mounted in a rigid postion-sensing gantry.
Images in cross-section, laterally, similar to an x-ray arterio-
gram, and in the anterio-posterior (AP) plane are easily obtained.

It is not necessary to move the patient or the gantry to
obtain these different images. Any vessel up to 6cm from the
skin surface can be scanned and imaging is much more rapid with
the earlier single channel systems.

Real Time B Mode Imaging

'Real Time' is a term used to describe any process in which
there is no time delay between the input and the output of signals.
In ultrasonic imaging the individual images are repeated sufficiently rapidly for a 'moving' picture to be perceived. A recent
development in real time ultrasonic imaging is the combination
of a real time B Scanner and pulsed Doppler Flowmeter (28). In
1979 the first applications of such "Duplex" scanners were reported
in studies of extracranial carotid artery disease (29).

These systems integrate pulse-echo and pulsed Doppler
techniques to form real time B-mode images with simultaneous
detection of blood flow velocity. The pulsed Doppler flow waveform
can be displayed next to the real time scan to reveal the actual
flow in its proper relationship to the vessel lumen and wall.
The ATL Duplex scanner* is a 5MHz mechanical real time scanner
with an incorporated pulsed Doppler flowmeter. Thirty B-mode
images are produced each second and the single-gated 5MHz pulsed
Doppler flowmeter can obtain the blood velocity waveform by
appropriate positioning of the sample volume. When a suitable
vessel is imaged it is possible to detect flow and measure its
qualitative characteristics.

CLINICAL APPLICATIONS

The ultimate place of ultrasonic imaging in the assessment
of the ischaemic lower limb is not yet defined. Techniques which
are developing include the assessment of profunda artery stenosis
(32) and studies of the natural history of implanted arterial
grafts (33 - 36). Their potential lies in the ability to
visualise the blood vessel lumen in three dimensions and to
analyse Doppler shifted signals from a known point in the blood-
flow.

Stenosis of, for example, the profunda femoris or the carotid
arteries can now be reliably detected with ultrasound. It may
draw attention to correctable stenoses which were not diagnosed
arteriographically.   Despite the clear demonstration by
Berne et al (1970) and Beales et al (1971) of the importance of
arteriographic views in several planes, single-plane arteriography remains commonplace (37). Inevitably some lesions which
are visible on lateral or oblique views, will be missed on single

---

* Advanced Technology Laboratories, Seattle, Washington, USA.

plane arteriograms. Application of femoral waveform analysis
can influence routine clinical practice by improving patient
selection for arteriography. Secondly, more significant proximal
disease may be more certainly detected so increasing accurate
patient selection for operation.

Apart from the progression of disease proximal or distal to
an arterial graft, factors influencing late graft patency include
proliferation of neointima leading to focal lesions or a gradual
silting up of the graft lumen (Figure 2), compliance mismatch
between artery and graft and rheological factors.

Both pulsed Doppler Mavis and Duplex ultrasound provide
useful physiological information about arterial grafts and can
identify many of these risk factors which, if uncorrected may
jeopardise lonterm graft patency.

In conclusion, the surgeon can apply these techniques to
confirm and localise arterial ischaemia, to help in deciding the
level of reconstruction in multisegment disease, and to study the
natural history of atherosclerosis.

References

1. C. Doppler. "Uber das Farbige Licht der Dopplelsterne and
         Einiger Anderer Gestirne des Himmels." Abh K Bohm Ges
         Wiss Prague 1842; 2: 465.
2. R.G. Gosling, D.H. King and J.P. Woodcock. Transcutaneous
         measurements of arterial blood velocity by ultrasound.
         Ultrasonics in Industry Conference Papers 1969; pp 16-23
3. R. Skidmore and J.P. Woodcock. "Physiological significance
         of arterial models derived using transcutaneous
         ultrasonic flowmeters." J. Physiol. 1978; 277: 29-30p
4. S.T. Yao, J.T. Hobbs and W.T. Irvine. "Pulse examination by
         an ultrasonic method." Br. Med. J. 1968; 4: 555-557.
5. S.T. Yao, J.T. Hobbs and W.T. Irvine. "Audible systolic
         pressure measurements in arterial disease affecting
         the lower extremities." Br. J. Surg. 1969; 56: 676-679.

6. D.E. Strandness and D.S. Sumner. "Non-invasive methods of
   studying peripheral arterial function". J. Surg. Res.
   1972; 12: 419-430.
7. T. Winsor. "Influence of arterial disease on the systolic
   blood pressure gradients of the extremity. Am. J. Med.
   Sci. 1950; 220: 117-126.
8. S.A. Carter. "Indirect systolic pressures and waves in
   arterial occlusive disease of the lower extremities".
   Circulation 1968; 27: 624-638.
9. J.K. Raines, R.C. Darling, J. Bath, D.C. Brewster and
   W.G. Austen. "Vascular laboratory criteria for the
   management of peripheral vascular disease of the lower
   extremities. Surgery 1976; 79: 21-29.
10. S.E. Heintz, G.E. Bone, E.E. Slaymaker, A.C. Hayes and
    R.W. Barnes. "Value of arterial pressure measurements
    in the proximal and distal part of the thigh in arterial
    occlusive disease". Surg. Gynae. and Obstet. 1978;
    146: 337-343.
11. R.B. Rutherford, D.H. Lowenstein and M.F. Klein. "Combining
    segmental systolic pressures and plethysomography to
    diagnose arterial occlusive disease of the legs." Am.
    J. Surgery. 1979; 138: 211-218.
12. A.E. Aburahma, E.B. Diethrich and M. Reiling. "Doppler
    testing in peripheral vascular occlusive disease."
    Surg. Gynae. and Obstet. 1980; 150: 26-28.
13. R.W. Barnes, G.D. Shanik and E.E. Slaymaker. "An index of
    healing in below knee amputation and leg blood pressure
    by Doppler ultrasound". Surgery 1976; 79: 13-20.
14. R.H. Dean, J.S.T. Yao, R.G. Thompson and J.J. Bergan.
    "Predictive value of ultrasonically derived arterial
    pressure in determination of amputation level." Am.
    Surgeon 1975; 41: 731-737.
15. F.W. Wagner. "Transcutaneous Doppler ultrasound in the
    prediction of healing and the selection of surgical
    level for dysvascular lesions of the toes and forefoot."
    Clinical Orthopaedics & Related Practice 1979; 142:
    110-114
16. T.F. O'Donnell. "Non-invasive intraoperative monitoring:
    a prespective study comparing Doppler systolic occlusion
    pressure and segmental plethysmography." Am. J.
    Surgery 1978; 135: 537-546.
17. A.D. Craxford and J. Chamberlain. "Pulse waveform transit
    ratios in the assessment of peripheral vascular disease."
    Br. J. Surgery 1977; 64: 449-452.
18. R.N. Baird, P.W. Davies and D.R. Bird. "Segmental air
    plethysmography during arterial reconstruction." Br.
    J. Surgery 1979; 66: 718-722.
19. R.N. Baird, B. Banninger and Davies et al. "Acute effects
    of cigarette smoking on main arteries of habitual
    smokers with arterial disease." J. Physiol. 1980;
    pp 51-52p.

20. R.G. Gosling, D.H. King and D.H. Newman. "Ultrasonic
    Angiology" in "Arteries and Veins". Ed. Harcus A.W.
    and Adamson L.   Edinburgh: Churchill Livingston 1975;
    pp 61-84.
21. R. Skidmore and J.P. Woodcock. "Physiological interpretation
    of Doppler-shift waveforms.   1.   Theoretical consider-
    ations".   Ultrasound Med. Biol. 1980; 6: 7-10.
22. R. Skidmore and J.P. Woodcock. "Physiological interpretation
    of Doppler-shift waveforms.   2.   Validation of the
    Laplace transform method for characterisation of the
    common femoral blood velocity/time waveform."
    Ultrasound Med. Biol. 1980; 6: 219-225.
23. R. Skidmore, J.P. Woodcock, P.N.T. Wells, D.R. Bird and
    R.N. Baird.   "Physiological interpretation of Doppler-
    shift waveforms.   3.   Clinical results."   Ultrasound
    Med. Biol. 1980; 6: 227-231.
24. P.C. Clifford, R. Skidmore, D.R. Bird, J.P. Woodcock, R.J.
    Lusby and R.N. Baird.   "Femoral artery doppler signal
    analysis in lower limb ischaemia."   J. Cardiovasc.
    Surg. 1981   In press.
25. R.W.T. Slack, P.C. Clifford, W.B. Campbell, P.J.B. Smith
    and R.N. Baird.   "Vasectomy and Smoking; cumulative risk
    factors in atherogenesis."   Br. J. Surg. 1981; in press.
26. P.J. Fish.   "Imaging blood vessels by ultrasound" in Blood
    flow measurement.   Ed. Roberts VC, Sector Publishing Ltd.,
    London 1972; pp 29-32.
27. D.J. Mozersky, D.W. Baker and D.E. Strandness.   "Ultrasonic
    arteriography."   Arch. Surg. 1971; 103: 663-667.
28. P.J. Fish, I.M. Wilson, B. Holt and D. Walter. "Multichannel
    pulsed Doppler imaging: measurement accuracy and beam
    vessel angle estimation."   In Ultrasound in Medicine,
    Ed. White D, Lyon EA. Plenum Press, New York 1978;
    4: 359-362.
29. F.E. Barber, D.W. Baker, A.W.C. Nation, D.E. Strandness Jr
    and J.M. Reid.   "Ultrasonic duplex echo-doppler scanner."
    IEEE Trans. Biomed. Engl. 1974; 21: 109-113.
30. W.M. Blackshear, D.J. Phillips, B.L. Thiele, J.H. Hirsch,
    P.M. Chikos, M.R. Marinelli, K.J. Ward and D.E. Strandness
    Jr.   "Detection of carotid occlusive disease by
    ultrasonic imaging and pulsed Doppler spectrum analysis.
    Surgery 1979; 86: 698-706.

31. P.C. Clifford, R. Skidmore, J.P. Woodcock et al. "Arterial
    grafts imaged using Doppler and real time ultrasound."
    Vasc. Diag. & Therapy 1981; 2: 43-57.
32. R.N. Baird, R.J. Lusby, Bird et al. "Pulsed Doppler
    angiography in lower limb arterial ischaemia."
    Surgery 1979; 96: 818-825.
33. A.H. Wolson, H.A. Kaupp and K. McDonald. "Ultrasound of
    arterial graft surgery complications." Am. J.
    Radiology 1979; 133: 869-875.
34. P.C. Clifford, R. Skidmore, D.R. Bird et al. "Pulsed
    Doppler and real time duplex imaging of dacron
    arterial grafts." Ultrasonic Imaging 1980; 2: 381-390.
35. P.C. Clifford, J.P. Woodcock and R.N. Baird. "The fate of
    the valves of autogenous vein grafts." Br. J. Radiology
    1981; 54: 348-350.
36. A.W. Gretchen, M.D. Gooding, D.J. Effeney and J. Goldstone.
    "The aortofemoral graft: Detection and identification
    of healing complications by ultrasonography."
    Surgery 1981: in press.
37. F.A. Berne, W.P. Lawrence and W.H. Carlton. "Roentgeno-
    graphic measurement of arterial narrowing." Am. J.
    Roentgenol 1970; 110: 757-759.
38. J.S.M. Beales, F.A. Adcock and J.S. Frawley et al. "The
    radiological assessment of disease of the profunda
    femoris artery." Br. J. Radiology 1971; 44: 854-859.
39. D.S. Macpherson, D.C. James and P.R.F. Bell. "Is aortography
    abused in lower limb ischaemia?" Lancet 1980; July
    80-82.

MYOCARDIAL LIPIDS IN RELATION TO CORONARY ARTERY DISEASE IN MAN

Sigmundur Gudbjarnason, Jonas Hallgrimsson and
Gudrun Skuladottir

Science Institute and Department of Pathology
University of Iceland, Reykjavik, Iceland

The purpose of this study was to examine the fatty acid
composition and content of phospholipids, and free fatty acids in
human heart muscle samples obtained at autopsy from people that
died suddenly in accidents and from people that died suddenly from
heart disease, with or without coronary artery disease.

Lipids play an important role in cardiovascular diseases, not
only by way of hyperlipemia and development of atherosclerosis,
but also by modifying the composition, structure and stability of
cellular membranes. The activity of membrane bound enzymes and
hormone receptors is markedly influenced by the composition of
membrane lipids, and the availability of specific fatty acids set
free from binding sites in membranes serve as rate limiting steps
in synthesis of important regulatory substances, such as prostaglandins. The activity of phospholipase A_2, which releases such
membrane bound fatty acids, can be modulated, for example stimulated
by catecholamines or inhibited by glucocorticoids, and may thus
have an important influence on the development of coronary artery
disease and myocardial response to ischemia.

Accelerated phospholipid degradation and accompanying membrane
dysfunction could produce irreversible cell injury and ultimately
cell death in ischemia, depending on the degree and duration of
ischemia. The normal function of the heart is dependent upon the
activities of numerous subcellular membrane systems which play
critical roles in the maintenance of intracellular ion distribution
modulating cardiac performance. During episodes of myocardial
ischemia, severe alterations in myocardial contractility and
electrical excitability are known to occur and ischemia-associated
defects in membrane systems which regulate calcium availability as

well as passive and active movement of sodium and potassium have been reported[1].

The polyene fatty acid composition of phospholipids in heart muscle is modified by dietary fat and catecholamine stress in rats[2,3]. Marked alterations in membrane composition affect the extent of cellular damage and mortality following excessive stimulation with the β-adrenergic agonist isoproterenol[4].

The observations made in this study show a significant diminution of linoleic acid in myocardial phospholipids in man during aging. Analyses of post-mortem heart muscle samples indicate that the stability or susceptibility of endogenous phospholipids to hydrolysis may be a function of the fatty acid composition, the most unsaturated fatty acids were released earlier than less unsaturated fatty acids. People who suffered a sudden cardiac death may be divided into several distinct groups according to different myocardial lipid abnormalities observed at autopsy and severity of coronary artery disease.

Material and Methods

Autopsy samples. Samples were obtained from human heart muscle at autopsy from people that died suddenly in accidents and from people who suffered a sudden cardiac death outside the hospital, at home or at their place of work. Sudden cardiac death was subdivided into instant death and delayed death, occurring within a few hours after onset of symptoms. Coronary atherosclerosis was graded on a scale from 0 to 6, grade 6 meaning total occlusion. Those that suffered instant cardiac death (n =12) has two or three vessel disease, with coronary stenosis of grades 4 to 6, whereas those that lived for up to a few hours after onset of symptoms (n = 12) had less severe coronary atherosclerosis, most having only one vessel disease with stenosis varying from grades 1 to 6. Delayed cardiac death was frequently associated with early stages of myocardial necrosis but the samples analyzed were selected from non-infarcted muscle. The samples were usually obtained 20-45 hours after death, packed in plastic bags and frozen at -20°C until analyzed. When the samples were prepared for analysis the outer layers were removed and discarded to avoid samples containing peroxidized lipids.

Analytical procedure. Lipid extraction, separation, and analyses were carried out as described previously[2,3]. Heart muscle samples, 2-3 g, were extracted with chloroform methanol and homogenized in an all glass tissue grinder. The antioxidant butylated hydroxytoluene (BHT) was added to the extraction medium at 5 mg/100 ml. Internal standards were added at this point to estimate recovery of free fatty acids and phospholipids. Dipentadecanoyl phosphatidyl choline served to estimate recovery of phospholipid

fatty acids. Heptadecanoic acid (17:0) served to estimate recovery
of free fatty acids.

Results and Discussion

I. Post-mortem degradation of myocardial phospholipids.

     Analyses of human autopsy material have to be viewed with
caution because of the autolytic changes that take place from the
time of death until the time of sampling. The autolytic changes
in heart muscle are relatively slow compared to those in many
other tissues, such as the liver. The post-mortem enzymatic
degradation of phospholipids in heart muscle may reveal features
relevant to phospholipid degradation in ischemia in vivo although
there would be differences with respect to reaction rates and
extent of hydrolysis. During the early phase of post-mortem
autolysis sphingolipids, cholesterol esters and triglycerides show
little change. The glycerol phospholipids are, however degraded
more rapidly and the free fatty acid level rises in proportion to
the extent of degradation of the phospholipids[5].

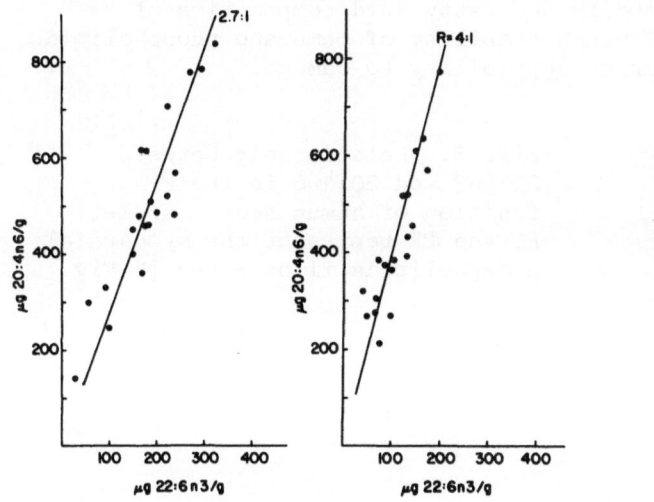

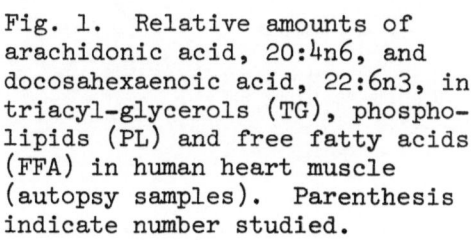

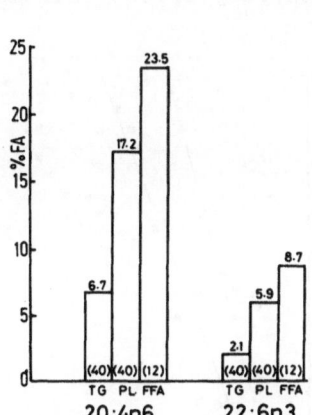

Fig. 1. Relative amounts of
arachidonic acid, 20:4n6, and
docosahexaenoic acid, 22:6n3, in
triacyl-glycerols (TG), phospholipids (PL) and free fatty acids
(FFA) in human heart muscle
(autopsy samples). Parenthesis
indicate number studied.

Fig. 2. Relationship between
22:6n3 and 20:4n6 in phosphatidyl
ethanolamine (PE), left, and
phosphatidyl choline (PC), right,
in human heart muscle.

The composition of free fatty acids found in autopsy samples
from human heart muscle indicated that these free fatty acids were
primarily derived from hydrolysis of phospholipids, i.e. glycerol
phospholipids. There was relatively more of the polyene fatty
acids, arachidonic acid, 20:4n6, and docosahexaenoic acid, 22:6n3
in the free fatty acids, than in the remaining phospholipids, Fig.
1. Those phospholipids that contain the above fatty acids were
thus more readily hydrolyzed by phospholipases than phospholipids
containing more saturated fatty acids. There also appeared to be
a faster breakdown of phospholipids containing 22:6n3 than those
containing 20:4n6[6]. There was a specific relationship between
20:4n6 and 22:6n3 in myocardial phosphatidyl choline (PC) and
phosphatidyl ethanolamine (PE), respectively, Fig. 2. The
relationship between these two fatty acids in myocardial free fatty
acids (FFA), mostly released from these two phospholipids, showed
that there was relatively more 22:6n3 than 20:4n6 in the FFA
fraction compaired to remaining PC and PE, illustrating that
endogenous phospholipids containing 22:6n3 were hydrolyzed more
readily than other phospholipids, Fig. 3.

These observations indicate that the stability of human
myocardial phospholipids is a function of the fatty acid composition.
The most unsaturated phospholipids are most unstable and the
resistance to hydrolysis increases with the saturation of the fatty
acids. Conditions which modify the fatty acid composition of
phospholipids may thus influence stability of membrane phospholipids
and thereby affect cellular susceptibility to damage.

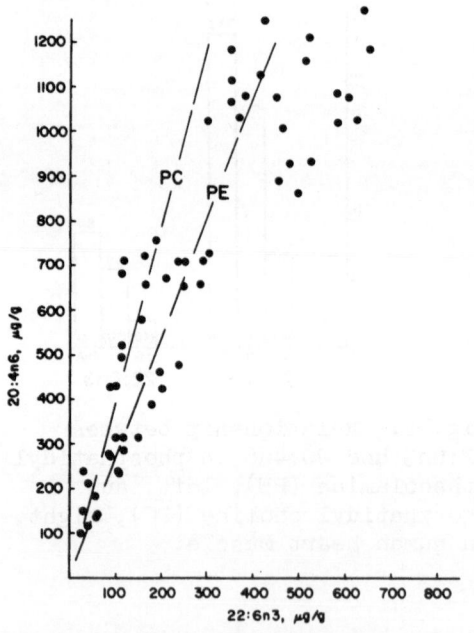

Fig. 3. Relationship between
22:6n3 and 20:4n6 in the FFA
fraction of human heart muscle.
PC and PE represent the myocardial
phospholipids illustrated in Fig.
2.

II. Fatty acid composition of myocardial phospholipids in normal
     and atherosclerotic hearts

The fatty acid composition of myocardial phospholipids in
absence or presence of severe coronary atherosclerotic stenosis is
shown in Table 1. There were no major differences observed in the
fatty acyl chain composition of myocardial phospholipids in hearts
with and without severe coronary artery disease except for a
significantly higher level of eicosapentaenoic acid (EPA), 20:5n3,
in atherosclerotic hearts.

EPA is derived primarily from fish and marine animals and may
have an important role to play in the cardiovascular system of
marine animals, such as the seal and the whale. EPA has been
considered a potential candidate for the treatment of cardiovascular
disease because this fatty acid is able to prevent platelet
aggregation[7].

Table 1

Fatty Acid Chain Composition of Myocardial Phospholipids
in Relation to Coronary Artery Disease.

| Fatty acid | Coronary artery stenosis, grades: | |
	0 - 2 n=14	5 - 6 n=14
16:0	14.33±0.21	15.06±0.44
18:0	15.18±0.68	14.38±0.74
18:1	11.46±0.29	10.03±0.58
18:2n6	19.83±1.14	19.74±1.00
20:4n6	18.60±0.34	17.82±0.57
20:5n3	1.06±0.15	2.69±0.58 (P<0.02)
22:5n3	1.74±0.11	1.46±0.10
22:6n3	6.28±0.51	7.25±0.57
mg/g	7.54±0.35	7.32±0.41
Age (years)	40.3±4.7 (18-72)	60.9±2.9 (46-78)
Time of sampling+	38.4±2.8	35.8±2.6

+Hours after death.

The mechanism responsible for this effect of 20:5n3 is not clear,
it has been proposed that 20:5n3 forms an inactive thromboxane A_3,
antiaggregating PGD_3 or inhibits thromboxane A_2 production. Long
term dietary intake of moderate amounts of cod liver oil may modify
the composition of blood lipids without, however, altering blood
coagulation in normal subjects[8]. The significantly higher level
of EPA in myocardial phospholipids of atherosclerotic hearts
observed in this study illustrates that there was no diminution in
myocardial tissue stores of this fatty acid in people with severe
coronary atherosclerosis.

        The role of EPA in the cardiovascular system may be more
complex than assumed thus far. EPA is major fatty acid (29%) in
PE of whale heart muscle, but a relatively minor fatty acid (3%)
in the coronary arteries of the whale heart[9]. In the seal and
presumably also the whale the coronary blood flow is reduced by
about 90% during diving[10] and in the whale the heart rate may at
the same time be reduced to 8-10 beats per min. Such a reduction
in coronary flow, resembling coronary vasospasm, would probably
cause ischemic damage and even death in man. It would be of great
interest to explore the role of 20:5n3 in the heart of these marine
animals. Although 20:5n3 is not present in large amounts in the
major coronary arteries of the whale this fatty acid might be
important for the microvasculature.

III.   Linoleic acid diminishes in the aging heart

        In the aging human heart there was a significant diminution
in linoleic acid content of phospholipids, accompanied by an
increase in docosahexaenoic acid[4], whereas arachidonic acid and the
saturated and monoene fatty acids remained unchanged. Changes in
composition of membrane lipids that come with age are likely to
influence cellular function and response to drugs. One of the
most striking physiological changes known to occur with age is a
decline in the hearts ability to respond to stress.

        Linoleic acid is a precursor of arachidonic acid, but the role
of linoleoyl chains in membrane phospholipids is not understood.
One phospholipid, cardiolipin, is particularely rich in linoleic
acid, with 70-80% of its fatty acyl chains consisting of this fatty
acid. Cardiolipin is required for the catalytic activity of
cytochrome oxidase and for electron transfer in complex I and III
in mitochondrial respiratory chain[11]. Cardiolipin is relatively
resistant to alterations in fatty acyl chain composition induced
in other phospholipids by diet[2] or stress[3].

        Linoleoyl chains may specifically modulate adenylate cyclase
in the plasma membrane. Linoleate incorporation into plasma
membrane phospholipids (PC and PE) activates adenylate cyclase.
Oleate incorporation was without effect whereas arachidonate

incorporation decreased adenylate cyclase activity[12].

The diminished effectiveness of adrenergic stimulation of the cardiovascular system, both myocardial and vascular tissue, during aging[13] may be associated with altered membrane composition reflected here in the diminution of linoleic acid in myocardial phospholipids.

IV. Free fatty acids in human heart muscle in relation to coronary artery disease

The free fatty acids found in autopsy samples are mostly released during post-mortem degradation of phospholipids. Differences in tissue levels of FFA reflect either differences in rates of degradation, i.e. activities of phospholipases, or differences in FFA levels existing in the tissue before death. The post-mortem increase in FFA tends thus to mask differences in FFA levels existing before death, except when these differences were extremely large.

Table II

Free Fatty Acids in Human Heart Muscle Autopsy Samples in Relation to Coronary Artery Disease.

	FFA mg/g ± SEM
I. *Hearts with no , mild or moderate coronary artery stenosis , grades 0-3 .*	3.72 ± 0.40 (n=28)
II. *Hearts with severe coronary artery stenosis , grades 4-6 .*	1.93 ± 0.21[+] (n=30)

Various   causes of death.

[+] $P < 0.001$

Despite these difficulties and limitations an attempt was made to detect differences in myocardial FFA levels accompanying sudden cardiac death. The tissue content and composition of FFA was determined in heart muscle from people that suffered a sudden cardiac death and in heart muscle from people that died suddenly in accidents.

Sudden cardiac death is most frequently due to ventricular fibrillation, a disorder usually but not exclusively secondary to inadequate myocardial blood flow. Other known causes of sudden cardiac death are for example congenital abnormality of conduction tissue and degeneration of the conduction system.

The role of high plasma free fatty acid levels in development of arrhythmias and death in patients with acute myocardial infarction has remained controversial since the hypothesis was proposed by Kurien and Oliver[14]. An association of elevated plasma FFA concentration, and presumably increased myocardial FFA levels, with an increased incidence of serious arrhythmias has important implications for treatment of patients with acute myocardial infarction. The possible arrhythmogenic effect of high plasma FFA concentrations has been studied extensively but with conflicting results.

Table III

Free Fatty Acids in Human Heart Muscle Autopsy
Samples in Accidental Deaths or Cardiac Deaths.

	FFA mg/g ± SEM
I. Sudden accidental death	3.37 ± 0.71 (n = 14)
II. Instant cardiac death	1.87 ± 0.37 [++] (n = 12)
III. Delayed cardiac death [+] (includes myocardial infraction)	3.34 ± 0.37 (n = 12)

+ Death within an hour or several hours after
  onset of symptoms of MI.

++ P < 0.01, group II. compared to group III.

The results in Table II show significantly lower post-mortem myocardial levels of FFA in hearts with severe coronary artery stenosis (grades 4-6) compared to hearts with no, mild or moderate coronary artery disease (grades 0-3). The results show furthermore that myocardial FFA levels of those that suffered instant cardiac death were significantly lower than in those that developed myocardial infarction and died several hours after onset of symptoms, i.e. delayed cardiac death, Table III. FFA levels observed in delayed cardiac death were similar to those observed following sudden death in accidents.

In hearts with severe coronary artery stenosis the free fatty acid composition in muscle samples showed a significantly lower content of arachidonic acid and oleic acid (18:1), but a higher content of eicosapentaenoic acid, 20:5n3, and docosahexaenoic acid, 22:6n3, Table IV. The relative release of arachidonic acid or the ratio of arachidonic acid to other major fatty acids, Table V, suggests a specific impairment in the release of arachidonic acid, i.e. a 30-40% diminution in arachidonic acid released compared to palmitic, stearic and linoleic acid and a 50% decrease compared to docosahexaenoic acid. Coronary artery disease in man did not seem to be associated with a diminution in tissue stores of any polyene fatty acid, Table I. In atherosclerotic hearts there appeared,

Table IV

Composition of Free Fatty Acids in Heart
Muscle in Relation to Coronary Artery Disease.

Fatty acid	Coronary artery stenosis, grades:	
	0 - 2 n=14	5 - 6 n=14
16:0	13.62 ± 0.97	15.99 ± 1.51
18:0	9.20 ± 0.52	11.86 ± 0.77
18:1	21.19 ± 1.46	15.03 ± 0.74 (P<0.001)
18:2n6	13.21 ± 1.01	14.83 ± 0.73
20:4n6	26.55 ± 1.78	20.88 ± 1.16 (P<0.02)
20:5n3	2.11 ± 0.44	3.92 ± 0.68 (P<0.02)
22:5n3	1.95 ± 0.21	1.78 ± 0.19
22:6n3	6.22 ± 0.66	9.95 ± 1.05 (P<0.01)
mg/g	3.00 ± 0.63	1.70 ± 0.33

however, to be a marked diminution in phospholipase activity and
a specific reduction in the release of arachidonic acid.

In heart muscle there may be two systems releasing arachidonic
acid from tissue phospholipids similar to the renal system[15]. The
first system is a hormone-insensitive system in which arachidonic
acid as well as other fatty acids are released. Nonspecific
stimuli, such as hypoxia, anoxia and mechanical trauma stimulate
this system to increase lipolysis and consequently, there is also
an increase in the formation of various prostaglandins and other
arachidonate-oxygenated products. The second system is a hormone-
activated system in which a hormone sensitive phospholipase
selectively releases arachidonic acid which is converted to tissue-
specific prostaglandin products. This system may be affected in
coronary artery disease in man and such a defect may be associated
with sudden cardiac death.

Impaired release of arachidonic acid means reduced availability
of the free precursor fatty acid which is the rate limiting step
in formation of prostacyclin, PGI_2, and other prostaglandins. The
most important source of cardiac PGI_2 is the vascular compartment
and the major site of action of PGI_2 in the heart is the coronary
vasculature[16], where PGI_2 relaxes coronary arteries and decreases
vascular resistance. In patients with ischemic heart disease there

Table V

Post-Mortem Myocardial Release of Arachidonic
Acid Relative to that of other Fatty Acids in
Relation to Coronary Artery Disease.

	Coronary artery stenosis, grades.		Changes in arachidonic acid release.
	0 - 2 n=14	5 - 6 n=14	
20:4n6 / 18:1	1.42±0.19	1.45±0.13	N.S.
20:4n6 / 16:0	2.11±0.21	1.44±0.13	-31.8% (P<0.02)
20:4n6 / 18:0	3.04±0.27	1.87±0.16	-38.5% (P<0.005)
20:4n6 / 18:2n6	2.33±0.38	1.43±0.08	-38.6% (P<0.05)
20:4n6 / 22:6n3	5.04±0.75	2.45±0.28	-51.4% (P<0.005)

is significantly reduced production of PGI_2[17], which may be relevant
to the apparent decrease in precursor availability suggested in
this study.

V. Myocardial free fatty acids and sudden cardiac death in absence of coronary atherosclerosis

We analyzed heart muscle samples from people who had died
suddenly from heart disease of other nature than atherosclerosis.
Lipid alterations in the heart muscle place these into three groups:
A, B and C.

A) A 58 year old male alcoholic with a history of heavy drinking
    for two weeks, but had sobered up. He died in his sleep. The
    heart showed grade 3 coronary atherosclerosis in 3 vessels and
    there was a slight focal interstitial myocardial fibrosis.
    The liver was fatty. A cause of death was not established by
    the autopsy dindings. Anterior and posterior heart muscle
    samples, taken 22 hours post-mortem, had very high levels of
    FFA 14.2 ± 2.3 mg/g. The composition of these FFA indicated
    that they were primarily plasma FFA, probably derived from
    glycerides or depot fat. Phospholipid levels were normal and
    there was no myocardial infarction. Assuming normal post-mortem
    release of FFA there might have been more than 10 mg FFA/g
    muscle before death, a highly toxic level. Normal levels in
    vivo can be assumed to range from 10-100 ug/g. It is thus
    probable that a 100-1000 fold increase in myocardial FFA would
    seriously impair energy production, energy transfer, activity
    of ion pumps, etc., and contribute to development of lethal
    arrhythmias. Sudden death related to alcoholic liver disease
    has been reported to be a relatively frequent event[18].

B) A 47 year old woman who died suddenly and unexpectedly in her
    sleep. There was no history of previous disease or an abuse
    of alcohol or medication. She was slightly obese. There was
    reason to believe that she was under considerable emotional
    stress. The heart showed coronary arteries without athero-
    sclerosis and normal myocardium on microscopic examination,
    except for focal interstitial fibrosis and a few chronic
    inflammatory cells in one section. The cause of death was not
    established at autopsy. Samples were taken 80 hours post-
    mortem, but post-mortem autolysis was not present as seen by
    microscopy of the heart.
    There was a moderate increase in levels of FFA, 6.2 ± 0.2 mg/g
    in both anterior and posterior muscle samples. In the anterior
    muscle sample the level of PE was low and very low levels of
    22:6n3 remaining in residual PE. These alterations could
    reflect membrane damage before or during the time of death.
    Degradation subsequent to death would have left 22:6n3 in the
    heart muscle where it would have been found.

C) In several cases of sudden cardiac death no significant

alterations in myocardial lipids could be detected. Two
examples will be described: 1) A 55 year old male who died
on the job. There was no previous medical history. The
autopsy revealed an enlarged heart, weighing 600 g, consistent
with dilated cardiomyopathy. Coronary atherosclerosis was of
grade 2 in three vessels and there was slight focal interstitial
myocardial fibrosis. The cause of death was established as
cardiomyopathy. Samples were taken 23 hours post-mortem. The
FFA levels were 4.82 mg/g in anterior sample and 4.31 mg/g in
posterior muscle sample. 2) A 10 year old girl who died
suddenly, apparently from cardiac arrhythmia while running at
play. Two years earlier she had suffered a similar attach but
had been resuscitated back to life. The only abnormal finding
at autopsy was an enlarged heart, weighing 200 grams, but
normal heart weight for her age is 120-150 g. The myocardium
was normal on microscopic examination. Samples were taken
23 hours post-mortem. The FFA levels were 3.87 mg/g in anterior
sample and 4.16 mg/g in posterior muscle.

The observations made in this study suggest that sudden cardiac
death may be due to several distinct biochemical abnormalities in
heart muscle. Myocardial ischemia and infarction may be caused by
several different pathological mechanisms and the response to acute
ischemia may differ depending on the absence or presence of severe
coronary atheroschlerosis and accompanying adaptive changes in
myocardial and vascular tissue.

Changes in myocardial metabolism due to acute experimental
coronary artery occlusion in normal animals may not reflect
accurately the response of the atherosclerotic human heart to acute
ischemia. This should be considered in the design of a meaningful
therapy of myocardial infarction in man.

Summary

The content and composition of free fatty acids and phospholipids were determined in heart muscle obtained at autopsy from
people that died suddenly in accidents and from people that suffered
a sudden cardiac death, with or without coronary artery disease.

Post-mortem degradation of myocardial phospholipids indicates
that the stability of phospholipids is a function of the fatty acid
composition, more unsaturated fatty acids were released more
readily than less unsaturated fatty acids.

The fatty acid composition of myocardial phospholipids was
similar in normal and atherosclerotic hearts, except for a significantly higher level of eicosapentaenoic acid, 20:5n3, in
atherosclerotic hearts.

There was a significant diminution of linoleic acid, 18:2n6, in phospholipids of the aging heart.

The content and composition of myocardial free fatty acids indicated reduced phospholipase activity and a specific impairment of arachidonic acid, (20:4n6), release in hearts with severe coronary atherosclerotic stenosis.

Sudden cardiac death in absence of severe coronary atherosclerosis could be divided into several groups according to myocardial lipid alterations: a) An extremely high level of myocardial FFA in an alcoholic subject, b) moderate increase in FFA but reduced level of specific phospholipids, and c) normal lipid profile of heart muscle.

References

1. A. Schwartz, J. M. Wood, J. C. Allen, E. P. Bornet, M. L. Entman, M. A. Goldstein, L. A. Sordahl, M. Suzuki, and R. M. Lewis, Biochemical and morphologic correlates of cardiac ischemia, I Membrane systems, Am. J. Cardiol., 32:46-61 (1973).

2. S. Gudbjarnason and G. Oskarsdottir, Modification of fatty acid composition of rat heart lipids by feeding cod liver oil, Biochim. Biophys. Acta, 487:1o-15 (1977).

3. A. Emilsson and S. Gudbjarnason, Changes in fatty acyl chain composition of rat heart phospholipids induced by noradrenaline. Biochim. Biophys. Acta, 664:82-88 (1981).

4. S. Gudbjarnason, G. Oskarsdottir, B. Doell and J. Hallgrimsson, Myocardial membrane lipids in relation to cardiovascular disease, Advances in cardiol., 25:130-144 (1978).

5. G. Rouser, G. I. Nelson and S. Fleischer, Lipid composition of animal cell membranes, organelles and organs, in: Biological Membranes, D. Chapman, ed., Academic Press, Vol., 1:5-69 (1968).

6. S. Gudbjarnason and I. Hallgrimsson, Cardiac lipids and ischemic tolerance, in: "Ischemic Myocardium and Antianginal Drugs", M. M. Winbury and Y. Abiko, ed., Raven Press p. 213-224 (1979).

7. J. Dyerberg, H. O. Bang, E. Stofferson, S. Moncada and J. R. Vane, Eicosapentaenoic acid and prevention of thrombosis and atherosclerosis, Lancet, 2:117-119 (1978).

8. R. Saynor and D. Verel, Effect of a marine oil high in eicosapentaenoic acid on blood lipids and coagulation, IRCS Medical Science, 8:378-379 (1980).

9. S. Gudbjarnason and A. Emilsson, Unpublished observations.

10. A. S. Blix, J. K. Kjekshus, I. Enge and A. Bergen, Myocardial blood flow in the diving seal, Acta Physiol. Scand., 96:277-280 (1976).

11. M. Fry and D. Green, Cardiolipin requirements for electron

transfer in complex I and III of the mitochondrial respiratory chain, J. Biol. Chem., 256:1874-1880 (1981).

12. O. Colard, A. Kervabon and C. Roy, Effects on adenylate cyclase
     activities of unsaturated fatty acid incorporation into rat
     liver plasma membrane phospholipids, Specific modulation by
     linoleate, Biochem. Biophys. Res. Comm., 95:97-102 (1980).

13. E. G. Lakatta, Age-related alterations in the cardiovascular
     response to adrenergic mediated stress, Fed. Proceed. Vol.,
     39:3173-3177 (1980).

14. V. A. Kurien and M. F. Oliver, A metabolic cause for
     arrhythmias during acute myocardial hypoxia, Lancet, 1:813-
     815 (1970).

15. M. Schwartzman, E. Liberman and A. Raz, Bradykinin and
     angiotensin II activation of arachidonic acid deacylation
     and prostaglandin E_2 formation in rabbit kidney, J. Biol.
     Chem., 256:2329-2333 (1981).

16. K. Schrör, Possible role of prostaglandins in the regulation
     of coronary blood flow, Basic Res. Cardiol., 76:239-249
     (1981).

FATTY ACID COMPOSITION OF PHOSPHOLIPIDS OF HEART MUSCLE IN

RELATION TO AGE, DIETARY FAT AND STRESS

S. Gudbjarnason, A. Emilsson and A. Gudmundsdottir

Science Institute, University of Iceland

Reykjavík, Iceland

The purpose of this study was to examine some of the factors that modify the fatty acid composition of myocardial membranes and thereby their structure, function and stability. The phospholipids play an important role in structure and function of membranes and the polyene fatty acyl chain composition of some of these phospholipids is readily modified. Changes in fatty acyl chain composition of phospholipids influence membrane permeability and other physical properties, influence properties of membrane bound enzymes and hormone receptors[1,2], influence transport pumps and probably ion channels as well, and the degree of peroxidation damage may depend on the fatty acid profile of membranes.

The functions of specific polyene fatty acyl chains in individual phospholipids are poorly understood. The role of certain polyene fatty acids released from phospholipids are better understood, such as the conversion of arachidonic acid to various prostaglandins and other important substances[3].

In the present study changes in the fatty acid composition of heart muscle lipids induced by aging, dietary lipids and stress were examined, but these factors have been implicated in the development of cardiovascular diseases. The relationship between oxidation of catecholamines to aminochromes and peroxidation of polyene fatty acids will be discussed, and its possible role in inactivation of β-receptor bound catecholamines and desensitization of β-recptors.

Material and methods

The experimental animals were male Wistar rats fed ad libidum. The rats were divided into various groups and fed the following diets:

I.   a standard diet (KFK, Viby, I., Denmark
II. a diet containing 10% (w/w) cod liver oil added to the standard
     feed[4], and
III. a diet containing 10% (w/w) corn oil (with 50% linoleic acid).

Rats subjected to catecholamine stress or repeated administration of norepinephrine were fed the standard diet. These rats
were injected daily for 15 days with increasing doses of norepinephrine bitartrate. During the first 3 days the rats received 1 mg./
kg., and then 2,3,4 and 5 mg./kg. for subsequent 3-day periods.
Mortality during the norepinephrine stress was about 50%. A control
group received daily injections of distilled water. The rats were
killed by decapitation, the hearts were excised and kept at -20° in
iceblock until analysed[4,5].

Results and Discussions

Aging and myocardial phospholipids

In rats the long-chain polyene fatty acyl composition of myocardial phospholipids changed markedly with age. The two major
phospholipids in heart muscle are phosphatidyl choline (PC) and
phosphatidyl ethanolamine (PE), these two phospholipids make up 75-
80% of total phospholipids in myocardial membranes.

In PC there was a progressive replacement of linoleic acid,
18:2n6, by arachidonic acid, 20:4n6, with age. Linoleic acid
decreased from 28.4% in 2 months old rats to 17% in 18 months old
rats. Arachidonic acid increased from 11.7% to 20.6% during the
same period.

In PE the linoleic acid was replaced by docosahexaenoic acid,
22:6n3, with age. Linoleic acid decreased from 15.0% at age 2 months
to 8.7% in 18 months old rats and docosahexaenoic acid increased
from 20.1% to 28.9% in the same period. In PE the relative content
of 20:4n6 remained constant during this time. The contents of
saturated and monoene fatty acyl chains in myocardial phospholipids
did not change significantly during this period.

Dietary fat and myocardial phospholipids

Dietary fat may cause extensive alterations in the composition
of myocardial phospholipids and thereby influence membrane properties.
Rats fed a diet containing 10% corn oil or 10% cod liver oil showed
significant alterations in fatty acyl chain composition of myocardial
glycerides and phospholipids. A diet containing 10% corn oil, rich
in linoleic acid, caused a marked and persistent diminution in 18:2n6
in myocardial PC, Fig. 1. The increased dietary intake of 18:2n6
in form of corn oil caused a marked elevation of arachidonic acid in
myocardial PC, Fig. 2, but linoleic acid serves as a precursor to
arachidonic acid.

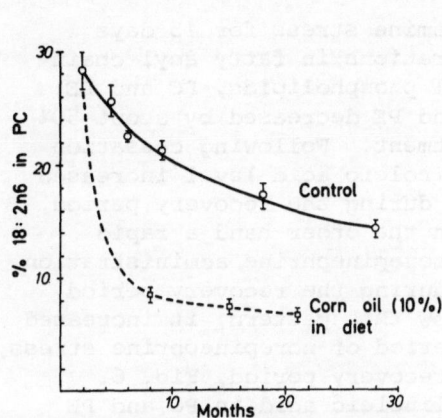

Fig. 1. Changes linoleic acid, 18:2n6, content of phosphatidyl choline with age and dietary corn oil (10% w/w).

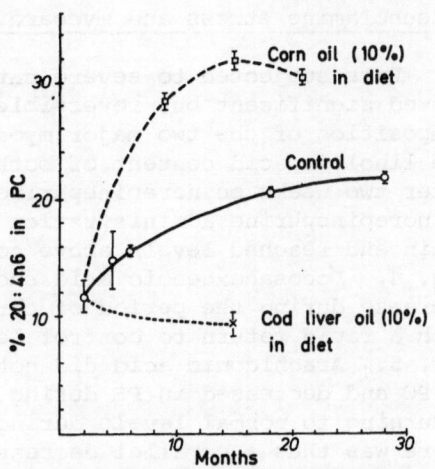

Fig. 2. Changes in arachidonic acid, 20:4n6, content of phosphatidyl choline with age and dietary corn oil (10% w/w) or cod liver oil (10% w/w).

A diet containing 10% cod liver oil which is rich in n3 fatty acids but poor in n6 fatty acids caused a marked reduction in arachidonic acid in PC, which normally increases with age, Fig. 2. Dietary cod liver oil caused a marked but transient increase in docosahexaenoic acid in myocardial phospholipids, primarily PE, Fig. 3. The level of 22:6n3 increased from 12% to 29% after 3 months of feeding the cod liver oil but it then returned to almost normal levels 6 months later. The adaptation to dietary fat varied depending on the particular fatty acid.

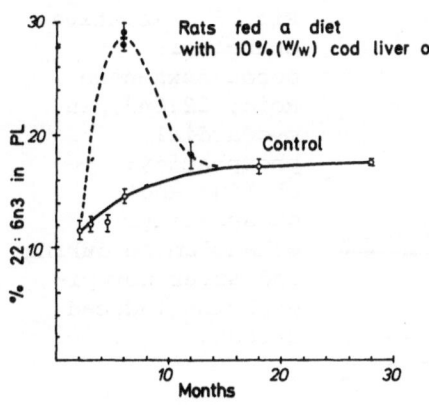

Fig. 3. Changes in docosahexaenoic acid, 22:6n3, content of myocardial phospholipids with age and adaptation to dietary cod liver oil.

Catecholamine stress and myocardial phospholipids

        Rats subjected to severe catecholamine stress for 15 days
showed significant but reversible alterations in fatty acyl chain
composition of the two major myocardial phospholipids, PC and PE.
The linoleic acid content of both PC and PE decreased by about 50%
after two weeks on norepinephrine treatment. Following cessation
of norepinephrine administration the linoleic acid level increased
again and reached levels above control during the recovery period,
Fig. 4. Docosahexaenoic acid showed on the other hand a rapid
increase during the period of chronic norepinephrine administration
with a rapid return to control levels during the recovery period,
Fig. 5. Arachidonic acid did not follow this pattern, it increased
in PC and decreased in PE during the period of norepinephrine stress,
returning to normal levels during the recovery period, Fig. 6.
There was thus a parallel decrease in linoleic acid in PC and PE
and a parallel increase in docosahexaenoic acid in PC and PE during
the period of stress. There was, on the other hand, an inverse
relationship between the arachidonic acid levels in PE and PC, i.e.
possibly a conversion of PE to PC by transmethylation.

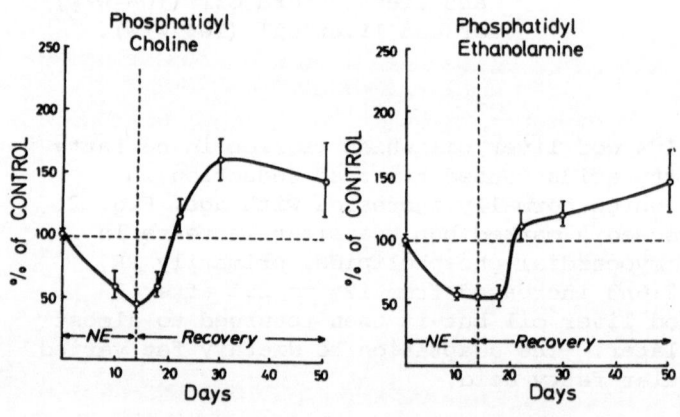

Fig. 4. Relative changes in linoleic acid, 18:2n6, in myocardial phosphatidyl choline and phosphatidyl ethanolamine during and after norepinephrine induced stress.

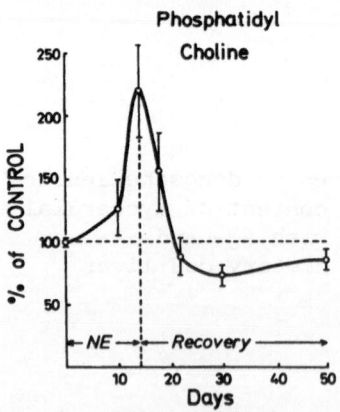 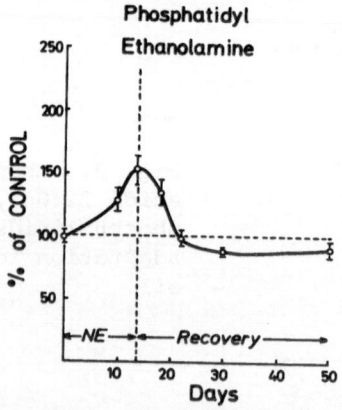

Fig. 5. Relative changes in docosahexaenoic acid, 22:6n3, in myocardial phosphatidyl choline and phosphatidyl ethanolamine during and after norepinephrine induced stress.

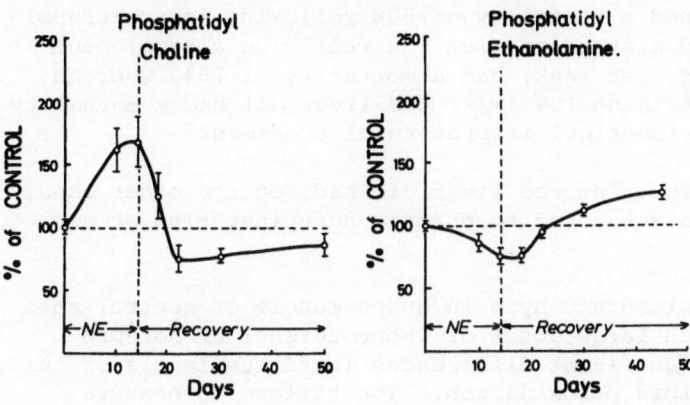

Fig. 6. Relative changes in arachidonic acid, 20:4n6, in myocardial phosphatidyl choline and phosphatidyl ethanolamine during and after norepinephrine induced stress.

Hirata and Axelrod[6] have postulated that catecholamine binding to β-adrenergic receptor on the cell surface activates methylation of PE to PC and that enzymatic methylation of phospholipids plays an important role in the transduction of receptormediated signals through the membrane. Phospholipid methylation, i.e. conversion of PE to PC increases membrane fluidity and enhances the lateral mobility and rotation of the β-adrenergic receptor. This should unmask hidden receptors and facilitate the coupling of the receptor on the outer surface with adenylate cyclase facing the cytoplasmic side of the membrane[6]. Our data are compatible with such a catecholamine induced conversion of PE, containing arachidonoyl chains to PC.

This process is possibly coupled to desensitization of cells when they are exposed to excessive amounts of hormones or transmitters. The phospholipid methylation is coupled to activation of phospholipase A_2 which appears to be involved in the desensitization of β-adrenergic receptors. This desensitization is probably mediated by one or more products of phospholipase A_2 activity, such as lysophosphatidyl choline, arachidonic acid or its prostaglandin metabolites[6].

Fatty acid profile, stress tolerance and lipid peroxidation

What are the consequences of major changes in the fatty acid profile of myocardial phospholipids? Do these changes affect stress tolerance or ischemic tolerance?

We have examined the influence of dietary cod liver oil and hydrogenated fish oil on the development of cardiac necrosis and mortality following isoproterenol stress[7]. Isoproterenol was given according to the method of Rona, 40 mg./kg., injected s.c. twice, the second injection 24 hours after the first one. Control animals fed a standard diet and animals fed a diet containing 10% or 20%

hydrogenated fish oil had a mortality of 50% following isoproterenol treatment. Animals fed a standard diet but receiving a supplement of vitamin E, 50 mg./kg. per week, had a mortality of 25%, whereas animals fed a diet containing 10% (w/w) cod liver oil had a mortality of 100%[7] following the identical isoproterenol treatment.

Control rats and rats fed cod liver oil had, on the other hand, the same mortality when subjected to chronic norepinephrine stress as described above.

Measurements of malondialdehyde in heart muscle of control rats and rats stimulated with large doses of isoproterenol or norepinephrine did not show significant differences in tissue levels of this product of excessive lipid peroxidation. The failure to observe elevated levels of malondialdehyde in heart muscle in vivo following overstimulation with catecholamines does not exclude excessive lipid peroxidation since malondialdehyde is very reacitve and may react rapidly in vivo and form Schiff's bases.

According to Meerson[8] emotional painful stress, accompanied by high plasma levels of glucocorticoids and catecholamines, increases myocardial lipid peroxidation which leads to multiple membrane damage and disturbances in cardiac metabolism, structure and function. In rats subjected to emotional stress there was a 3-fold increase in myocardial lipid hydroperoxides and a 5-fold increase in Schiff's base formation, i.e. reaction products of malondialdehyde. Meerson concluded that the observed disturbances in contractile function of the heart during emotional painful stress and the decrease in adreno-reactivity or catecholamine sensitivity of the heart were the result of damage to the sarcoplasmic reticulum and sarcolemma induced by increased production of lipid hydroperoxides during stress[8].

Catecholamines and lipid peroxidation

There is a complex relationship between oxidation of catecholamines to aminochromes and peroxidation of polyene fatty acids. Hirata and Axelrod[6] observed that catecholamines stimulated methylation of phospholipids and coupling of the β-adrenergic receptor to adenylate cyclase was accompanied by activation of phospholipase A_2 and subsequent desensitization of the receptors by arachidonic acid or other reaction product. It is possible that lipid peroxidation may play a role in desensitization of β-adrenergic receptors.

Polyene fatty acids, either arachidonic acid or docosahexaenoic acid, stimulated oxidation of epinephrine to adrenochrome by heart muscle microsomes[7]. Subsequently, i.e. following a lag time of few minutes, there was a progressive peroxidation of the polyene fatty acid as estimated from the oxygen consumption and disappearance or utilization of the polyene fatty acid. Addition of adrenochrome stimulated the microsomal peroxidation or oxygenation of the polyene

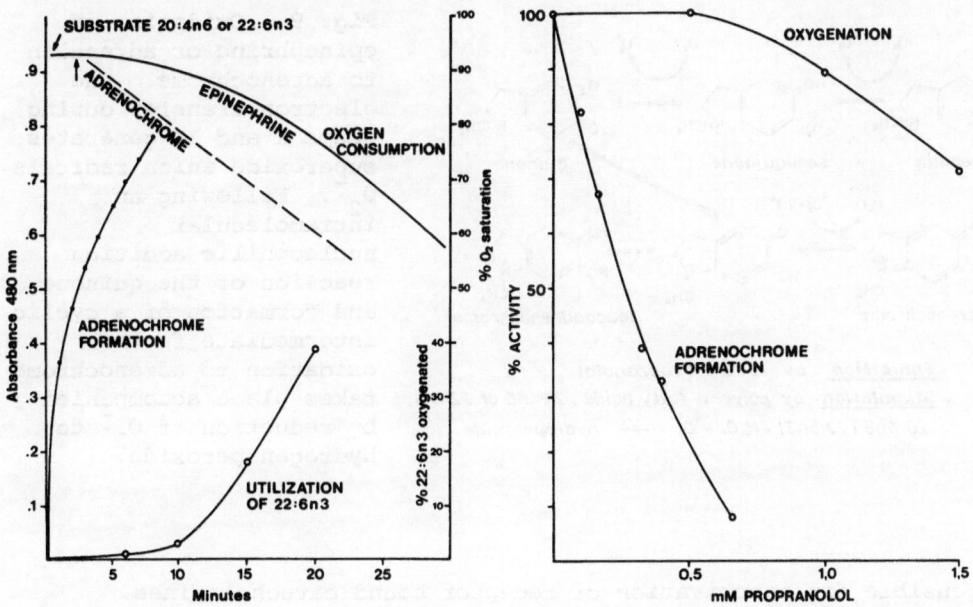

Fig.7. Polyene fatty acid stimulated oxidation of epinephrine
to adrenochrome and epinephrine
stimulated peroxidation or
oxygenation of polyene fatty
acids. Assay conditions: As
described in ref. 7.

Fig. 8. Inhibition of 22:6n3
stimulated adrenochrome formation
and epinephrine stimulated oxygenation of 22:6n3 with propranolol.
Assay conditions: As described in
ref. 7.

fatty acids, eliminating the time lag, Fig. 7. The oxidation of
epinephrine to adrenochrome was inhibited by the β-adrenergic antagonist propranolol whereas the peroxidation was inhibited subsequently
to the inhibition of adrenochrome formation by propranolol, Fig. 8.

What purpose do these reactions serve in the cell, if any?
The oxidation of epinephrine to adrenochrome may serve to inactivate
receptor-bound catecholamines. The oxidation does not take place
if the receptor is occupied by the antagonist propranolol. The
mechanism responsible for inactivation of receptor-bound catecholamines is not known. The two recognized enzymes which can inactivate
adrenergic agonists are MAO, monoamine oxidase, and COMT, catechol-
O-methyltransferase. MAO is an intracellular enzyme and does not
appear to have a primary role in removing catecholamines from the
region of receptors. COMT is also an intracellular enzyme in non-
neuronal cells, and a membrane transport system appears to be
required for movement of catecholamines into these cells. Neuronal
uptake appears to be the principal mechanism for removing agonists
from the region of the receptor, but this mechanism may not be

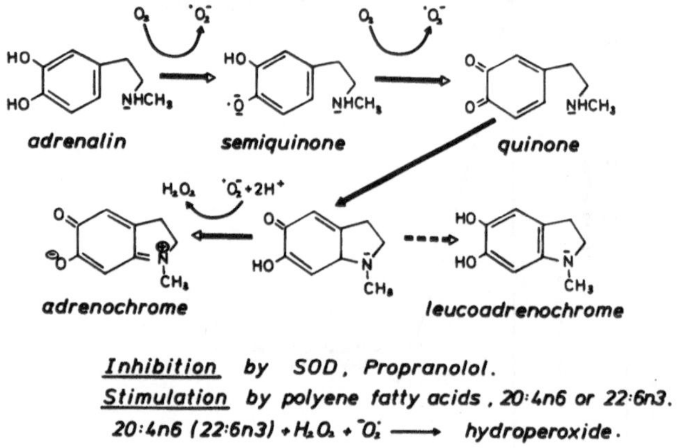

adrenalin   semiquinone   quinone

adrenochrome   leucoadrenochrome

Inhibition by SOD, Propranolol.
Stimulation by polyene fatty acids , 20:4n6 or 22:6n3.
20:4n6 (22:6n3) + H_2O_2 + O_2^- ⟶ hydroperoxide.

Fig. 9. Oxidation of epinephrine or adrenalin to adrenochrome. One electron transfer during steps I and II generates superoxide anion radicals O_2^-. Following an intramolecular nucleophilic addition reaction of the quinone and formation of a cyclic intermediate further oxidation to adrenochrome takes place accompanied by reduction of O_2^- to hydrogen peroxide.

responsible for inactivation of receptor bound catecholamines.

The oxidation of epinephrine to adrenochrome appears to be due to the superoxide anion radical which is also generated during epinephrine oxidation, Fig. 9. Superoxide dismutase, SOD, breaks down the O_2^- and inhibits the reaction whereas a reaction with catalase liberates O_2 and indicates that H_2O_2 is a product of the reaction[9]. The first step in the reaction appears to be a one electron transfer to give the semiquinone, which is then oxidized to the open-chain quinone, Fig. 9. The reaction stops at this stage in strongly acidic solution which rapidly removes O_2^- by spontaneous dismutation. In slightly acidic or neutral solution the quinone undergoes 1.4-Michael addition reaction presumably to give an inter-mediate which can by directly converted to the aminochrome or give a leucoaminochrome, which is oxidized to aminochrome[10]. During the epinephrine oxidation epinephrine may serve both as a source of O_2^- and as a scavenger of O_2^- requiring O_2^- for adrenochrome formation and peroxide production[9].

In this manner increased levels of catecholamines might lead to production of both O_2^- and H_2O_2, which in turn generate the potent oxidant hydroxyl radical by the reaction: $H_2O_2 + O_2^- \rightarrow O_2 + OH^- + \cdot OH$. This radical initiates lipid peroxidation and formation of products, which either directly (prostaglandins) on indirectly, through perturbation of membrane microarchitecture, facilitate uncoupling of the β-receptor adenylate cyclase complex and desensitization.

During anoxia and ischemia the inactivation of receptor bound catecholamines by oxidation to aminochromes would be delayed facilitating continued stimulation of glycogen breakdown and glycolytic energy production which should enhance cellular viability.

Excessive levels of catecholamines could thus stimulate peroxidations beyond the level of useful, defensive regulation and to the point of destructive peroxidations. The aminochromes derived from catecholamines are oxidized further to melanins, generating still more radicals[11]. The increase in myocardial lipid hydroperoxides and Shciff's bases observed during emotional stress[8] and the favorable effect of the antioxidant α-tocopherol on survival of rats during overstimulation with isoproterenol[7] indicate that excessive and harmful lipid peroxidations may accompany certain forms of stress.

Summary

Alterations in fatty acid composition of phospholipids in rat heart muscle were examined in relation to age, dietary fat and catecholamine stress.

Aging was accompined by replacement of linoleic acid (18:2n6) by arachidonic acid (20:4n6) in phosphatidyl choline (PC) and replacement of linoleic acid by docosahexaenoic acid (22:6n3) in phosphatidyl ethanolamine (PE).

Dietary corn oil (10% w/w) increased arachidonic acid in PC at the expense of linoleic acid, whereas dietary cod liver oil (10% w/w) increased docosahexaenoic acid replacing the n6 fatty acids.

Repeated administration of norepinephrine caused significant but reversible alterations in polyene fatty acid composition of PC and PE. A decrease in linoleic acid and an increase in docosahexaenoic acid was observed in these phospholipids during stress, whereas arachidonic acid decreased in PE and increased in PC during the same period.

Dietary cod liver oil increased mortality during overstimulation with isoproterenol whereas dietary hydrogenated fish oil was without effect. Control rats had significantly lower mortality during isoproterenol stress when receiving vitamin E supplements.

Polyene fatty acids stimulated oxidation of epinephrine to adrenochrome by heart muscle microsomes, and this reaction was inhibited by the β-adrenergic antagonist propranolol. It is suggested that the polyene fatty acid stimulated oxidation of catecholamines to aminochromes may serve to inactivate β-receptor bound catecholamines. The reaction products induce peroxidation of the polyene fatty acids which in turn could facilitate uncoupling and desensitization of β-receptors.

References

1. L. E. Hokin and T. C. Hexum, Studies on the characterization of
    the $(Na^+ + K^+)$ transport adenosine triphosphatase IX, On the
    role of phospholipids in the enzyme, Archiv. Biochem. Biophys.,
    151:453-463 (1972).
2. R. J. Lefkowitz, Catecholamine stimulated myocardial adenylate
    cyclase: effects of phospholipase digestion on the role of
    membrane lipids, J. Molec. Cell, Cardiol, 7:27-37 (1975).
3. B. Samuelsson, G. C. Folco, E. Granström, H. Kindahl, and C.
    Malmsten, Prostaglandins and thromboxanes: Biochemical and
    physiological considerations, in: Advances in Prostaglandin
    and Thromboxane Research Vol. 4, B. Samuelsson, and R.
    Paoletti, Raven Press, N.Y. pp. 1-25 (1978).
4. S. Gudbjarnason, and G. Óskarsdóttir, Modification of fatty acid
    composition of rat heart lipids by feeding cod liver oil,
    Biochim. Biophys. Acta 487:10-15 (1977).
5. A. Emilsson, and S. Gudbjarnason, Changes in fatty acyl chain
    composition of rat heart phospholipids induced by
    noradrenalin, Biochim. Biophys. Acta 664:82-88 (1981).
6. F. Hirata, and I. Axelrod, Phospholipid methylation and
    biological Transmission, Science 209:1082-1090 (1980).
7. S. Gudbjarnason, G. Óskarsdóttir, B. Doell, and I. Hallgrímsson,
    Myocardial membrane lipids in relation to cardiovascular
    disease, Adv. in Cardiol, 25:130-144 (1978).
8. F. Z. Meerson, Disturbances of metabolism and cardiac function
    under the action of emotional painful stress and their
    prophylaxis, Basic Res. in Cardiol, 75:479-500 (1980).
9. H. P. Misra, and I. Fridovich, The role of superoxide anion in
    the autoxidation of epinephrine and a simple assay for
    superoxide dismutase, J. Biol. Chem., 247:3170-3175 (1972).
10. R. A. Heacock, and W. S. Powell, Aminochrome and related
    compounds, Progr. Med. Chem., 9:275-339 (1972).
11. R. C. Sealy, C. C. Felix, J. S. Hyde, and H. M. Schwartz,
    Structure and reactivity of melanins: influence of free
    radicals and metal ions, in: Free Radicals in Biology, Vol.
    IV:209-259 (1980).

BIOCHEMICAL ALTERATIONS IN THE ISCHEMIC AND INFARCTED HEART

FOLLOWING CORONARY ARTERY OCCLUSION

Sigmundur Gudbjarnason

Science Institute
University of Iceland
Reykjavik, Iceland

I. Substrate utilization by the normal heart

The heart utilizes the energy of substrate fuels primarily to perform mechanical work. The metabolism of the heart, and consequently the extraction of oxygen and substrates, depends on the muscular activity of the heart and when the performance of work increases the rate of metabolism rises.

The pioneering studies of Bing showed the usefulness of measurements of arteriovenous differences across the heart[1]. The human heart uses primarily glucose, lactate and fatty acids and their utilization is a function of their arterial concentration. In the resting, fasted state, the uptake of glucose could, if fully oxidized, account for 30% of the concomitant oxygen uptake, lactate could account for 10% and free fatty acids (FFA) for 60%. After a light low-fat breakfast, the increased uptake of glucose accounts for 68% and that of lactate for 28% the oxygen uptake. Thus the balance between carbohydrate and lipid substrates is altered by the nutritional state of the body. In the fasted state, high circulating FFA and low insulin levels, lead to increased uptake of FFA by the heart, whereas high insulin and low FFA after a low-fat meal lead to increased glucose uptake.

Glucose uptake and its metabolism is controlled at several levels. Glucose uptake is increased by an increased circulating glucose concentration, by increased insulin activity, by increased heart work, by decreased uptake of competing substrates (such as lactate and FFA), by anoxia and uncoupling of mitochondrial metabolism. These agents are thought to act directly on the transmembrane transport of glucose or to stimulate glucose uptake secondary to increased glycolytic flow.

125

Free fatty acids taken up from the circulation are the major
fuel in the fasted state, but triglyceride fatty acids can account
for another 10%. The uptake of triglyceride fatty acids is
regulated in part by the activity of the lipoprotein lipase
(clearing factor lipase) which may be located on the vascular
endothelium. Once TG fatty acids are removed and liberated as
fatty acids, the fatty acids are thought to follow the same pathway
as FFA taken up by the heart from circulating albumin, uptake of
FFA is governed by the arterial concentration and at very high
rates of uptake the supply of coenzyme A or of carnitine can be
rate limiting, limiting the activation of FFA or transport of
activated FFA into mitochondria[2].

Usually we only consider carbohydrates and FFA as substrates
for energy production in the heart, but these substrates have other
important functions as well. Carbohydrates are not only fuels for
the heart but carbohydrates are also intimately associated with the
plasma membrane or sarcolemma, covalently linked to proteins or
lipids forming glycoproteins and glycolipids. Little is known
about the chemical structure and distribution of these polysaccharides in heart muscle.

The fatty acids are not only an important fuel for the heart
muscle, but certain polyunsaturated fatty acids, such as arachidonic acid, serve as substrates for synthesis of important
regulatory substances, such as prostaglandins, etc. Most of the
fatty acids in heart muscle are present in the esterfied form, in
phospholipids and triglycerides. The phospholipids play an
important role in structure and function of membranes and the
fatty acid composition of these phospholipids is continuously
modified by external and internal factors, such as diet or hormones[3].
The myocardial levels of triglycerides are normally low, but in
certain conditions, such as hypoxia and ischemia there may be an
accumulation of triglycerides in heart muscle.

II.   Metabolism of ischemic heart muscle

Ischemia is defined as reversible alterations in metabolism
due to insufficient O_2 supply, whereas infarction represents
irreversible changes, damage and death of heart muscle cells.

Myocardial energy metabolism may be divided into 4 phases and
these are all profoundly affected by myocardial ischemia. The
experimental data reported here were obtained in studies on myocardial infarction produced in dogs by coronary artery ligations.
The biochemical alterations observed in this model may be relevant
to some forms of myocardial infarction in man. Gradual development
of coronary artery stenosis in man may, however, be accompanied by

adaptive changes in heart muscle and microvessels, which might significantly alter the response of the myocardium to acute ischemia compared to the response of a normal heart in absence of coronary artery disease.

Energy liberation or substrate oxidation

When insufficient supply of O_2 impairs energy metabolism or when energy production is inadequate for other reasons there is stimulation of anaerobic glycolytic metabolism, an emergency system for ATP production in heart muscle. One of the best known consequences of ischemia is early anaerobic glycolysis, i.e. conversion of glucose to lactate and release of lactate by the myocardium, Fig. 1.

Since myocardial release of lactate or diminished myocardial uptake of lactate is often used as an aid in diagnosis of coronary artery disease it is important to keep in mind that glycolysis and lactate formation are not only due to ischemia but may also be the result of an energy deficit due to other causes[4].

The energy liberated by oxidation of substrates to CO_2 is carried by NADH to the respiratory chain. During the transfer of this energy along the respiratory chain by coenzymes and cytochromes part of the energy is stepwise conserved in the formation of high energy phosphate bonds and the electrons are finally transferred to O_2, which is reduced to H_2O.

Energy concervation or oxidative phosphorylation

The energy derived from the substrates is transferred from electron donors of higher redox potential or electron pressure to electron acceptors of lower redox potential, Fig. 2. The decrease in redox potential is directly related to the change in free energy which can be used to phosphorylate ADP to ATP. Every molecule of NADH oxidized requires one atom of oxygen and we may gain up to three molecules of ATP. We would thus have a P/O ratio of 3.

In the ischemic myocardium the oxygen becomes limiting, the NADH can not be oxidized and consequently the ATP formation is sharply reduced. Ischemia can also inhibit ATP production indirectly because of an accumulation of FFA or acyl-CoA, which may impair ATP formation[5,6].

Energy transfer or ATP-ADP translocation across the mitochondrial membrane may be a physiological control step in myocardial energy metabolism, Fig. 3. This transport of ATP is stimulated by Ca^{2+} and K^+ and inhibited by fatty acyl-CoA derivatives, e.g. oleoyl-CoA[6,7].

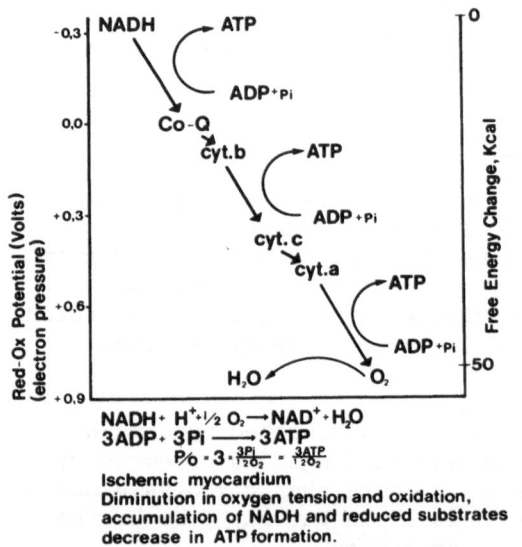

NADH+ H$^+$+1/2 O$_2$ → NAD$^+$·H$_2$O
3ADP+ 3Pi → 3ATP
P/o · 3 · $\frac{3Pi}{1/2O_2}$ - $\frac{3ATP}{1/2O_2}$
Ischemic myocardium
Diminution in oxygen tension and oxidation,
accumulation of NADH and reduced substrates
decrease in ATP formation.

Fig. 1. Energy liberation or
         substrate oxidation in
         normal and ischemic
         heart muscle.

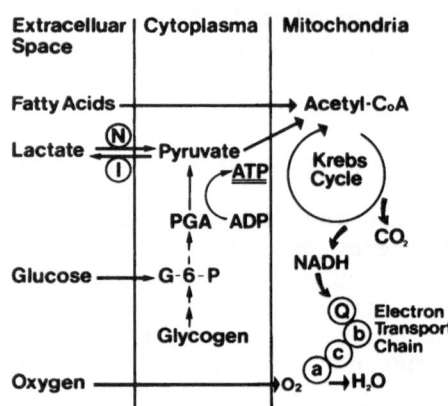

Normal substrates: FA, glucose, lactate

Ischemic myocardium: Early increase in anaerobic
glycolysis, increased uptake of glucose and conversion
to lactate. Glycolysis results in increased formation
of lactate and [H$^+$] and release of these products
from the myocardium.

Fig. 2. Energy conservation or
         oxidative phosphorylation
         in mitochondria of normal
         and ischemic myocardium.

Following coronary occlusion there is an early inhibition of
ATP-utilization in the presence of unimpaired utilization of
creatine phosphate (CP) stores. This corresponds to an inhibition
of ATP transport from mitochondria, but unimpaired utilization of
extramitochondrial ATP and energy reserves in form of CP[8,9]. Fig.
4 shows the correlation between CP and ATP in ischemic and non-
ischemic muscle of the heart following coronary artery occlusion.
When the CP levels are reduced below 7 μmole/g in non-ischemic
muscle then ATP levels are also reduced[8]. The survival limits and
lowest levels able to maintain muscle contraction in non-ischemic
muscle is 1.5 - 2.0 μmole ATP and 3 μmole CP per gram tissue[8,10].

In the ischemic myocardium there is early inhibition of ATP-
utilization in the presence of unimpaired utilization of CP stores.
The ischemic muscle stops contracting at an ATP level of 4.5 μmole/
g, when only about 20% of the ATP has been utilized[8,9].

Energy utilization in heart muscle is primarily for contractile
activity. Cardiac contraction is normally triggered by cellular
depolarization, influx of Ca^{2+} and liberation of intracellular
Ca^{2+}. The Ca^{2+}-ions bind to troponin resulting in a conformational
change in the troponin-tropomyosin-actin complex making a cross-
bridge formation with myosin possible with subsequent hydrolysis
of ATP, sliding of filaments and muscle shortening.

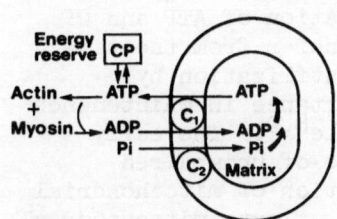

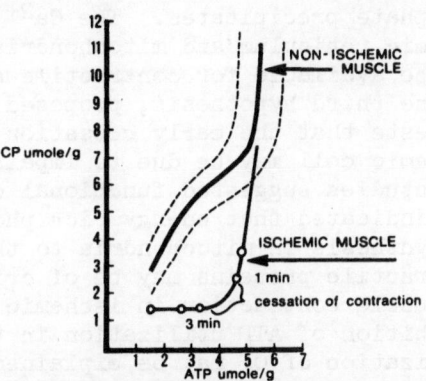

When the creatine phosphate (CP) is reduced below 7 umole/g the ATP content is also reduced. The survival limits and lowest levels able to maintain muscle contraction in non-ischemic muscle are 1.5 umole/g ATP and 3 umole/g CP.

ISCHEMIC MYOCARDIUM

Early inhibition of ATP utilization in the presence of unimpaired utilization of CP stores. Muscle contraction stops at an ATP level of 4.5 umole/g.

Fig. 3. Energy transfer or
ADP-ATP transloca-
tion in normal and
ischemic myocardium.

Fig. 4. The correlation between
tissue content of CP and
ATP in normal and
ischemic heart muscle.

Relaxation represents the removal of Ca^{2+} and subsequent inhibition of the actin-myosin interaction.

Why does contractile activity stop at relatively high ATP levels in the ischemic muscle when the non-ischemic muscle can maintain contractile activity at much lower ATP levels? At least three hypothesis have been offered to explain the early cessation of contractile activity in ischemic cardiac muscle. Two of these hypothesis suggest that early diminution and cessation of contractile activity in the ischemic myocardium may be due to an interference with the function of Ca^{2+} in the contractile process.
a) The increase in intracellular H^+ concentration accompanying anaerobic glycolysis depresses the responsiveness of contractile proteins to Ca^{2+}. Katz and Hecht[11] have suggested that H^+ and Ca^{2+} compete for troponin binding sites. The increase in H^+ concentration causes a displacement of the Ca^{2+} bound to troponin reducing the number of troponin molecules bound to Ca^{2+} during systole. The result would be fewer points of release of the inhibition of the actin-myosin interaction, i.e. diminution in Ca^{2+} induced reversal of the tropomyosin-troponin inhibition of the myosin-actin interaction and reduced contractility.
b) A second hypothesis, by Kübler and Katz[12], proposes that the early loss of contractile function in the ischemic myocardium may be due to removal of free intracellular Ca^{2+} because of a large rise in cellular phosphate and formation of insoluble calcium-

phosphate precipitates. The Ca^{2+} would be trapped in the sarcoplasmic reticulum and mitochondria of the ischemic myocardium and
not be available for contractile activity.
c) The third hypothesis, proposed by Gudbjarnason et al.[8,9],
suggests that the early cessation of contractile activity in the
ischemic cell may be due to impaired intracellular energy transfer.
The studies suggested functional compartmentation of ATP and CP
and indicated that energy rich phosphate transfer from the site
of synthesis in mitochondria to the site of utilization by
contractile proteins may be of critical importance in maintenance
of muscle contraction in ischemic heart muscle[8,9]. The early
inhibition of ATP utilization in the presence of unimpaired
utilization of CP may be explained by inhibition of mitochondrial
adenine nucleotide translocase and depletion of extramitochondrial
energy stores. Primary impairment in contractile activity by
inhibition of Ca^{2+}- troponin interaction would not be expected to
lead to such selective utilization of CP and leave 80% of cellular
ATP intact.

Subsequently Bricknell and Opie[13] proposed that a subcompart-
ment of ATP, produced by glycolysis, might be of particular
importance for maintenance of membrane integrity and the production
of the normal action potential. Inhibition of mitochondrial ATP-
ADP translocase by long chain acyl-CoA accumulating in the ischemic
muscle has been reported by Shug et al.[14] and extensive studies on
intracellular energy transfer in heart muscle have been carried
out in recent years by Saks et al.[15]

The early events following acute coronary artery occlusion
can be summarized as follows:
    1. Diminution in myocardial oxygen tension,
       50% decrease in 15 sec.
    2. Activation of anaerobic glycolysis,
       15 sec. after coronary occlusion.
    3. Inhibition of ATP utilization, 15-30 sec.
    4. Impaired contractile activity, 15-30 sec.
    5. Depletion of creatine phosphate, 30-60 sec.
    6. Diminution in rate of anaerobic glycolysis, 30-60 sec.
    7. Cessation of contractile activity, 60-90 sec.
Following diminution in myocardial oxygen tension the mitochondrial
energy production is impaired. The emergency system, i.e. anaerobic
glycolytic energy production is turned on and the rate of glycolysis
increases rapidly during the first 30 sec. and is subsequently
reduced again[8,16]. During the rise in anaerobic glycolysis ATP
utilization is markedly reduced, but at the same time there is an
early depletion of CP and inhibition of muscle contraction.

The cellular response to acute ischemia is thus to turn off
the most energy consuming process or muscle contraction, preserving
70-80% of cellular ATP. The early and marked increase in glycolysis

may serve as a signal to turn off contractile activity, to preserve mitochondrial ATP and glycolysis provides additional extramito-chondrial ATP for maintenance of membrane structure and essential cellular functions for survival.

The early increase in lactate production and H^+ concentration may initially serve to protect the ischemic cell from excessive entry of Ca^{2+} since mild acidosis may protect the hypoxic cell because H^+ and Ca^{2+} can compete for sarcolemmal or superficial binding sites[17,18]. Severe acidosis is, however, harmful to the cell, leading to damage and cell death.

Various cellular functions preserving cell structures gradually deplete the energy or ATP reserves during the period of reversible ischemia. Among such energy requiring processes are ion transfer and reacylation of membrane lipids which may be deacylated during the period of ischemia. If coronary flow is not restored within 20-30 minutes the cells become depleted of ATP below the level required for survival. The degree of ATP depletion can thus be viewed as an index of the severity of ischemic damage.

The rapidity of cellular damage appears to depend on the functional state of the ischemic muscle. Non-functioning ischemic muscle survives longer than, for example, electrically stimulated muscle.

III. Metabolism of infarcted heart muscle during healing and tissue repair

When the ischemic myocardium enters the state of irreversible damage and death of muscle cells the heart develops myocardial necrosis with subsequent tissue repair and replacement of necrotic muscle by connective tissue.

The metabolic activity of necrotic, infarcted muscle observed 1 to 10 days following coronary artery occlusion represents primarily the activity of invading leucocytes, fibroblasts and other cells involved in removal of dead cells and formation of new connective tissue. Two opposite processes take place in the infarcted tissue, the degradation and removal of dead muscle cells and the proliferation of fibroblasts and formation of collagen and scar tissue. The biosynthetic processes and cellular proliferation in the infarcted area require energy that cannot be provided by aerobic metabolism, but must be provided by more primitive metabolism.

Catabolic and anabolic activity

The alteration in activity of lysosomal enzymes in the necrotic muscle is a reflection of the rate of catabolic processes, i.e.

removal of necrotic muscle. During the early stage of myocardial
necrosis, the autolytic phase of cell destruction takes place by
release of hydrolytic enzymes from endogenous lysosomes originating
in heart muscle cells and local connective tissue cells. This
period is characterized by an early increase in free and a decrease
in particle-bound enzyme activity[19]. The second stage of tissue
degradation, the hydrolytic phase, is characterized by an influx
of phagocytic cells and a continuous increase in the activity of
free lysosomal enzymes which reach a maximum 2 to 8 days after
infarction (in the dog). During the period of highest activities
of soluble hydrolytic enzymes the major task of tissue degradation
and removal of debris takes place[19]. The diminution in activity of
free lysosomal enzymes 6-10 days after infarction is paralleled by
an increase in activity of particle bound enzymes and diminution in
catabolic activity.

Changes in DNA metabolism of infarcted tissue reflect these
opposite catabolic and anabolic processes, Fig. 5. The rate of
DNA synthesis in proliferating fibroblasts increases 2 days after
infarction, i.e. the incorporation of ^{14}C-glycine into purine
rings of DNA, and at the same time the tissue content of DNA
increases, coinciding with an increase in number of fibroblasts[20].
The degradation of dead muscle cells begins immediately after death
of these cells. The particle bound or lysosomal DNase is released
and the amount of free and soluble DNase increases in the necrotic
muscle. The activity of DNase reaches a maximum 4 days after
infarction and at this time DNA content has diminished somewhat
despite continuous synthesis of new DNA, Fig. 5. This means that
the degradation of DNA from dead muscle cells proceeds faster than
synthesis of fibroblastic DNA. Subsequently the catabolic activity
diminishes and the DNA content increases further. The catabolic
activity continues at a slower rate and six weeks after coronary
occlusion the DNA content has returned to normal levels[20].

The synthesis of collagen and changes in the proline content
of infarcted muscle provide similar information. The collagen
formation in the infarcted tissue is reflected in the increase in
hydroxyproline in the necrotic muscle[21]. A rapid rise in
hydroxyproline content in the infarcted area during the first 10
days after infarction represents the fibroblastic proliferation
during this period and rapid synthesis of collagen. A subsequent
period of slower increase in hydroxyproline content reflects not
only collagen formation but also the increase in density of the
developing scar tissue[21].

The discontinuous increase in proline content of infarcted
muscle probably reflects the balance between degradation of
necrotic muscle and synthesis of new scar tissue, Fig. 6. The
proline content failed to increase significantly from the fourth
to the eigth day after infarction. This period represents the

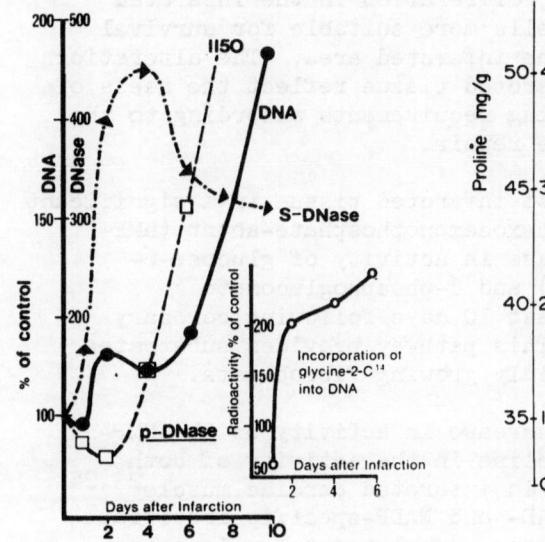

Fig. 5. Changes in DNA content, activity of particle bound DNase (p-DNase), free- or soluble-DNase (s-DNase) and incorporation of glycine-2-C^{14} into purine rings of DNA (DNA synthesis) in infarcted heart muscle.

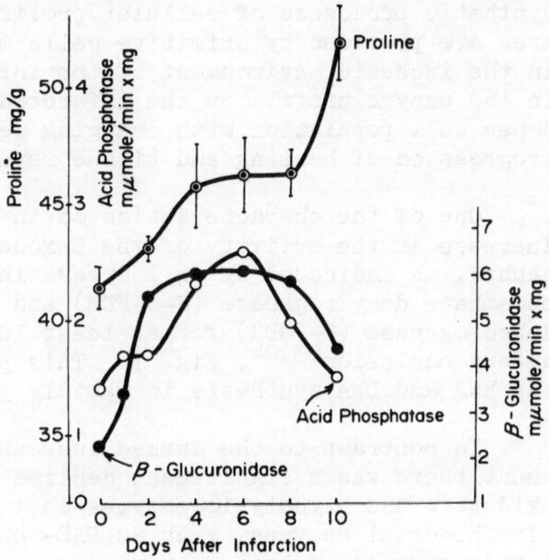

Fig. 6. Changes in proline content, β-glucuronidase, and acid phosphatase activity in infarcted heart muscle.

time of maximum lysosomal activity, as illustrated in the change in β-glucuronidase and acid phosphatase, Fig. 6. When the activities of these hydrolytic enzymes decrease the proline content of the tissue protein increases reflecting a greater rate of scar tissue formation compared to tissue degradation[19,21].

The lysosomal enzymes released into the necrotic tissue are transported by lymph and blood vessels into the circulatory system. Significant changes in the serum activity of lysosomal enzymes such as γ-glutamyl transpeptidase have been observed in patients with myocardial infarction[22]. In contrast to enzymes, such as CPK, LDH and GOT, which indicate acute cellular damage and necrosis, changes in serum γ-glutamyl transpeptidase activity may yield information on reparative processes and cellular replacement in the necrotic myocardium[22].

Energy and substrate metabolism

The energy and substrates required for the anabolic, bio-

synthetic processes of cellular proliferation in the infarcted
area are provided by primitive cells more suitable for survival
in the ischemic environment of the infarcted area. The alterations
in the enzyme profile in the infarcted tissue reflect the needs of
a new cell population with changing requirements according to the
progression of healing and tissue repair.

One of the characteristics of infarcted tissue is a significant
increase in the activity of the hexosemonophosphate-shunt (HMP-
shunt), as indicated by an increase in activity of glucose-6-
phosphate dehydrogenase (G-6-PDH) and 6-phosphogluconate
dehydrogenase (6-PGDH) for at least 10 days following coronary
artery occlusion[23,24], Fig. 7. This pathway provides substrates
for RNA and DNA synthesis in rapidly growing fibroblasts.

In contrast to the marked increase in activity of the HMP-
shunt there was a significant decline in the activity of both
oxidative and glycolytic enzymes in infarcted cardiac muscle[23,25].
Mitochondrial enzymes, such as NAD- and NADP-specific isocitrate
dehydrogenases, malate dehydrogenase and glutamate oxaloacetate
transaminase reached the lowest level in the centre of the
infarcted tissue ten days after infarction with 8 to 13% of normal
activity, Fig. 7.

The activity of glycolytic enzymes was also significantly
reduced. Aldolase and lactate dehydrogenase (LDH) activity
decreased to 14 and 21% of original activity respectively, whereas
the activity of glyceraldehyde phosphate dehydrogenase (GAPDH)
was reduced to 32% of control ten days after infarction[23,25], Fig.
7. The relatively high activity of GAPDH remaining in infarcted
tissue indicates that the glycolytic phosphorylation of ADP to
ATP can continue in the infarcted area during healing and scar
formation. The quantitative decrease in LDH activity of infarcted
muscle was also accompanied by qualitative changes in the isoenzyme
pattern. The ischemic environment of the infarcted tissue, with
its low oxygen tension, favours synthesis of M-LDH[26], the form
best suited for anaerobic metabolism and this increase in synthesis
of M-LDH is illustrated in the increase in isoenzyme IV (HM_3) and
isoenzyme V (M_4) in the infarcted heart muscle[23,26,27].

IV. Reversible biochemical and functional changes in non-infarcted
     heart muscle following myocardial infarction

It is normally assumed that metabolism and function of the
non-infarcted myocardium remote from the infarcted area will remain
unimpaired. Biochemical and functional abnormalities in the non-
infarcted remote myocardium would be of great importance because
the ability of the heart to compensate for the loss of muscle and
to survive is largely determined by the metabolic and functional
integrity of the non-infarcted muscle.

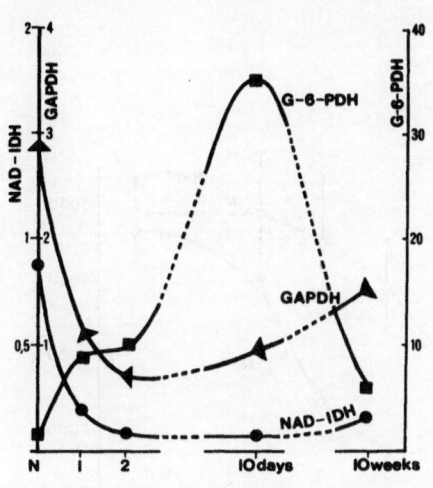

Fig. 7. Changes in specific
activities (µmoles sub-
strate per min mg protein)
of NAD-specific isocitrate
dehydrogenase (NAD-IDH),
glyceraldehydephosphate
dehydrogenase (GAPDH) and
glucose-6-phosphate
dehydrogenase (G-6-PDH)
in infarcted heart muscle
during the postinfarction
period.

During the post-infarction period significant biochemical and
functional alterations were observed in the non-infarcted myocardium:
   a) Diminution in ATP and CP levels of functioning muscle.
   b) Impairment in left ventricular function, stroke work (SW) and
      left ventricular pressure rise (dp/dt).
   c) Reduction in myocardial norepinephrine levels.
   d) Increase in protein synthesis, i.e. development of
      compensatory hypertrophy.

Fig. 8 illustrates a correlation between the diminution in
ATP content of non-infarcted muscle and the impairment in left
ventricular function, i.e. decrease in SW, following myocardial
function. One day after myocardial infarction stroke work (SW)
was significantly diminished, accompanied by a marked reduction in
ATP levels of the muscle[28]. Protein synthesis, reflecting compensatory increase in functioning muscle mass, increased immediately
after infarction and death of muscle cells in the infarcted area,
Fig. 8. Improvement in cardiac function and an increase in high
energy phosphate levels were observed during development of
compensatory hypertrophy. The restoration of normal function and
normal myocardial energy levels depends upon the development of
compensatory processes[28].

The reasons for the diminution in ATP and CP stores in non-
infarcted myocardium during the post-infarction period are not
clear, they may be related to the increase in workload and increased
energy utilization per unit of surviving muscle mass, which may not
be proportional to the rate of synthesis. Corday et al[29] observed
following early experimental coronary occlusion that the nonoccluded
zone responds with hypercontraction in about 50% of cases, whereas

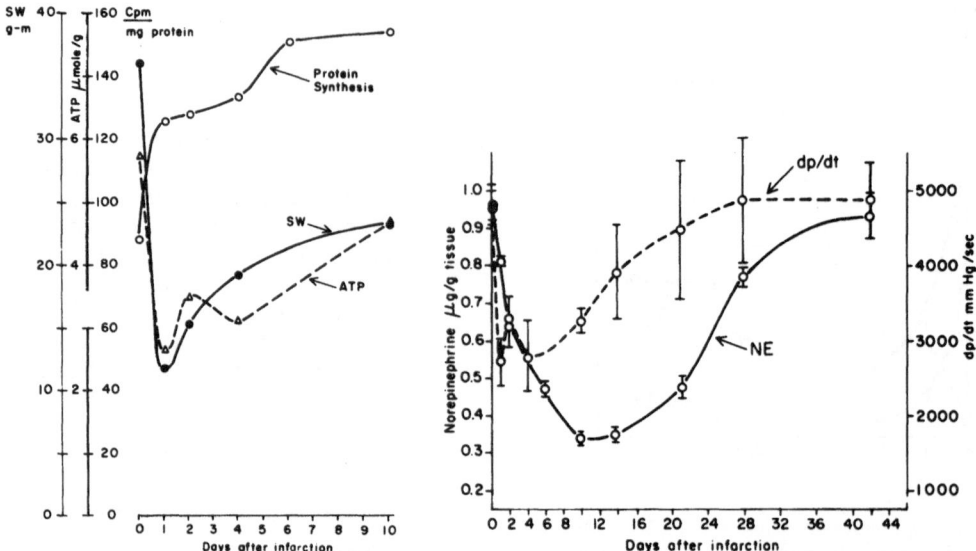

Fig. 8. Changes in stroke work (SW), ATP levels and protein synthesis or glycine-2-C[14] incorporation into protein in non-infarcted heart muscle following myocardial infarction.

Fig. 9. Changes in left ventricular function (dp/dt) and tissue content of norepinephrine (NE) in non-infarcted left ventricular muscle following myocardial infarction.

there was hypocontraction or normal contraction in the remaining instances. Other studies have confirmed the presence of metabolic and functional abnormalities in the non-infarcted area of the infarcted heart[30,31].

The impairment in left ventricular function was followed by a significant reduction in norepinephrine (NE) content of the non-infarcted muscle[32,33]. The infarcted tissue lost its NE-content entirely after 48 hours, and a rapid decline in the NE-content of the functioning myocardium was observed, Fig. 9. The endogenous level of NE fell from a control value of 0.99μg to 0.35μg NE/g in the non-infarcted portion of the left ventricle 10 days after infarction. The NE-levels rose gradually after the 2nd week and reached control values again 6 weeks after infarction. The decreases in NE-stores did not correlate with changes in energy-rich phosphates or with changes in myocardial function. The changes in NE-stores could not be related to ischemia, edema or fibrosis of non-infarcted muscle, and the uptake, accumulation or subcellular distribution of norepinephrine -7-^{14}C in non-infarcted muscle was not affected by the coronary artery occlusion[32,33].

An increase in NE-release due to the increased activity of the sympathetic nervous system following myocardial infarction appears to be the major factor responsible for the temporary reduction in myocardial NE-stores[34]. Following completion of compensatory processes and restoration of myocardial function, the activity of the sympathetic nervous system returns to normal and subsequently the NE-levels are restored.

Recently Baumann has observed a specific impairment of sarcolemmal β-receptor function in non-ischemic myocardium induced by increased levels of circulating catecholamines. Treatment with β-blocking agents during the post-infarction period can prevent the loss of β-receptors and reduced affinity of remaining receptors in the non-ischemic muscle[35].

V. Attempts to influence infarct size, healing and compensatory processes.

Attempts to influence healing and infarct size following myocardial infarction have been made during the past 15 years. The earliest studies attempting to stimulate healing and reduce the size of the developing scar employed anabolic agents such as growth hormone, anabolic steroids, insulin and other agents expected to stimulate healing and repair[36].

In a recent review Opie[37] describes the following interventions most frequently studied in an attempt to limit infarct size: a) Catecholamine antagonists, i.e. beta-blocking agents; b) increased collateral flow or diffusion to ischemic zone with nitrates or hyaluronidase; c) metabolic measures, i.e. glucose-insulin-potassium treatment, increased provision of oxygen, or stabilization of membranes (steroids); d) relief of load on the heart with nitrates or nitroprussid; e) relief of vascular obstruction with antithrombotic agents, antiplatelet agents, or by relief of spasm with Ca^{2+}-antagonists.

These interventions have been most thoroughly studied by Braunwald, Maroko et al[38,39]. This discussion will be limited to two largely ignored aspects of metabolic support for the infarcted heart muscle: a) the role of diet and dietary protein intake during the post-infarction period, and b) the reduction of scar size and stimulation of healing and compensatory hypertrophy in the infarcted heart by treatment with anabolic steroids and other anabolic agents.

The role of diet in healing of an infarct.

When dogs were fed a protein-free diet for one week before coronary artery ligations and then further during the post-infarction period the animals frequently developed left ventricular

aneurysm with thin scars, delayed healing, impaired development of
compensatory hypertrophy in non-infarcted muscle and a significant.
increase in mortality rate[21,36,40]. Animals fed the protein-free
diet had significantly lower ATP levels in infarcted and non-
infarcted muscle 10 days after myocardial infarction[21]. These
observations suggest that it might be worth while to examine
further the role of diet in repair and recovery of the infarcted
heart.

Anabolic agents and stimulation of recovery

Treatment with various agents such as growth hormone, insulin,
anabolic steroids (methandrostenolone or norbolethone) or ascorbic
acid stimulated protein synthesis in infarcted muscle and tissue
repair[21,36,40]. Treatment with anabolic steroids (norboloethone,
2 mg/kg per day for 10 days) stimulated compensatory processes in
non-infarcted muscle, increased formation of new muscle mass and
significantly increased ATP and CP levels of non-infarcted muscle
10 days after myocardial infarction. The ATP level increased from
4.65 μmole/g in untreated animals to 5.9 μmole/g in animals treated
with the anabolic steroid[21], Fig. 1o.

Treatment with anabolic steroids increases the rate of protein
synthesis, but appears to reduce scar formation in the necrotic
area. Table 1 illustrates attempts to determine the effect of the
anabolic steroid upon the size of the scar 3 weeks after myocardial
infarction. The first column shows the relative weight of the
damaged tissue or developing scar tissue, i.e. per cent of the
left ventricle that is infarcted, in control and treated animals.
The second column shows the collagen content, as estimated from
hydroxyproline determinations, in cross-sections of the previously
ischemic area[21]. The treatment appeared to reduce scar size or
collagen content by about 25%. These data suggest further
experiments with anabolic agents since these agents might also

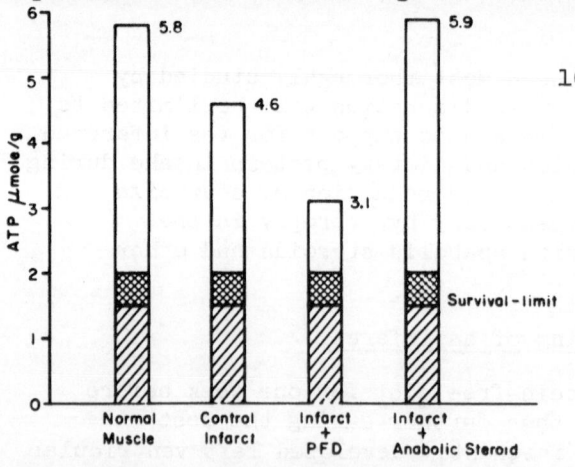

10. Effect of an anabolic
     steroid (norbolethone,
     2 mg/kg BW per day) or
     protein free diet (PFD)
     on ATP levels of non-
     infarcted heart muscle
     10 days after coronary
     occlusion.

Table I. Effect of Anabolic Steroids upon Infarct Size and Scar Formation 3 Weeks After Myocardial Infarction

	Size of Infarcted Area (Scar) % of left Ventricle	Collagen Content of Infarcted area mg/g
Control Untreated Animals N = 8	20,6% ± 1,2	160,7 ± 8,7
Steroid-Treated Animals N = 8	15,6% ± 0,6	119,2 ± 5,9
Decrease in Infarct Size or Collagen Content	24,3%	25,8%

stimulate compensatory processes and recovery of the infarcted heart.

Catabolic steroids have been used experimentally and clinically in treatment of myocardial infarction. The catabolic steroids reduced infarct size, but impaired healing and were frequently associated with development of thin scars and left ventricular aneurysm[39,41]. There should therefore be a clear distinction between the use of catabolic and anabolic steroids in treatment of myocardial infarction.

Summary

The purpose of this review is to draw attention to the following questions:
1. What is the mechanism responsible for cessation of contractile activity in ischemic heart muscle before cellular energy stores are depleted?
2. How can we stimulate healing and tissue repair in the infarcted heart muscle?
3. How can we stimulate compensatory processes in non-infarcted remote muscle and enhance functional recovery of the infarcted heart?

References

1. R. J. Bing, A. Siegal, A. Vitale, F. A. Balboni, E. Sparks
    M. Klapper and S. Edwards, Metabolic studies on the human
    heart in vivo, Am. J. Med., 15:284-296 (1953).
2. L. H. Opie, Role of carnitine in fatty acid metabolism of
    normal and ischemic myocardium, Am. Heart, J., 97:375-388
    (1979)
3. S. Gudbjarnason, G. Oskarsdottir, B. Doell and J. Hallgrimsson,
    Myocardial membrane lipids in relation to cardiovascular
    disease, Adv. in Cardiol, 25:130-144 (1978).
4. S. Gudbjarnason, The use of glycolytic metabolism in the
    assessment of hypoxia in human hearts, Cardiol., 57:35-46
    (1972).
5. A. Lochner, J. C. N. Kotzé, L. Benade and W. Gevers,
    Mitochondrial oxidative phosphorylation in low-flow
    hypoxia, role of free fatty acids, J. Molec. Cell. Cardiol,
    10:857-875 (1978).
6. S. V. Pande and M. C. Blancher, Reversible inhibition of
    mitochondrial adenosine diphosphate phosphorylation by
    long chain acyl Coenzyme A esters, J. Biol. Chem.
    246:402-411 (1971).
7. R. A. Harris, B. Farmer and T. Ozawa, Inhibition of the
    mitochondrial adenine nucleotide transport system by oleoyl
    CoA, Archiv. Biochem. Biophys., 150:199-209 (1972).
8. S. Gudbjarnason, P. Mathes and K. G. Ravens, Functional
    compartmentation of ATP and creatine phosphate in heart
    muscle, J. Molec. Cell. Cardiol, 1:325-339 (1970).
9. S. Gudbjarnason, Inhibition of energy transfer in ischemic
    heart muscle, in: Recent advances in studies on cardiac
    structure and metabolism, E. Bajusz and G. Rona, ed.,
    University Park Press, Baltimore, 1:17-26 (1972).
10. W. Kübler and P. G. Spieckermann, Regulation of glycolysis in
    the ischemic and anoxic myocardium, J. Molec. Cell. Cardiol.,
    1:351-377 (1970).
11. A. M. Katz and H. H. Hecht, The early "pump" failure of the
    ischemic heart, Am. J. Med., 47:497-502 (1969).
12. W. Kübler and A. M. Katz, Mechanism of early "pump" failure
    of the ischemic heart: Possible role of adenosine
    triphosphate depletion and inorganic phosphate accumulation,
    Am. J. Cardiol., 40:467-471 (1977).
13. O. I. Bricknell and L. H. Opie, Glycolytic ATP and its
    production during ischemia in isolated Langendorff-perfused
    rat hearts, in: Recent advances in studies on cardiac
    structure and metabolism, T. Kobayashi, T. Sano and N. S.
    Dhalla ed., University Park Press, Baltimore, 11:505-519
    (1978).
14. A. L. Shug, E. Shrago, N. Bittar, J. D. Folts and J. R. Kokes,
    Long chain fatty acyl CoA inhibition of adenine nucleotide
    translocase in the ischemic myocardium, Am. J. Physiol.,

228:689-692 (1975).

15. V. A. Saks, N. V. Lipina, V. N. Smirnov and E. I. Chazov, Studies of energy transport in heart cells. The functional coupling between mitochondrial creatine phosphokinase and ATP-ADP translocase, kinetic evidence, Archives Biochem. Biophys., 173:34-41 (1976).

16. J. R. Neely, M. J. Rovetto, J. T. Whitmer and H. E. Morgan, Effects of ischemia on function and metabolism of the isolated working rat heart, Am. J. Physiol., 225:651-658 (1973).

17. P. A. Poole-Wilson, Is early decline in cardiac function in ischemia due to carbon dioxide retention, Lancet, 2:1285-1287 (1975).

18. J. R. Williamson, M. L. Woodrow and A. Scarpa, Calcium binding to cardiac sarcolemma, in: Recent advances in studies on cardiac sturcture and metabolism, A. Fleckenstein, and N. S. Dhalla, ed., University Park Press, Baltimore 61-71 (1975).

19. K. G. Ravens and S. Gudbjarnason, Changes in the activities of lysosomal enzymes in infarcted canine heart muscle, Circul. Res., 24:851-856 (1969).

20. S. Gudbjarnason, C. De Schryver, C. Chiba, J. Yamanaka, and R. J. Bing, Protein and nucleic acid synthesis during the reparative processes following myocardial infarction, Circul. Res., 15:320-326 (1964).

21. S. Gudbjarnason, K. G. Ravens and P. Mathes, Metabolic changes in infarcted and non-infarcted myocardium during the postinfarction period, in: Recent advances in studies on cardiac structure and metabolism, E. Bajusz and G. Rona, ed., University Park Press, Baltimore, 1:439-446 (1972).

22. K. G. Ravens, S. Gudbjarnason, C. Cowan and R. J. Bing, Gamma-glutamyl-transpeptidase in myocardial infarction, Circul., 39:693-700 (1969).

23. S. Gudbjarnason, C. Cowan, W. Braasch and R. J. Bing, Changes in enzyme pattern of infarcted heart muscle during tissue repair, Cardiologia, 51.148-159 (1967).

24. S. Gudbjarnason, C. Cowan and R. J. Bing, Increase in hexosemonophosphate shunt activity during tissue repair, Life Sciences, 6:1093-1097 (1967).

25. S. Gudbjarnason, W. Braasch, C. Cowan and R. J. Bing, Metabolism of infarcted heart muscle during tissue repair, Am. J. Cardiol., 22:360-369 (1968).

26. S. Gudbjarnason and D. Priver, LDH-isoenzymes in infarcted heart muscle, Life Sciences, 7:623-627 (1968).

27. D. M. Dawson, T. L. Goodfriend and N. O. Kaplan, Lactic dehydrogenases-functions of the two types, rates of synthesis, Science 143:929-933 (1964).

28. S. Gudbjarnason, P. S. Puri and P. Mathes, Biochemical changes in non-infarcted heart muscle following myocardial infarction, J. Molec. Cellul. Cardiol., 2:253-276 (1971).

29. E. Corday, L. Kaplan, S. Meerbaum, J. Brasch, C. Constantini,
     T. W. Lang, H. Gold, S. Rubins and I. Osher, Consequences
     of coronary arterial occlusion on remote myocardium:
     Effects of occlusion and reperfusion, Am. J. Cardiol.,
     36:385-393 (1975).

30. A. M. Vikhert and N. M. Cherepachenko, Changes in metabolism
     of undamaged sections of myocardium following infarction,
     Circul. Res. 34, Suppl III, 182-191, (1974).

31. H. L. Wyatt, J. S. Forrester, P. L. da Luz, G. A. Diamond,
     R. Chagrasulis and H. J. Swan, Functional abnormalities
     in nonoccluded regions of myocardium after experimental
     coronary occlusion, Am. J. Cardiol. 37:366-372 (1976).

32. P. Mathes and S. Gudbjarnason, Changes in norepinephrine
     stores in the canine heart following experimental
     myocardial infarction, Am. Heart J., 81:211-219 (1971).

33. P. Mathes, C. Cowan and S. Gudbjarnason, Storage and
     metabolism of norepinephrine after experimental myocardial
     infarction, Am. J. Physiol, 220:27-32 (1971).

34. R. F. Klein, W. G. Troyer, H. K. Thompson, M. D. Bogdonoff
     and A. G. Wallace, Catecholamine excretion in myocardial
     infarction, Arch. Int. Med., 122:476-482 (1968).

35. G. Baumann, Abstract 8, in: Catecholamines and the heart,
     recent advances in experimental and clinical research.,
     Munich, (1981).

36. S. Gudbjarnason, J. C. Fenton, P. L. Wolf and R. J. Bing,
     Stimulation of reparative processes following experimental
     myocardial infarction, Archiv. Int. Med., 118:34-40 (1966).

37. a) L. H. Opie, Myocardial infarct size, Part 1, Basic
        consideratons, Am. Heart J., 100:355-372 (1980).
     b) Myocardial infarct size, Part 2, Comparison of antiinfarct
        effects of beta-blockade, glucose-insulin-potassium
        nitrates and hyaluronidase, Am. Heart J., 100:531-550 (1980).

38. P. R. Maroko and E. Braunwald, Effects of metabolic and
     pharmacologic interventions on myocardial infarct size
     following coronary occlusion, Circul. 53 Suppl. I, 162-168
     (1976).

39. P. R. Maroko, R. A. Kloner, T. Yasuda, L. G. T. Ribeiro, D.
     Maclean and E. Braunwald, Recent investigations on attempts
     to limit infarct size, in: Acute and long-term management
     of myocardial ischemia, A. Hjalmarsson and L. Wilhelmsen,
     ed., A. Lindgren and Söner AB, Mölndal, Sweden, 203-220
     (1978).

40. S. Gudbjarnason, W. Braasch and R. J. Bing, Protein synthesis
     in cardiac hypertrophy and heart failure, in: Heart
     failure, Pathophysiological and clinical aspects,
     H. Reindell, J. Keul and E. Doll, ed, George Thieme Verlag,
     Stuttgart, 184-189 (1968).

41. R. Robert, V. de Mello and B. E. Sobel, Deleterious effects of
     methylprednisolone in patients with myocardial infarction,
     Circul. Res. Suppl. I, 1-204 (1976).

THE APOLIPOPROTEINS - TAXONOMY AND FUNCTIONS

Peter N. Herbert and Linda L. Bausserman

Brown University Program-in-Medicine, Division of
Nutrition and Metabolism, The Miriam Hospital
164 Summit Avenue, Providence, Rhode Island U.S.A. 02906

Our selection of the material included in this chapter was
based largely on the specific requests of the students attending the
NATO Advanced Study Institute on Arterial Pollution. A brief overview of lipoprotein physiology introduces sections summarizing
current knowledge of the chemistry, functions, and distributions of
the apolipoproteins.

THE LIPOPROTEINS

Lipoproteins are often inappropriately referred to as "molecules", whereas they in fact are particles comprised of many molecules that are not covalently bound. All lipoproteins have their
origins in the liver and/or intestine, but after release into the
circulation may acquire lipids from other tissues. Their structure
appears to be pseudomicellar[1]. The neutral lipids, cholesteryl
esters and triglycerides, constitute the core oil droplet which is
surrounded by a monolayer of phospholipids, unesterified cholesterol, and apolipoproteins. Thus, lipoproteins accomplish the
solubilization (or suspension) and transport of neutral lipids and
other hydrophobic biochemicals.

Chylomicrons

This term is appropriately applied to both large and small
triglyceride-rich lipoproteins (Fig. 1) elaborated by the intestinal mucosa. Fatty acids and monoglycerides derived from dietary
fat are resynthesized to triglycerides and receive a surface
monolayer of unesterified cholesterol, phospholipid, and apolipo-

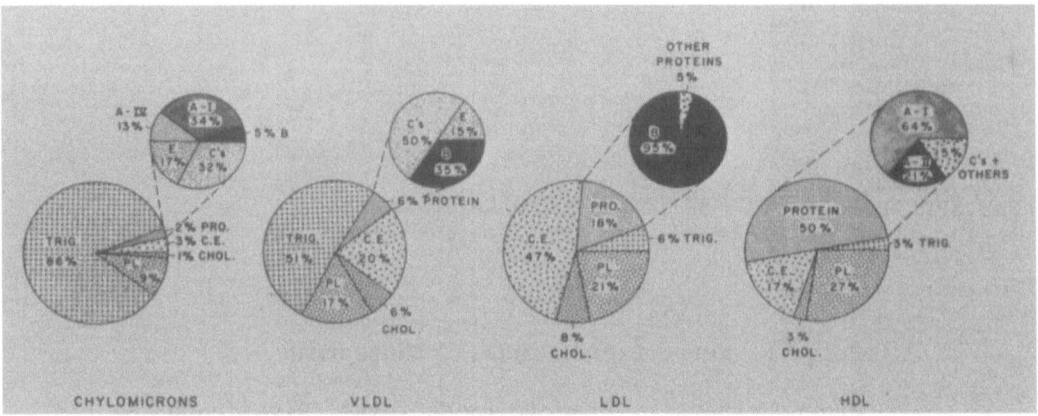

Fig. 1. Lipid and apolipoprotein composition of the major classes
         of plasma lipoproteins. Phospholipid and protein, the
         surface components, constitute 80% of the mass of HDL.
         Lipoprotein core components, triglycerides and cholesteryl
         esters, account for most of the mass of the lower density
         lipoproteins.

protein before secretion as chylomicrons into the mesenteric
lymphatics. Chylomicron formation by the small intestine is
necessary not only for normal absorption of triglyceride but also
for the fat soluble vitamins: A, D, E, and K.

     Protein synthesis is required for chylomicron secretion[2] and
immunochemical methods have demonstrated a striking increase in the
apoB, apoA-I, and apoA-IV content of intestinal epithelium during
active fat absorption[3-7]. The C-apolipoproteins comprise about
30% and 55% of the apoprotein of chylomicrons in mesenteric lymph
and plasma, respectively. However, the intestine appears to synthesize only negligible amounts of the C-apoproteins[8-12] and these
are acquired from other lipoproteins in the mesenteric lymph and
circulation.

     Chylomicron triglyceride is hydrolyzed by lipoprotein lipase
at the capillary endothelium of adipose and muscle tissues. Normally, chylomicrons survive in the circulation for only 5-15
minutes; and in lower species, at least, chylomicron remnants are
rapidly and quantitatively extracted from plasma by the liver[13,14].
As discussed below, much of the chylomicron surface lipids and proteins may be transferred to HDL as hydrolysis of triglyceride
ensues.

Very Low Density Lipoproteins (VLDL)

The availability of excess calories, irrespective of source, and of free fatty acids leads to VLDL secretion by the liver. Triglycerides are the major VLDL lipid (Fig. 1) and apoB and apoE are the principal newly synthesized apolipoproteins in VLDL derived from liver Golgi bodies[15]. As in the case of chylomicrons, plasma HDL transfer C-apoproteins to VLDL after their secretion by hepatocytes and C-apoproteins comprise 50% or more of the protein in VLDL.

VLDL are normally cleared from the circulation within two hours[16]. They are progressively degraded to short-lived intermediate density lipoproteins (IDL) and finally to low density lipoproteins (LDL). Lipoprotein lipase is responsible for most of the triglyceride hydrolysis and hepatic triglyceride hydrolase may be involved in the final conversion of IDL to LDL[17]. As VLDL triglycerides are progressively hydrolyzed, excess surface lipid and C-apoproteins from VLDL appear to be transferred to HDL[18].

Low Density Lipoproteins (LDL)

Seventy percent or more of the plasma cholesterol is contained in the LDL. As noted, these lipoproteins are largely end products of VLDL catabolism although some may be directly secreted by the liver. They are not known to serve any essential function. Cholesteryl esters account for about 50% of the mass of LDL (Fig. 1) and apoB comprises over 90% of the LDL protein.

Studies in the rat have suggested that direct hepatic degradation accounts for only a minor fraction of the LDL cleared from plasma[19]. Most LDL is thought to be catabolized by extrahepatic tissues, approximately a third by a highly specific receptor-mediated process and the remainder by a receptor independent pathway[20]. Most of the chemical components of LDL can be degraded by peripheral tissues, but the cholesterol must eventually either accumulate intracellularly or be transferred back to the extracellular fluid for transport to the liver.

High Density Lipoproteins (HDL)

The intestine and liver both appear to synthesize apoA-I and apoA-II, the major HDL apoproteins. Studies in the rat indicate that newly secreted HDL of hepatic and intestinal origin are disc-shaped particles containing protein, phospholipid, and cholesterol but little cholesteryl ester[21,22]. Newly secreted HDL from rat livers, like the discoidal HDL of familial lecithin: cholesterol acyltransferase (LCAT) deficiency, contain primarily apoE[21] rather than apoA-I. ApoA-I, in contrast, is the major protein in the disk-shaped HDL produced by the intestine[22].

The conversion of discoidal nascent HDL to the spherical micellar particles normally found in plasma is presumably effected by LCAT acting in the plasma compartment. It is hypothesized that LCAT also promotes the incorporation into HDL of lecithin and cholesterol from the surface of chylomicrons and VLDL. The marked reductions in HDL levels that characterize states with defective catabolism of VLDL and chylomicrons probably reflect the importance of this latter pathway in HDL formation.

Studies in which radiolabeled HDL have been perfused through isolated rat liver suggest that direct uptake by this organ is not a major path of HDL catabolism[23]. Other possible mechanisms of HDL clearance are discussed in the chapter dealing with "Determinants of Plasma High Density Lipoprotein Concentrations".

THE APOLIPOPROTEINS

The major apolipoproteins (Table 1) are here discussed in alphabetical-numerical order. We use the ABC nomenclature system suggested by Alaupovic; it should be viewed as noncommittal with respect to evolutionary origins, functions in lipoprotein structure or metabolism, and interrelationships of these proteins.

The definition of an apolipoprotein is a vexing problem. We formerly considered two operational criteria to be adequate. First, an apolipoprotein should associate in plasma with neutral and charged lipid. This would effectively exclude serum albumin, sterol binding proteins, and others. Second, an apolipoprotein should quantitatively distribute with the plasma lipoprotein fraction that has buoyant density less than 1.21 g/ml.

The appropriateness of these criteria is not certain. Ultracentrifugation, for example, may dissociate apolipoproteins from lipoproteins[25,26]. This appears to be true for apoE[27] and apoproteins A-IV and D may be similarly affected (Table 2). The cholesteryl ester exchange protein[28] may one day be elected to the apolipoprotein elite, but it quantitatively distributes with the lipoprotein-free plasma fraction. Finally, the capacity of many putative apolipoproteins to bind both neutral and charged lipid has not been directly demonstrated.

The conformation or physical state of both biochemicals is usually changed when apolipoproteins interact with lipid. As described below, these proteins are not particularly enriched in apolar amino acids; and where primary structures are known they do not have long linear sequences of hydrophobic amino acids. Rather, specific lipid-binding domains are "induced" in the

Table 1. Selected Properties of the Human Apolipoproteins

Apoprotein	Plasma Concentration (mg/dl)	Molecular Weight	Terminal Residues NH2	Terminal Residues COOH	Isoelectric Points[a]	Carbohydrate
A-I	90-130	28,300	asp	gln	5.3-5.7	-
A-I$_{Milano}$	35-74	28,000	?	?	5.0-5.5	?
A-II	30-50	17,000	PCA[b]	gln	4.2	-
A-IV	16	46,000	glu/gln	?	5.15	?
B$_{100}$	80-100	549,000	?	?	?	+
B$_{48}$	<5	264,000	?	?	?	+
C-I	4-7	7,000	thr	ser	6.5	-
C-II	3-8	8,800	thr	glu	4.8-5.0	-
C-III-0,1,2	8-15	8,800	ser	ala	4.5-5.1	+
"D$_2$"	?	7,000	leu	ser	?	-
D	5-6	32,500	?	ser	5.2,5.08,5.00	+
E	3-6	39,000	lys	ala	5.5,5.6,5.75	+
F	3	26,000-32,000	?	?	3.7	?

a) Several of the apoproteins have two or more isoelectric forms and ranges are presented for these.

b) PCA = pyrrolidone carboxylic acid.

Table 2.   Ultracentrifugal Distribution of Apolipoproteins

	Lipoproteins (d<1.21 g/ml)	Lipoprotein-Free Plasma (d>1.21 g/ml)
A-I	90%	10%
A-II	>98%	<2%
A-IV	2%	98%
B	∿100%	∿0%
C's	∿99%	<1%
D	64%	36%
E	75-80%	20-25%

proteins on exposure to lipid. Amphipathic helixes are formed in which polar, water-soluble amino acids are located on one face of the cylinder while the nonpolar water-insoluble residues occupy the opposite face. The polar surface is perceived as interacting with the aqueous environment and perhaps the polar head groups of phospholipids. The apolar surface, in contrast, is suited for interaction with the fatty acyl chains of phospholipids and perhaps the sterol nucleus of cholesterol. Such amphipathic helixes theoretically can be formed by all five of the apolipoproteins whose primary structure is known[29].

Not well elucidated are the lipid specificities which are integral to the functions of the apolipoproteins (Table 3). The composition or organization of surface lipids must somehow account for the distribution of A-apoproteins almost exclusively to HDL and for the preferential association of C-apoproteins with chylomicrons and VLDL. A few apolipoproteins may function primarily in a structural role to stabilize the lipoprotein micelle. Most, however, probably have very specific functions in intracellular assembly, transcellular transport, enzyme activation, and cell-surface receptor binding.

Apolipoprotein A-I (apoA-I)

ApoA-I is the major protein in all primate HDL (Figs. 1 and 2), accounting for about 30% of the lipoprotein mass. It is a single chain protein of 243-245 residues that contains no cystine, cysteine, leucine or carbohydrate (Table 4). Two major and several minor species with different isoelectric points (Table 1) have been observed in normal human plasma[37,38]. Unlike the apoE isoelectric heterogeneity described below, that for apoA-I appears

Table 3. Apolipoprotein Origins and Functions

Apoprotein	Tissue Origin	Function
A-I	Liver and Intestine	Formation and structural integrity of HDL; activator of LCAT
A-II	Liver and Intestine	Unknown; ?activation of hepatic triglyceride hydrolase
A-IV	Intestine; ?Liver	Unknown
B-100	Liver	VLDL formation and transcellular transport; receptor mediated uptake of LDL
B-48	Intestine and Liver	Chylomicron (and VLDL) formation and transcellular transport; ?receptor mediated lipoprotein clearance
C-I	Liver; ?Intestine	Activator of LCAT; probably other functions
C-II	Liver; ?Intestine	Activator of lipoprotein lipase
C-III	Liver; ?Intestine	Unknown; ?essential to stability and modulates hydrolysis of chylomicrons and VLDL
D	Unknown	Unknown; possible LCAT cofactor
E	Liver	Receptor mediated uptake of chylomicron and VLDL remnants by apoB/E and apoE receptors

quantitatively similar among individuals[38].

Two laboratories have reported primary structure analyses of apoA-I. There are 25 differences in the reported sequences (Figs. 3 and 4). Eight of the discrepancies involve amide/dicarboxylic amino acid assignments (positions 49, 60, 61, 67, 71, 72, 149, and 150 in Fig. 3). Six represent simple reversals of three pairs of adjacent residues (69-70; 84-85; and 189-190 in Fig. 3); and the tryptophan placed at residue 48 in Fig. 3 is at 50 in Fig. 4. A 5 amino acid tryptic peptide (residues 77-81 in

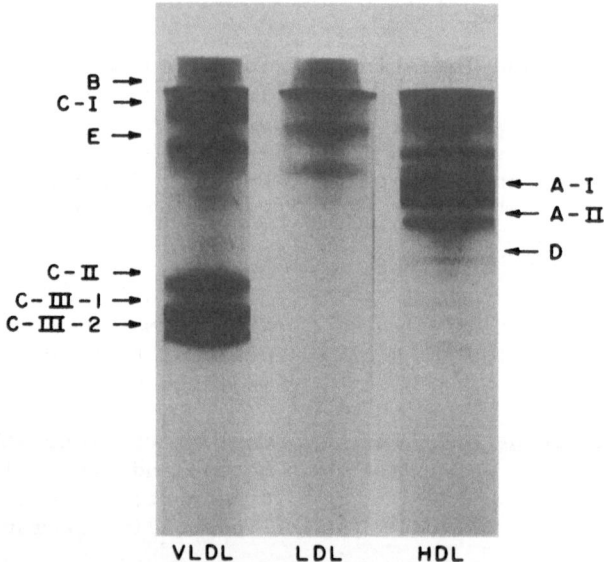

Fig. 2.   The major apoproteins of human plasma VLDL, LDL, and HDL
          demonstrated by polyacrylamide gel electrophoresis in a
          urea-containing alkaline system.

Fig. 3) is absent in the more recently described sequence (Fig. 4).
The dipeptide (aspartic acid-serine) at positions 51-52 in Fig. 4
is absent from Fig. 3; and Fig. 4 describes "insertions" of a
glutamic acid between positions 114 and 115 (Fig. 3) and lysine
between 241 and 242 (Fig. 3) in otherwise identical segments.
Finally, the glutamine at residue 74 in Fig. 3 is absent from the
sequence in Fig. 4.

     A variant form of apoA-I containing cysteine (Table 4),
apoA-I$_{Milano}$, was recently discovered[32]. By virtue of the presence
of cysteine, apoA-I$_{Milano}$ is capable of forming intermolecular
disulfide bonds. The HDL from carriers of this mutation were
found to contain proteins with relative molecular weights of
55,000, 35,000 and 28,000. The 55,000 and 28,000 molecular weight
species are dimers and monomers, respectively, of apoA-I$_{Milano}$.
The protein of $M_r \sim 35,000$ contained two different subunits,
A-I$_{Milano}$ and apoA-II in a mixed disulfide. Unpublished studies
cited elsewhere[37] demonstrate the presence of normal apoA-I in

Table 4.　Amino Acid Compositions of the A Apolipoproteins

	A-I[a]		A-I Milano	A-II	A-IV		
Literature Reference	30	31	32	33	34	35	36
	(moles/100 moles amino acid)						
aspartic acid/asparagine	8.3 (21)[b]	8.6 (21)	9.1	3.9 (3)	10.0	9.7	9.3
threonine	4.0 (10)	4.0 (10)	4.3	7.8 (6)	3.6	4.6	5.8
serine	5.8 (14)	6.2 (15)	7.0	7.8 (6)	5.1	7.3	9.2
glutamic acid/glutamine	19.8 (47)	19.1 (46)	19.1	20.8 (16)	23.0	22.5	17.4
proline	3.8 (10)	4.4 (10)	4.6	5.2 (4)	3.7	3.4	3.8
glycine	3.9 (10)	4.3 (10)	6.6	3.9 (3)	4.7	6.2	4.5
alanine	7.5 (19)	7.9 (19)	8.0	6.5 (5)	8.2	8.3	9.4
½ cystine	0 (0)	0 (0)	0.8	1.3 (1)	N.D.[c]	N.D.	N.D.
valine	5.0 (13)	5.6 (13)	4.9	7.8 (6)	4.6	5.1	6.2
methionine	1.1 (3)	1.3 (3)	0.2	1.3 (1)	0.7	1.2	1.9
isoleucine	0 (0)	0 (0)	0.6	1.3 (1)	1.5	2.0	1.6
leucine	15.6 (39)	15.6 (37)	14.2	10.4 (8)	13.6	11.5	10.0
tyrosine	2.6 (7)	2.9 (7)	2.7	5.2 (4)	2.2	1.6	2.9
phenylalanine	2.4 (6)	2.4 (6)	2.6	5.2 (4)	3.0	3.1	4.4
histidine	1.9 (5)	1.9 (5)	1.7	0 (0)	2.0	2.2	1.4
lysine	7.8 (21)	8.8 (21)	7.9	11.7 (9)	6.8	5.9	8.0
tryptophan	1.4 (4)	N.D. (4)	N.D.	0 (0)	N.D.	N.D.	N.D.
arginine	6.1 (16)	6.6 (16)	5.7	0 (0)	6.2	5.3	4.0

a) Compositions are based on the two different published sequences.　b) Numbers in parentheses are the calculated number of residues in each protein molecule.　c) N.D. = not determined.

P. N. HERBERT AND L. L. BAUSSERMAN

NH₂ - Asp - Glu - Pro - Pro - Gln - Ser - Pro - Trp - Asp - Arg - Val - Lys - Asp - Leu - Ala - (15)

Thr - Val - Tyr - Val - Asp - Val - Leu - Lys - Asp - Ser - Gly - Arg - Asp - Tyr - Val - (30)

Ser - Gln - Phe - Gln - Gly - Ser - Ala - Leu - Gly - Lys - Gln - Leu - Asn - Leu - Lys - (45)

Leu - Leu - Trp - Asp - Asp - Val - Thr - Ser - Thr - Phe - Ser - Lys - Leu - Arg - Gln - (60)

Glu - Leu - Gly - Pro - Val - Thr - Gln - Glu - Trp - Phe - Asn - Asp - Leu - Gln - Glu - (75)

Lys - Leu - Asn - Leu - Glu - Lys - Thr - Gly - Gly - Leu - Arg - Gln - Glu - Glu - Met - (90)

Ser - Lys - Asp - Leu - Glu - Val - Val - Lys - Ala - Lys - Val - Gln - Pro - Tyr - Leu - (105)

Asp - Asp - Phe - Gln - Lys - Lys - Trp - Gln - Glu - Met - Glu - Leu - Tyr - Arg - Gln - (120)

Lys - Val - Glu - Pro - Leu - Arg - Ala - Glu - Leu - Gln - Glu - Gly - Ala - Arg - Gln - (135)

Lys - Leu - His - Glu - Leu - Gln - Glu - Lys - Leu - Ser - Pro - Leu - Gly - Glu - Glu - (150)

Met - Arg - Asp - Arg - Ala - Arg - Ala - His - Val - Asp - Ala - Leu - Arg - Thr - His - (165)

Leu - Ala - Pro - Tyr - Ser - Asp - Glu - Leu - Arg - Gln - Arg - Leu - Ala - Ala - Arg - (180)

Leu - Glu - Ala - Leu - Lys - Glu - Asn - Gly - Gly - Ala - Arg - Leu - Ala - Glu - Tyr - (195)

His - Ala - Lys - Ala - Thr - Glu - His - Leu - Ser - Thr - Leu - Ser - Glu - Lys - Ala - (210)

Lys - Pro - Ala - Leu - Glu - Asp - Leu - Arg - Gln - Gly - Leu - Leu - Pro - Val - Leu - (225)

Glu - Ser - Phe - Lys - Val - Ser - Phe - Leu - Ser - Ala - Leu - Glu - Glu - Tyr - Thr - (240)

Lys - Leu - Asn - Thr - Gln - COOH   (245)

Fig. 3.   Primary structure of human apolipoprotein A-I as described by Baker and co-workers.[30] Compare with that in Fig. 4.

NH$_2$ - Asp - Glu - Pro - Pro - Gln - Ser - Pro - Trp - Asp - Arg - Val - Lys - Asp - Leu - Ala - (15)

Thr - Val - Tyr - Val - Asp - Val - Leu - Lys - Asp - Ser - Gly - Arg - Asp - Tyr - Val - (30)

Ser - Gln - Phe - Gln - Gly - Ser - Ala - Leu - Gly - Lys - Gln - Leu - Asn - Leu - Lys - (45)

Leu - Leu - Asp - Asn - Trp - Asp - Ser - Val - Thr - Ser - Thr - Phe - Ser - Lys - Leu - (60)

Arg - Glu - Gln - Leu - Gly - Pro - Val - Thr - Gln - Glu - Phe - Trp - Asp - Asn - Leu - (75)

Glu - Lys - Glu - Thr - Glu - Gly - Leu - Arg - Gln - Glu - Met - Ser - Lys - Asp - Leu - (90)

Glu - Glu - Val - Lys - Ala - Lys - Val - Gln - Pro - Tyr - Leu - Asp - Asp - Phe - Gln - (105)

Lys - Lys - Trp - Gln - Glu - Glu - Met - Glu - Leu - Tyr - Arg - Gln - Lys - Val - Glu - (120)

Pro - Leu - Arg - Ala - Glu - Leu - Gln - Glu - Gly - Ala - Arg - Gln - Lys - Leu - His - (135)

Glu - Leu - Gln - Glu - Lys - Leu - Ser - Pro - Leu - Gly - Glu - Gln - Met - Arg - Asp - (150)

Arg - Ala - Arg - Ala - His - Val - Asp - Ala - Leu - Arg - Thr - His - Leu - Ala - Pro - (165)

Tyr - Ser - Asp - Glu - Leu - Arg - Gln - Arg - Leu - Ala - Ala - Arg - Leu - Glu - Ala - (180)

Leu - Lys - Glu - Asn - Gly - Gly - Ala - Arg - Leu - Ala - Glu - Tyr - His - Ala - Lys - (195)

Ala - Thr - Glu - His - Leu - Ser - Thr - Leu - Ser - Glu - Lys - Ala - Lys - Pro - Ala - (210)

Leu - Glu - Asp - Leu - Arg - Gln - Gly - Leu - Leu - Pro - Val - Leu - Glu - Ser - Phe - (225)

Lys - Val - Ser - Phe - Leu - Ser - Ala - Leu - Glu - Glu - Tyr - Thr - Lys - Lys - Leu - (240)

Asn - Thr - Gln - COOH (243)

Fig. 4. Primary structure of human apolipoprotein A-I as described by Brewer and co-workers.[31] Compare with that in Fig. 3.

the plasma of patients having apoA-I$_{Milano}$. Vertical transmission of apoA-I$_{Milano}$ has been shown and this mutant thus constitutes the first example of apoA-I allelism.

ApoA-I has an alpha-helix content of about 55% in the lipid-free state, which increases to about 75% on association with phospholipid. It has been postulated that the protein contains a basic unit of 22 residues (made of 2 similar 11 residue halves), repeated eight times; and that these units reflect a single ancestral chain which, by gene duplication, has generated a repeating unit[39]. These units have close sequence homology and are thought to represent the lipid-binding regions of the protein.

ApoA-I activates lecithin:cholesterol acyltransferase (LCAT), the plasma enzyme catalyzing the conversion of cholesterol and phosphatidylcholine to cholesteryl esters and lysophosphatidyl-choline[40-42]. Recent studies with small (10-43 amino acid) synthetic peptides with high alpha-helical structure and phospholipid affinity suggested the possibility that LCAT activation may be effected by the domains of apoA-I that bind phospholipid. The cyanogen bromide fragments corresponding to the COOH-terminal 94 residues and the NH$_2$-terminal 89 residues each maximally activated LCAT about 25% as well as the whole protein[41]. A synthetic peptide corresponding to residues 121-164 (Fig. 3) had 17% alpha-helix content and was 30% as active as apoA-I in stimulating LCAT[43].

ApoA-I is synthesized by both intestine and liver, and a higher molecular weight precursor has been identified in organ culture media from intestinal mucosal cells and liver[38]. It has been suggested that posttranslational modification reduces the protein size and renders it more acidic[38]. There is little information on mechanisms controlling apoA-I synthesis in either the liver or intestine. Active fat absorption, for example, diverts intestinal apoA-I from venous blood into mesenteric lymph without increasing apoA-I synthesis[12].

Apolipoprotein A-II (apoA-II)

About a third of the total protein and 15% of HDL mass is accounted for by apoA-II (Figs. 1 and 2). This protein contains no histidine, arginine, or tryptophan (Table 3). It occurs primarily as a dimer of two identical chains of 77 residues linked covalently at cysteine 6 by a disulfide bond (Fig. 5). Monomeric species of apoA-II have been identified in plasma and account for about 10% of the total[44]. ApoA-II can form a mixed disulfide with apoE[45] and theoretically with any other cysteine containing protein (as in apoA-I$_{Milano}$ cited above).

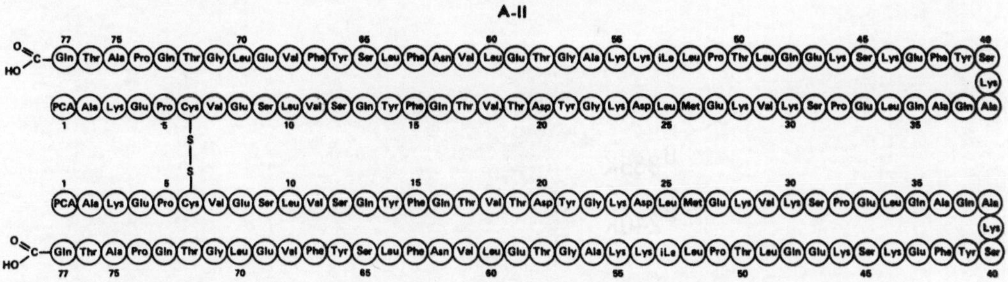

Fig. 5.   Primary structure of human apolipoprotein A-II reported
          by Brewer and co-workers.[33]

Both the monomeric and dimeric forms are able to complex with
phosphatidylcholine or sphingomyelin. Interaction with phospholipid increases the alpha-helical content of apoA-II from 40 to
65%.[46] After treatment of apoA-II with cyanogen bromide to cleave
the protein at its single methionine (position 26, Fig. 5), only
the COOH-terminal peptide of 51 amino acids retains the capacity
to interact with phosphatidylcholine.[47] A synthetic peptide fragment corresponding to residues 40-77 bound 44 moles of dimyristoylphosphatidylcholine per mole of peptide, whereas a fragment
corresponding to positions 56-77 failed to complex with phospholipid.[48]

ApoA-II is synthesized by the intestine[49] and the liver.[50]
It is a quantitatively minor HDL apoprotein in subhuman species
and its specific function in lipid transport is not known. Activation of hepatic triglyceride hydrolase by apoA-II, normal plasma,
HDL, and LDL has been described in a preliminary report.[51] This
observation is at variance with data demonstrating hepatic lipase
inhibition by HDL.[52]

Apolipoprotein A-IV (apoA-IV)

A protein of about 46,000 molecular weight, first recognized
as a major component of rat chylomicrons and HDL[53] (Fig. 6), has
been identified in human plasma and lymph[34-36]. The human protein
appears rich in glutamic acid/glutamine residues, but reported
amino acid compositions (Table 4) are moderately discordant. The
NH_2-terminus of human apoA-IV has been reported to be glutamate or
glutamine[35] (Table 1).

In contrast to the dog[34] and rat, apoA-IV in the human is not
a major apoprotein of any class of lipoproteins. After preparative
ultracentrifugation, however, more than 95% of the total in plasma

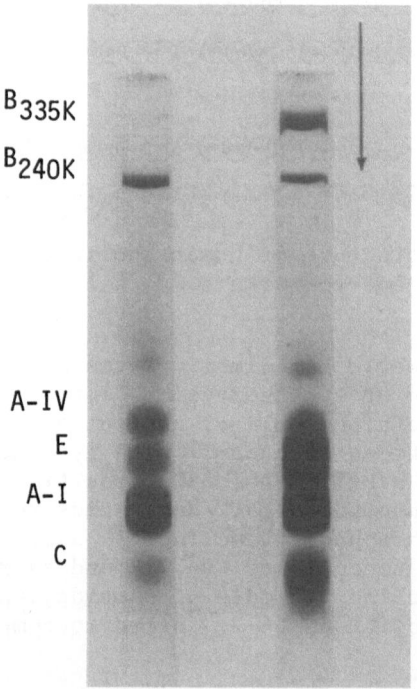

Mesenteric   Plasma
Lymph

Fig. 6.   Apolipoprotein patterns in the total lipoproteins
           (<1.21 g/ml) isolated from rat mesenteric lymph and
           plasma.   Electrophoresis was on 4% polyacrylamide gels
           containing 0.1% sodium dodecyl sulfate.   The larger B_{335K}
           species is not apparent in the lymph but both apoB species
           are readily identified in plasma.   Compare with the pattern
           in human plasma where little of the lower molecular apoB
           form is demonstrable (Fig. 7). (Reproduced with permission
           of Herbert G. Windmueller and The Journal of Biological
           Chemistry).[61]

is found in the lipoprotein-free fraction of plasma.   While there
is some evidence that human apoA-IV is amphipathic[35], the apparently low affinity of this protein for lipoproteins is puzzling.   It
would be of interest to determine if human and rat apoA-IV differed
in their ability to bind to homologous and heterologous HDL.

     Human intestinal epithelial cells contain apoA-IV as judged
by immunofluorescence,[36] and studies in the rat suggest that about
half of the plasma apoA-IV is synthesized in the liver.[12]   This

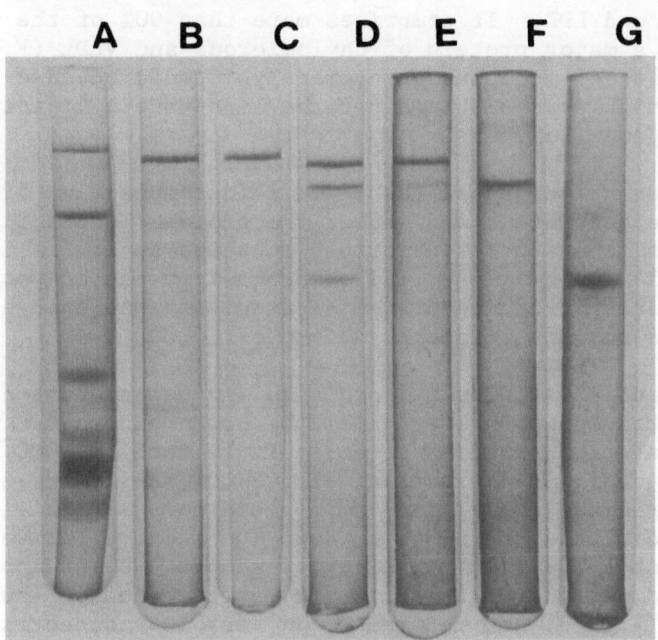

Fig. 7.   Apolipoprotein in human lymph and serum lipoproteins.
          The gels demonstrate patterns in thoracic duct lymph chy-
          lomicrons (A), plasma VLDL (B), and two preparations of
          plasma LDL (C and D). Gels E, F, and G show the B_{100},
          B_{76}, and B_{24} species isolated from the LDL shown in
          gel D. The second band from the top in gel A is the B_{48}
          protein which is also present in gel D. Lower bands in
          gel A are the proline-rich apolipoprotein and apolipopro-
          teins E, A-I, and C's. Electrophoresis was in gels con-
          taining 3% polyacrylamide and 0.1% sodium dodecyl sulfate.
          (Photograph provided by John P. Kane and reproduced with
          permission of the publishers, Proceedings of the National
          Academy of Sciences, U.S.A.).[57]

protein accounts for 10-30% of human chylomicron protein[36] but is
rapidly lost when chylomicrons reach the plasma compartment. The
function of apoA-IV is unknown.

Apolipoprotein B (apoB)

ApoB is probably the only apolipoprotein that is absolutely
required for the formation and transcellular transport of chylomicrons, VLDL and LDL. It comprises more than 90% of the protein
of LDL and is a major protein of chylomicrons and VLDL (Fig. 1).
Characterization of apoB has been greatly impeded because it aggregates and is highly insoluble after the lipoprotein lipids are removed with organic solvents.

Earlier descriptions of the amino acid composition of apoB
(Table 5) were consistent and showed the protein lacked distinctive
features. Two laboratories described subunits as low as 10,000-
30,000 molecular weight[58,59]; and evidence from the composition and
terminal residues of cyanogen bromide fragments was thought compatible with a subunit molecular weight of 30,000.

Very recently, studies in both rats and humans have convincingly demonstrated apoB heterogeneity. Human plasma LDL was
found to contain apoB species of molecular weight 549,000, 407,000,
and 126,000[57] designated, respectively, B-100, B-74, and B-26.
Based on their size (Fig. 7) and amino acid compositions (Table 5)
it was concluded that the B-74 and B-26 species are derived from
the predominant B-100 form. A distinct second type of apoB, of
$M_r \sim 265,000$ and designated B-48, is a major component of human lymph
chylomicrons (Fig. 7) and is present in very low concentrations in
human plasma LDL.

Analogous forms of apoB have been identified in the rat. Rat
small intestine produces primarily a smaller form of apoB of
$M_r \sim 240,000$ (B_{240K}) while liver synthesizes forms of $M_r \sim 335,000$
(B_{335K}) as well as B_{240K}.[61] Chylomicrons containing B_{240K} are
very short-lived in the circulation. Hepatic lipoproteins containing B_{240K} have somewhat longer turnover times; and unlike the
human B-48 species, the B_{240K} apoprotein is readily identifiable
among rat plasma lipoproteins (Fig. 6). The circulation half-life
of the larger B_{335K} is much longer than that of B_{240K},[61-63]
suggesting that they are not incorporated into the same lipoprotein
particles. This apoB heterogeneity, therefore, may provide a
structural basis for the rapid turnover of apoB in chylomicrons
relative to that in most VLDL and LDL particles.

Receptor mediated uptake of LDL in both liver and extrahepatic
tissues is a process specific for lipoproteins containing apoB or
apoE. Chemical modification of the lysine or arginine residues of
apoB can abolish LDL binding and uptake by both fibroblasts[64] and
hepatocytes[65] in vitro. Moreover, alteration of apoB arginine
residues with cyclohexanedione prolongs the life of LDL in the
circulation of man,[66,67] providing additional evidence for a role

Table 5. Amino Acid Compositions of B Apolipoproteins

	B			B_{100}	B_{74}	B_{26}	B_{48}
Literature Reference	54	55	56	57	57	57	57
			(moles/100 moles amino acids)				
aspartic acid/asparagine	10.7	11.1	10.6	10.7	11.2	9.1	10.6
threonine	6.6	6.7	6.4	6.6	6.4	6.7	6.9
serine	8.7	8.9	8.2	8.6	9.0	8.1	9.1
glutamic acid/glutamine	12.2	11.9	12.4	11.6	11.6	12.3	10.0
proline	4.7	3.4	3.8	3.9	3.4	4.8	3.9
glycine	4.8	4.5	4.8	4.7	4.5	5.5	5.6
alanine	6.2	6.3	6.1	6.1	5.9	6.5	6.5
½ cystine	0.8	0.7	0.7	0.4	0.3	0.9	6.3
valine	5.0	5.1	6.1	5.6	5.5	5.8	5.1
methionine	1.7	1.4	1.8	1.6	1.4	2.4	2.1
isoleucine	5.4	5.4	6.1	6.0	6.4	5.2	4.8
leucine	11.9	11.4	11.8	11.8	11.9	12.0	11.6
tyrosine	3.3	3.3	3.0	3.4	3.4	3.0	3.4
phenylalanine	5.0	5.0	5.3	5.0	5.4	3.9	4.4
histidine	2.0	2.2	2.5	2.6	2.8	2.0	2.6
lysine	7.9	8.2	6.7	8.0	7.9	7.9	7.8
tryptophan	N.D.[a]	1.5	0.6	N.D.	N.D.	N.D.	N.D.
arginine	3.0	3.0	3.2	3.4	3.2	3.9	3.9

a) N.D. = not determined.

of apoB in LDL clearance as well as formation.

Apolipoprotein C-I (apoC-I)

ApoC-I accounts for about 10% of the protein in VLDL and 2%
of that in HDL. It is the most basic of the apolipoproteins with
lysine and arginine accounting for more than 20% of its amino acids
(Table 6). ApoC-I contains no cystine, cysteine, tyrosine, or
histidine. It is a single chain protein without glycosidic
linkages (Fig. 8). This protein self-associates in aqueous solution at neutral pH where its secondary structure is highly concentration dependent.[73] Alpha-helical content increases to 73% when
apoC-I is combined with vesicles of phosphatidylcholine.[74] Cyanogen
bromide cleavage at the single methionine yields a 38 residue
amino-terminal peptide and a 19 residue carboxyl-terminal fragment.
Both peptides increase their α-helicity on combining with phosphatidylcholine.[74]

ApoC-I is able to activate LCAT in vitro but is less effective
than apoA-I when unsaturated acyl donors, like those in plasma
phosphatidylcholine, are used.[75,76] The relative importance of
apoA-I and apoC-I in the physiological activation of LCAT is
unresolved. ApoA-I is probably most important since LCAT appears
to circulate in association with this apoprotein.[77] ApoC-I
was also reported to activate lipoprotein lipase[78] but this
observation could not be confirmed in our laboratory.

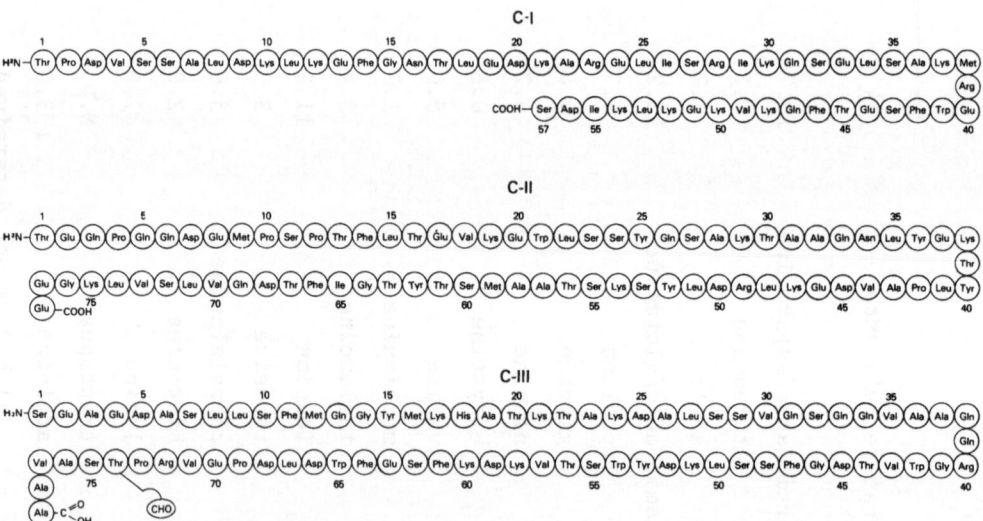

Fig. 8. Primary structures of apolipoproteins C-I,[68] C-II,[69]
         and C-III.[71]

Table 6. Amino Acid Composition of the C-Apoproteins and of Apoprotein D

	C-I	C-II	C-III		D	
Literature Reference	68	69,70	71	100	101	102
			(moles/100 moles amino acid)			
aspartic acid/asparagine	9.2 (5)a	7.1 (5)	8.9 (7)	11.6	10.0	13.0
threonine	4.7 (3)	100 (9)	6.3 (5)	6.2	5.5	6.6
serine	12.1 (7)	10.5 (8-9)	13.9 (11)	4.9	10.7	4.5
glutamic acid/glutamine	16.4 (9)	18.8 (14)	12.7 (10)	13.8	17.4	11.6
proline	1.5 (1)	4.8 (4)	2.5 (2)	9.3	4.3	7.0
glycine	2.1 (1)	2.8 (2)	3.8 (3)	4.7	9.1	4.5
alanine	5.6 (3)	8.3 (6)	12.7 (10)	7.0	5.9	6.2
½ cystine	0 (0)	0 (0)	0 (0)	1.3	0	3.2
valine	3.7 (2)	5.4 (4)	7.6 (6)	7.0	6.5	7.1
methionine	1.5 (1)	2.2 (2)	2.5 (2)	0.9	1.2	1.2
isoleucine	5.1 (3)	0.9 (1)	0 (0)	5.2	2.1	5.6
leucine	11.3 (6)	10.3 (8)	6.3 (5)	7.8	8.2	8.7
tyrosine	0 (0)	6.2 (5)	2.5 (2)	3.6	2.9	3.9
phenylalanine	5.6 (3)	2.5 (2)	5.1 (4)	4.0	3.4	4.2
histidine	0 (0)	0 (0)	1.3 (1)	1.5	8.1	1.4
lysine	5.8 (9)	7.9 (6)	7.6 (6)	8.2	1.7	1.6
tryptophan	N.D.b (1)	1.0 (1)	3.8 (3)	0.4	N.D.	2.0
arginine	5.5 (3)	1.4 (1)	2.5 (2)	2.4	3.0	2.7

a) Values in parentheses are the numbers of residues in each protein molecule based on primary structure analysis.   b) N.D. = not determined.

ApoC-I is probably synthesized primarily by the liver but this postulate is based on analogy with the other two C-apoproteins.[9] Like the other C-apoproteins it has a high affinity for chylomicrons and VLDL but is present in relatively greater proportions in HDL (Fig. 9).

Apolipoprotein C-II (apoC-II)

This protein of approximately 9,000 M.W. accounts for about 10% of the protein of VLDL, 1 to 2% of that in HDL_2 (1.063-1.125

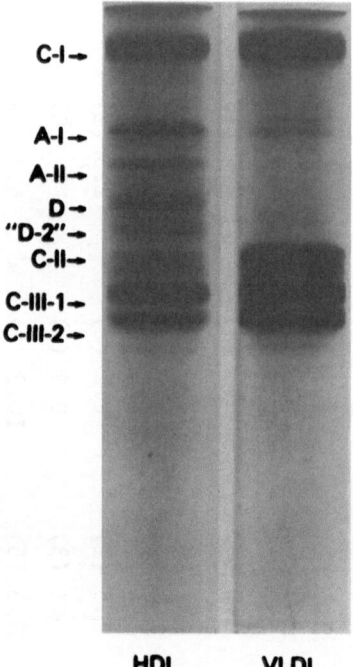

C-Proteins

Fig. 9.   Polyacrylamide gel electrophoresis patterns of the low molecular weight fractions of human apoVLDL and apoHDL. These contain primarily the C-apoproteins. The bands designated A-I and A-II in apoHDL may represent SAA_4 and SAA_5. Note that the relative proportion of apoC-II is much greater in VLDL while "D-2"[72] and D are absent from the VLDL. Electrophoresis was in an anionic-urea system with gels containing $7\frac{1}{2}$% polyacrylamide.

g/ml) and less than 1% in HDL_3 (1.125-1.21 g/ml).[79] ApoC-II contains no histidine (Table 6) or carbohydrate. It is a single chain protein of 78-79 residues[69,70] and a preliminary report of its sequence has been published[69] (Fig. 8). Isoelectric heterogeneity of apoC-II has been noted[80] but the chemical basis of this polymorphism is not known.

ApoC-II has three domains theoretically capable of α-helix formation[81]: residues 13 to 22, 28 to 38, and 42 to 51 (Fig. 8). The first 10 residues and the COOH-terminal 30 amino acids probably cannot form a helix.[81] The circular dichroic spectrum of apoC-II suggests a 30% α-helical content in the lipid-free state,[81] increasing to 45% α-helix when combined with phospholipid.[131]

This protein is a potent activator of lipoprotein lipase with which it forms a stable complex[82] with a 1:1 molar ratio and a dissociation constant probably less than 10^{-8} M.[83] The NH_2-terminal 50-51 residues of apoC-II, which bind phospholipid, do not activate lipoprotein lipase whereas the 29 COOH-terminal resiudes have maximal activity as great as native apoC-II.[84,85] A synthetic peptide corresponding to residues 60-78 (Fig. 8) is about one-third as active as apoC-II whereas a synthetic fragment of residues 55-78 is virtually fully active.[86] The physiological importance of this lipase activating function was unequivocally documented when one form of severe familial hypertriglyceridemia was shown secondary to an absolute deficiency of apoC-II.[88]

ApoC-II is synthesized primarily if not exclusively in the liver[9,50] and the newly synthesized form does not differ from that in plasma.[50] ApoC-II appears to turn over quite rapidly with an estimated half-life of about 1.5 days.[87]

Apolipoprotein C-III (apoC-III)

This most abundant of the C-apoproteins accounts for about 50% of the protein in VLDL and about 2% of that in HDL. It is a single chain protein of 79 residues (Fig. 8). Galactose and galactosamine are attached in a glycosidic linkage at the threonine in position 74.[89] ApoC-III exists in at least three polymorphic forms containing two (apoC-III-2), one (apoC-III-1), or no (apoC-III-0) sialic acid residues at the end of the carbohydrate chain.[90,91]

The secondary structure of lipid-free apoC-III is mostly disordered. The addition of phosphatidylcholine causes the content of α-helix to increase from 22 to 54%.[92] Thrombin cleaves apoC-III into two peptides of equal size. The amino-terminal fragment of 40 residues does not bind phospholipid whereas the carboxyl-terminal

39 residue peptide forms a stable complex while increasing its
α-helicity from 13 to 38%.[93]

ApoC-III is synthesized in the liver.[9,50] In normal plasma
about 25% is in VLDL and 60% in HDL. More than 50% of the total
may be associated with VLDL in hypertriglyceridemic serum.[94] The
monosialylated apoC-III-1 is absent from plasma in abetalipoproteinemia,[95] a defect that is comparable to that seen in the rat
when orotic acid is used to block VLDL release from the liver.[96]
It has been argued from these observations that the sialic acid-rich
form of apoC-III, apoC-III-2, is normally secreted with HDL.[97]
Conversely, apoC-III-1 may usually be elaborated with VLDL.

Under appropriate in vitro conditions, apoC-III can diminish
lipoprotein lipase activity.[98,99] This property, however, is not
unique to apoC-III and is of uncertain physiologic significance.
A specific function of apoC-III in lipoprotein metabolism has not
yet been defined.

Apolipoprotein D (apoD)

Three laboratories have reported the purification of apoD
(originally designated apoA-III[101]) from human HDL.[100-102]
Molecular weight estimates have ranged from 20,000[101,103] to
35,000[102,104] and there are significant differences in the amino
acid compositions which have been described (Table 6). It is estimated that this glycoprotein may contain up to 18% carbohydrate by
weight.[103]

The primary structure of apoD is not known and its lipid-
binding properties have not been defined. Less than 5% of the
apoD in plasma is associated with heparin-manganese precipitable
lipoproteins,[102] about 65% is in the HDL density range, and up to
35% is in the 1.21 g/ml ultracentrifugal infranatant fraction.[105]
The site of apoD synthesis is unknown.

ApoD was originally thought to stimulate LCAT,[106] but this
property was not observed in other studies.[107,108] Recently it
has been suggested that apoD effects transfer of cholesteryl esters
and triglycerides between lipoproteins,[104] and that a complex of
apoA-I:apoD:LCAT (1:2:1) occurs naturally in plasma catalyzing
both esterification and transfer of cholestesteryl esters.[109]
Others, however, have reported that the cholesteryl ester transfer
protein is not apoD,[110] and that immunoadsorption of all plasma
apoD does not quantitatively remove LCAT activity.[102]

Apolipoprotein E (apoE)

ApoE comprises 10-20% of VLDL protein and immunochemical techniques have demonstrated its presence in all lipoprotein density classes. Reported molecular weights range from 33,000-38,000.[111,112] Most of the protein occurs in plasma as a single chain but trimers[113] and mixed disulfides with apoA-II[45,114,115] have also been identified. The protein is rich in arginine and glutamic acid/glutamine residues (Table 7). When rabbit apoE forms complexes with dimyristoylphosphatidylcholine its α-helical content increases from 45 to 65%.[153]

Heterogeneity of apoE, demonstrated by isoelectric focusing in polyacrylamide gels (Fig. 10), has been reproducibly demonstrated[118-122]. The polymorphism is perhaps most elegantly shown and interpreted when isoelectric focusing and SDS polyacrylamide gel electrophoresis are combined to analyze the apoE pattern in VLDL[123] (Fig. 11). Differences in sialic acid content, and hence posttranslational modification, account for much of the apparent polymorphism. Treatment of apoVLDL with neuraminidase eliminates the higher molecular weight forms of apoE and individual subjects are then found to have either one or two apoE isoforms[123]. These are shown diagramatically in Fig. 12. The three major isoforms of apoE (E-4, E-3, and E-2) are thought to be the products of three alleles at a single genetic locus[123,124]. The α-pattern (Fig. 11) reflects heterozygosity, the β-pattern homozygosity.

Very recently data relevant to the primary structural differences between the major E-isoforms have been provided. It was reported that the E-4 isoform (Utermann designation Fig. 12) contains one more arginine than is contained in E-3, and that E-3 contains one arginine less than E-2.[117] The arginines appear to be replaced by cysteine residues resulting in loss of 0, 1, and 2 positive charge units (and greater anodic mobility, Fig. 12) for E-4, E-3 and E-2 respectively. These differences in amino acid composition (Table 7) and cysteine-arginine substitutions were confirmed by sequence analysis of 2 cyanogen bromide fragments of E-2 and E-3.[117]

Lipoproteins containing primarily apoE accumulate in the plasma of cholesterol-fed dogs, and these lipoproteins bind with higher affinity to the B-receptor of cultured skin fibroblasts than do LDL themselves.[125] The liver also has receptors for apoE-containing lipoproteins[126] and hepatic uptake and catabolism of apoE appear to preferentially involve the more basic E-3 and E-4 isoforms. Recognition of these isoproteins by hepatic receptors may provide a link in the normal conversion of VLDL remnants to LDL.[127]

The importance of these observations in vitro and in animals relates to the observation that subjects homozygous for apoE-2 (E-D or βIV pattern, Fig. 12) may have an inability to normally

Table 7.   Amino Acid Composition of Unfractionated ApoE and Three of the ApoE Isoproteins

	E		E-4	E-3	E-2
Literature Reference	116	111	117	117	117
		(moles/100 moles amino acids)			
aspartic acid/asparagine	5.7	6.8	4.5	4.3	4.3
threonine	5.1	4.6	3.7	3.6	3.6
serine	7.6	6.0	4.7	4.7	4.7
glutamic acid/glutamine	23.8	17.9	24.4	24.3	24.2
proline	3.7	3.8	2.9	3.0	3.1
glycine	5.9	6.7	6.2	6.1	6.2
alanine	9.1	10.4	11.9	12.3	12.3
½ cystine	0	0	0.1	0.4	0.7
valine	6.0	7.4	7.3	7.5	7.6
methionine	1.1	0.7	2.1	2.2	2.0
isoleucine	1.1	1.8	0.7	0.6	0.7
leucine	10.5	12.0	12.7	12.6	12.6
tyrosine	1.7	1.8	1.2	1.2	1.2
phenylalanine	1.9	2.1	1.1	1.1	1.1
histidine	1.2	0.8	0.7	0.7	0.7
lysine	4.6	4.9	4.3	4.1	4.2
tryptophan	N.D.[a]	3.2	N.D.	N.D.	N.D.
arginine	9.3	9.1	11.5	11.2	10.9

a) N.D. = not determined.

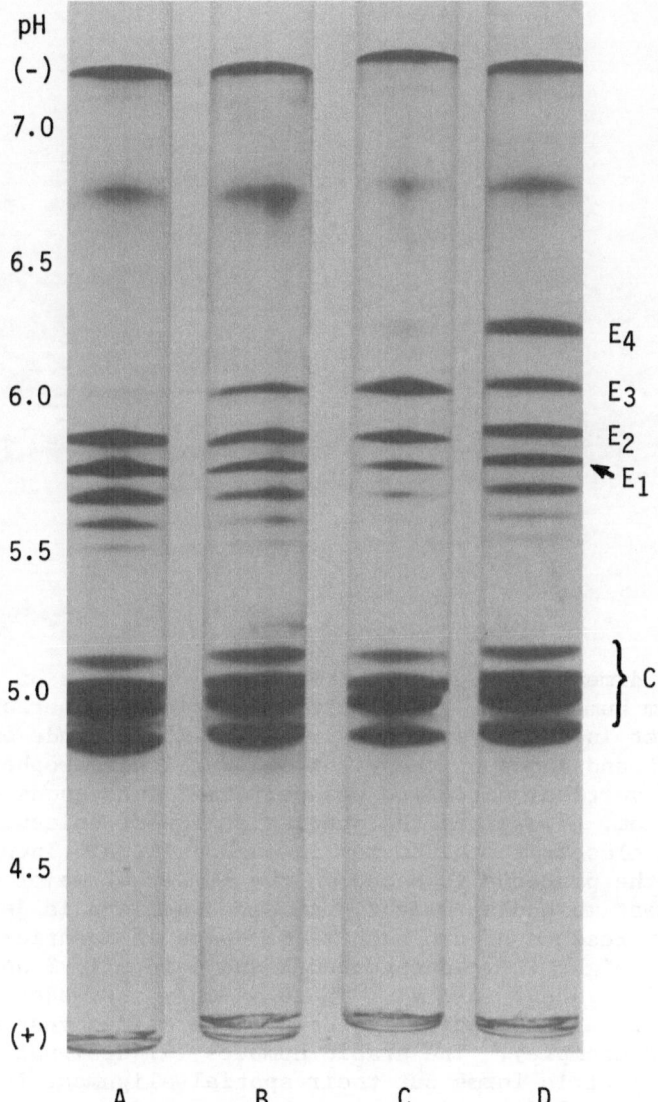

Fig. 10.   Heterogeneity of apoE demonstrated by isoelectric focusing
           in 7.5% polyacrylamide gels.   Gel A demonstrates apoVLDL
           from a subject with type 3 hyperlipoproteinemia who lacks
           the more basic E4 and E3 isoforms.   Gels B and C show
           common patterns from normolipemic individuals and apoVLDL
           in gel D contains the E4 isoform (Photograph courtesy of
           G. Russell Warnick and reproduced with permission from
           the publishers of Clinical Chemistry).[118]

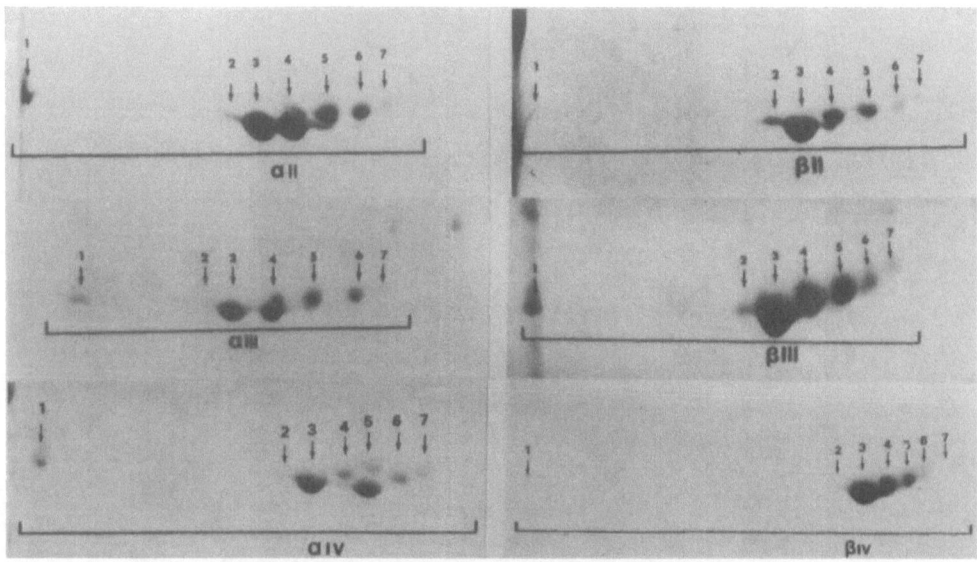

Fig. 11. Two dimensional gel electrophoresis patterns of apoE
          from human VLDL. Isoelectric focusing was performed
          first in the horizontal direction with cathode on the
          left and anode on the right. SDS gel electrophoresis in
          the vertical direction was performed with anode on the
          bottom. Therefore the species of lowest molecular weight
          are closest to the bottom in each pattern. Interpretation
          of the patterns is based on the number of major spots of
          lowest molecular weight. An alpha pattern is defined by
          the presence of two such major spots of identical molecu-
          lar weight (here designated 3 and 4 in αII, 3 and 4 in
          αIII, 3 and 5 in αIV). There is only one major low mole-
          cular weight species in the β pattern (designated 3 in
          each example). The arabic numbers 1→7 designate different
          isoelectric forms but their spatial alignment in the
          horizontal direction cannot be compared since the apoVLDL
          for each pattern was run separately. (Photograph kindly
          provided by Vassilis I. Zannis and reproduced with per-
          mission from the publishers of the American Journal of
          Human Genetics).[124]

convert VLDL to LDL. They sometimes exhibit a variety of hyperlipoproteinemia termed type 3 or dysbetalipoproteinemia. ApoE from
subjects with type 3 hyperlipoproteinemia indeed is removed from
plasma at a slower than normal rate in control subjects as well as
type 3 patients.[128] Homozygosity for apoE-2, however, appears
necessary but not sufficient to produce this disorder. Other factors such as simultaneous inheritance of another disorder affecting
lipoprotein metabolism or hypothyroidism are critical to the phenotypic expression of the E-2 homozygous state. This topic is discussed by Dr. Assmann elsewhere in this volume.

ApoE is synthesized by the liver and not by the intestine.[8]
Diet has only a moderate effect on plasma apoE concentrations.[122]
Serum levels correlate highly with triglyceride concentrations[129]
and highest levels are found in type 3 hyperlipoproteinemia.[121,130]

Other Apolipoproteins

In addition to the apolipoproteins already mentioned, a number
of other serum proteins have been identified in lipoproteins isolated by ultracentrifugation. The status of many of these is uncertain but they are briefly described for other technicians in this
field who are constantly encountering new species of apolipoproteins.

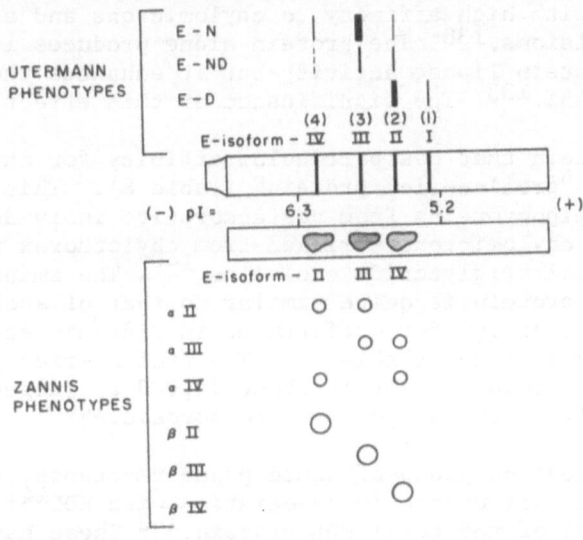

Fig. 12. Relationship between one and two dimensional systems for
          displaying apoE polymorphism. Note that in the two pheno-
          typing systems only isoform 3 is equivalent. A typical
          subject with type 3 hyperlipoproteinemia would be classi-
          fied as E-2 homozygous or E-D in the Utermann system.
          The same pattern is designated βIV or E-IV homozygous in
          the Zannis system.

The appellation "D-2" was applied to a protein of $M_r \sim 7,000$ that is consistently identified among the low molecular weight proteins of HDL[72] (Fig. 9). This protein contains cystine or cysteine, is relatively rich in lysine (Table 8), and has carboxyl-terminal serine and amino-terminal leucine. Another minor HDL apoprotein, designated apoF, is highly acidic.[133] ApoF of $M_r \sim 30,000$, also contains cystine or cysteine and is relatively poor in basic amino acids (Table 8). In anionic polyacrylamide gel electrophoresis systems it has mobility similar to apoD (Fig. 2). Functions for apoF and "D-2" have not been suggested.

An apoprotein provisionally designated apoG[134] has been isolated from HDL and is also reported to have electrophoretic mobility similar to apoD (Fig. 2). It is reported to have a molecular weight of about 72,000, contains glucosamine, and does not have a distinctive amino acid composition (Table 8).

The apoprotein most recently receiving a letter,[135] apoH, appears identical to the plasma β_2-glycoprotein I.[136] This protein contains, by weight, 82% protein, 7% hexoses, 6% acetyl hexosamine, and 4% sialic acid.[137] It has electrophoretic mobility[136] and size ($M_r \sim 40,000$) similar to apoE. At least 70% of the apoH in plasma is not lipoprotein bound; about 15% is associated with HDL and trace amounts are present in all lipoprotein fractions.[136] It appears to bind with high affinity to chylomicrons and artificial triglyceride emulsions.[138] The protein alone produces little stimulation of lipoprotein lipase activity but it enhances the activation with apoC-II by 45%.[135] The significance of this effect is unknown.

Another protein that has particular affinity for chylomicrons is the so-called "proline-rich protein" (Table 8). This protein is not found in lipoproteins from postabsorptive individuals, has been detected in chylomicrons purified from chylothorax fluid, and binds to artificial triglyceride emulsions.[140] The amino acid composition of this protein is quite similar to that of apoH, the β_2-glycoprotein I, except for differences in glutamic acid/glutamines, lysine and arginine (Table 8). The proline-rich protein, however, had a molecular weight of about 74,000 as judged by mobility in SDS polyacrylamide gel electrophoresis.[140]

A very interesting group of acute phase reactants, the serum amyloid A proteins, circulate in association with HDL[141] and may comprise up to 25% of the total HDL protein.[142] These have molecular weights of around 11,000, occur in at least six polymorphic forms,[142] contain no carbohydrate, and are distinctly poor in threonine and valine while being relatively enriched in arginine (Table 8). The two major SAA polymorphs, SAA4 and SAA5, have mobilities almost identical to apoA-I and apoA-II in anionic-urea polyacrylamide gel electrophoresis[142] (Fig. 2).

Table 8. Amino Acid Composition of Some Minor and Novel Apolipoproteins

Literature Reference	D-2 72	F 133	G 134	H 139	PRP[a] 140	SAA[b]$_1$ 142	SAA$_5$ 142
	(moles/100 moles amino acids)						
aspartic acid/asparagine	4.9	9.5	12.4	8.0	9.0	15.9	16.3
threonine	6.6	6.0	4.7	7.1	7.2	1.3	0
serine	7.5	8.1	4.8	10.1	9.1	7.0	6.4
glutamic acid/glutamine	19.9	13.6	13.0	9.4	12.7	9.5	10.4
proline	5.4	2.5	6.3	9.0	8.9	4.0	4.2
glycine	5.0	11.8	6.5	9.5	8.7	14.1	14.3
alanine	6.7	12.2	8.6	5.8	4.1	15.4	16.8
½ cystine	1.7	7.4	N.D.[c]	N.D.	3.4	0	0
valine	7.0	1.4	7.1	4.9	4.6	1.3	1.1
methionine	1.0	1.7	tr	1.1	0.6	1.8	1.9
isoleucine	1.4	3.8	3.9	3.4	4.0	3.0	3.0
leucine	10.2	9.4	10.3	5.7	6.4	5.5	3.4
tyrosine	4.6	4.3	2.5	4.4	3.8	6.0	5.4
phenylalanine	4.9	5.7	4.7	4.6	3.8	5.8	8.5
histidine	0.2	3.2	2.6	1.7	2.7	2.7	3.1
lysine	11.6	4.5	8.5	8.6	5.9	5.0	4.4
tryptophan	1.3	0	N.D.	N.D.	N.D.	2.3	2.4
arginine	0.6	2.3	4.1	3.2	5.1	11.6	9.9

a) PRP = proline-rich protein
b) SAA = serum amyloid A
c) N.D. = not determined

Finally, it must be recognized that other proteins not considered here are frequently isolated in association with the plasma lipoproteins and may play important roles in lipid transport. There is one in which three amino acids - serine, glutamic acid/glutamine, and glycine - account for more than 55% of the total residues;[143] and there are others. Currently our skills in isolation and characterization of quantitatively minor "apolipoproteins" have outdistanced our physiological insights. This apparent gap, however, is being progressively narrowed.

Acknowledgments: Work described herein performed in the authors' laboratory was supported in part by a grant from Reynolds Industries, The Miriam Hospital Cardiology and Atherosclerosis Trust, and N.I.H. grant HL 26156. We gratefully appreciate the assistance of Mrs. Mildred Moverman in preparing the manuscript. Herbert Windmueller, Vassilis Zannis, John Kane, and Russell Warnick were most generous in providing materials that may make this paper a useful reference source.

REFERENCES

1. T. Sata, R. J. Havel, and A. L. Jones, Characterization of subfractions of triglyceride-rich lipoproteins separated by gel chromatography from blood plasma of normolipemic and hyperlipemic humans, J. Lipid Res. 13:757 (1972).
2. R. M. Glickman, K. Kirsch, and K. J. Isselbacher, Fat absorption during inhibition of protein synthesis: Studies of lymph chylomicrons, J. Clin. Invest. 51:356 (1972).
3. R. M. Glickman, J. Khorana, and A. Kilgore, Localization of apolipoprotein B in intestinal epithelial cells, Science 193: 1254 (1976).
4. R. M. Glickman and P. H. R. Green, The intestine as a source of apolipoprotein A_1, Proc. Natl. Acad. Sci. U. S. A. 74:2569 (1977).
5. D. Rachmilewitz, J. J. Albers, D. R. Saunders, and M. Fainaru, Apoprotein synthesis by human duodenojejunal mucosa, Gastroenterology 75:677 (1978).
6. G. Schonfeld, E. Bell, and D. H. Alpers, Intestinal apoproteins during fat absorption, J. Clin. Invest. 61:1539 (1978).
7. P. H. R. Green, R. M. Glickman, J. W. Riley, and E. Quinet, Human apolipoprotein A-IV. Intestinal origin and distribution in plasma, J. Clin. Invest. 65:911 (1980).
8. A.-L. Wu and H. G. Windmueller, Relative contributions by liver and intestine to individual plasma apolipoproteins in the rat, J. Biol. Chem. 254:7316 (1979).
9. H. G. Windmueller, P. N. Herbert, and R. I. Levy, Biosynthesis of lymph and plasma lipoprotein apoproteins by isolated perfused rat liver and intestine, J. Lipid Res. 14:215 (1973).

10. K. Imaizumi, R. J. Havel, M. Fainaru, and J.-L. Vigne, Origin and transport of the A-I and arginine-rich apolipoproteins in mesenteric lymph of rats, J. Lipid Res. 19:1038 (1978).

11. A. -L. Wu and H. G. Windmueller, Identification of circulating apolipoproteins synthesized by rat small intestine in vivo, J. Biol. Chem 253:2525 (1978).

12. H. G. Windmueller and A. -L. Wu, Biosynthesis of plasma apo- lipoproteins by rat small intestine without dietary or biliary fat, J. Biol. Chem. 256:3012 (1981).

13. S. H. Quarfordt and D. S. Goodman, Metabolism of doubly- labeled chylomicron cholesteryl esters in the rat, J. Lipid Res. 8:264 (1967).

14. A. D. Cooper and P. Y. S. Yu, Rates of removal and degradation of chylomicron remnants by isolated perfused rat liver, J. Lipid Res. 19:635 (1978).

15. L. L. Swift, N. R. Manowitz, G. D. Dunn, and V. S. Lequire, Isolation and characterization of hepatic Golgi lipoproteins from hypercholesterolemic rats, J. Clin. Invest. 66:415 (1980).

16. G. Sigurdsson, A. Nicoll, and B. Lewis, Conversion of very low density lipoprotein to low density lipoprotein. A metabolic study of apolipoprotein B kinetics in human subjects, J. Clin. Invest. 56:1481 (1975).

17. T. Murase and H. Itakura, Accumulation of intermediate density lipoprotein in plasma after intravenous administration of hepatic triglyceride lipase antibody in rats, Atherosclerosis 39:293 (1981).

18. J. R. Patsch, A. M. Gotto, Jr., T. Olivecrona, and S. Eisenberg, Formation of high density lipoprotein$_2$-like particles during lipolysis of very low density lipoproteins in vitro, Proc. Natl. Acad. Sci. 75:4519 (1978).

19. G. Sigurdsson, S. -P. Noel, and R. J. Havel, Catabolism of the apoprotein of low density lipoproteins by the isolated per- fused rat liver, J. Lipid Res. 19:628 (1978).

20. J. Shepherd, S. Bicker, A. R. Lorimer, and C. J. Packard, Re- ceptor-mediated low density lipoprotein catabolism in man, J. Lipid Res. 20:999 (1979).

21. R. L. Hamilton, M. C. Williams, C. J. Fielding, and R. J. Havel, Discoidal bilayer structure of nascent high density lipopro- teins from perfused rat liver, J. Clin. Invest. 58:667 (1976).

22. P. H. R. Green, A. R. Tall, and R. M. Glickman, Rat intestine secretes discoid high density lipoprotein, J. Clin. Invest. 61:528 (1978).

23. G. Sigurdsson, S. -P. Noel, and R. J. Havel, Quantification of the hepatic contribution to the catabolism of high density lipoproteins in rats, J. Lipid Res. 20:316 (1979).

24. P. Alaupovic, Conceptual development of the classification sys- tems of plasma lipoproteins, in:"Protides of the Biological Fluids," H. Peeters, ed., Pergamon, Oxford, England (1971).

25. P. N. Herbert, T. M. Forte, R. S. Shulman, M. J. La Piana,
    E. L. Gong, R. I. Levy, D. S. Fredrickson, and A. V. Nichols,
    Structural and compositional changes attending the ultra-
    centrifugation of very low density lipoproteins, Prep.
    Biochem. 5:93 (1975).

26. M. Fainaru, R. J. Havel, and K. Imaizumi, Apoprotein content
    of plasma lipoproteins of the rat separated by gel chroma-
    tography or ultracentrifugation, Biochem. Med. 17:347 (1977).

27. C. B. Blum, L. Aron, and R. Sciacca, Radioimmunoassay studies
    of human apolipoprotein E, J. Clin. Invest. 66:1240 (1980).

28. D. B. Zilversmit, L. B. Hughes, and J. Balmer, Stimulation of
    cholesterol ester exchange by lipoprotein-free rabbit plasma,
    Biochim. Biophys. Acta 409:393 (1975).

29. J. T. Sparrow, J. D. Morrisett, H. J. Pownall, R. L. Jackson,
    and A. M. Gotto, Jr., The mechanism of lipid binding by the
    plasma lipoproteins: synthesis of model peptides, in:
    "Peptides: Chemistry, Structure and Biology," R. Walter and
    J. Meienhofer, eds., Ann Arbor Science, Ann Arbor (1975).

30. H. N. Baker, T. Delahunty, A. M. Gotto, Jr., and R. L. Jackson,
    The primary structure of high density apolipoprotein-gluta-
    mine-I, Proc. Natl. Acad. Sci. U. S. A. 71:3631 (1974).

31. H. B. Brewer, Jr., T. Fairwell, A. LaRue, R. Ronan, A. Houser,
    and T. J. Bronzert, The amino acid sequence of human apo-I,
    an apolipoprotein isolated from high density lipoproteins,
    Biochem. Biophys. Res. Commun. 80:623 (1978).

32. K. H. Weisgraber, T. P. Bersot, R. W. Mahley, G. Franceschini,
    and C. R. Sirtori, A-I-Milano apoprotein. Isolation and
    characterization of a cysteine-containing variant of the
    A-I apoprotein from human high density lipoproteins, J. Clin.
    Invest. 66:901 (1980).

33. H. B. Brewer, Jr., S. E. Lux, R. Ronan, and K. M. John, Amino
    acid sequence of human apoLp-Gln-II (apoA-II), an apolipo-
    protein isolated from the high density lipoprotein complex,
    Proc. Natl. Acad. Sci. U. S. A. 69:1304 (1972).

34. K. H. Weisgraber, T. P. Bersot, and R. W. Mahley, Isolation and
    characterization of an apoprotein from the d<1.006 lipopro-
    teins of human and canine lymph homologous with the rat A-IV
    apoprotein, Biochem. Biophys. Res. Commun. 85:287 (1978).

35. U. Beisiegel and G. Utermann, An apolipoprotein homolog of rat
    apolipoprotein A-IV in human plasma, Eur. J. Biochem. 93:601
    (1979).

36. P. H. R. Green, R. M. Glickman, C. D. Saudek, C. B. Blum, and
    A. R. Tall, Human intestinal lipoproteins. Studies in
    chyluric subjects, J. Clin. Invest. 64:233 (1979).

37. P. N. Herbert, G. Assmann, A. M. Gotto, Jr., and D. S. Fredrick-
    son, Familial lipoprotein deficiency (Abetalipoproteine-
    mia and Tangier disease), in:"The Metabolic Basis of
    Inherited Disease." J. B. Stanbury, J. B. Wyngaarden, D. S.
    Fredrickson, J. L. Goldstein, and M. S. Brown, eds.,
    (In press).

38. V. I. Zannis, J. L. Breslow, and A. J. Katz, Isoproteins of human apolipoprotein A-I demonstrated in plasma and intestinal organ culture, J. Biol. Chem. 255:8612 (1980).

39. A. D. McLachlin, Repeated helical pattern in apolipoprotein A-I, Nature 267:465 (1977).

40. C. J. Fielding, V. G. Shore, and P. E. Fielding, A protein cofactor of lecithin:cholesterol acyltransferase, Biochem. Biophys. Res. Commun. 46:1493 (1972).

41. A. K. Soutar, C. W. Garner, H. N. Baker, J. T. Sparrow, R. L. Jackson, A. M. Gotto, and L. C. Smith, Effect of the human plasma apolipoproteins and phosphatidylcholine acyl donor on the activity of lecithin:cholesterol acyltransferase, Biochemistry 14:3057 (1975).

42. J. J. Albers, Lecithin:cholesterol acyltransferase, Artery 5:61 (1979).

43. D. Fukushima, S. Yokoyama, D. J. Kroon, F. J. Kezdy, and T. Kaiser, Chain length-function correlation of amphiphilic peptides, J. Biol. Chem. 255:10651 (1980).

44. T. A. Musliner, P. A. Garner, L. O. Henderson, and Peter N. Herbert, Radioimmunoassay of apolipoprotein A-II, Submitted for publication.

45. K. H. Weisgraber and R. W. Mahley, Apoprotein (E-A-II) complex of human plasma lipoproteins. I. Characterization of this mixed disulfide and its identification in a high density lipoprotein subfraction, J. Biol. Chem. 253:6281 (1978).

46. R. L. Jackson, S. J. T. Mao, and A. M. Gotto, Jr., Effects of maleylation on the lipid-binding and immunochemical properties of human plasma high density apolipoprotein A-II, Biochem. Biophys. Res. Commun. 61:1317 (1974).

47. S. E. Lux, K. M. John, S. Fleischer, R. L. Jackson, and A. M. Gotto, Jr., Identification of the lipid-binding cyanogen bromide fragment from the cystine-containing high density apolipoprotein, apolp-gln-II, Biochem. Biophys. Res. Commun. 49:23 (1972).

48. S. J. T. Mao, J. T. Sparrow, E. B. Gilliam, A. M. Gotto, Jr., and R. L. Jackson, Mechanism of lipid-protein interaction in the plasma lipoproteins: lipid-binding properties of synthetic fragments of apolipoprotein A-II, Biochemistry 16:4150 (1977).

49. D. Rachmilewitz, J. J. Albers, D. R. Saunders, and M. Fainaru, Apoprotein synthesis by human duodenojejunal mucosa, Gastroenterology 75:677 (1978).

50. V. I. Zannis, D. N. Kurnit, and J. L. Breslow, Synthesis of apolipoproteins by human fetal intestine and liver in organ culture, Fed. Proc. 40:1635 (1981).

51. C. Jahn, J. C. Osborne, Jr., E. J. Schaefer, and H. B. Brewer, Jr., Activation of the enzymatic activity of hepatic lipase (HTGL) by apoA-II, Circulation 64:IV-229 (1981)

52. G. Bengtsson and T. Olivecrona, The hepatic heparin releasable lipase binds to high density lipoproteins, FEBS Letters 119:290 (1980).

53. J. B. Swaney, H. Reese, and H. A. Eder, Polypeptide composition of rat high density lipoprotein: characterization by SDS-gel electrophoresis, Biochem. Biophys. Res. Commun. 59:513 (1974).

54. A. M. Gotto, W. V. Brown, R. I. Levy, M. E. Birnbaumer and D. S. Fredrickson, Evidence for the identity of the major apoprotein in low density and very low density lipoproteins in normal subjects and patients with familial hyperlipoproteinemia, J. Clin. Invest. 51:1486 (1972).

55. J. L. Granda and A. Scanu, Solubilization and properties of the apoproteins of the very low- and low-density lipoproteins of human serum, Biochemistry 5:3301 (1966).

56. S. Margolis and R. G. Langdon, Studies on human serum β_1-lipoprotein. I. Amino acid composition, J. Biol. Chem. 241:469 (1966).

57. J. P. Kane, D. A. Hardman, and H. E. Paulus, Heterogeneity of apolipoprotein B: Isolation of a new species from human chylomicrons, Proc. Natl. Acad. Sci. U. S. A. 77:2465 (1980).

58. J. P. Kane, E. G. Richards and R. J. Havel, Subunit heterogeneity in human serum beta lipoprotein, Proc. Natl. Acad. Sci. 66:1075 (1970).

59. C. -H. Chen and F. Aladjem, Subunit structure of the apoprotein of human serum low density lipoproteins, Biochem. Biophys. Res. Commun. 60:549 (1974).

60. W. A. Bradley, M. F. Rohde, A. M. Gotto, Jr., and R. L. Jackson, The cyanogen bromide peptides of the apoprotein of low density lipoprotein (apoB): Its molecular weight from a chemical view, Biochem. Biophys. Res. Commun. 81:928 (1978).

61. A. -L. Wu and H. G. Windmueller, Variant forms of plasma apolipoprotein B. Hepatic and intestinal biosynthesis and heterogeneous metabolism in the rat, J. Biol. Chem. 256:3615 (1981).

62. J. Elovson, Y. O. Huang, N. Baker, and R. Kannan, Apolipoprotein B is structurally and metabolically heterogeneous in the rat, Proc. Natl. Acad. Sci. U. S. A. 78:157 (1981).

63. C. E. Sparks and J. B. Marsh, Metabolic heterogeneity of apolipoprotein B in the rat, J. Lipid Res. 22:519 (1981).

64. R. W. Mahley, K. H. Weisgraber, G. W. Melchior, T. L. Innerarity, and K. S. Holcombe, Inhibition of receptor-mediated clearance of lysine and arginine-modified lipoproteins from the plasma of rats and monkeys, Proc. Natl. Acad. Sci. U. S. A. 77:5923 (1980).

65. A. D. Attie, R. C. Pittman, and D. Steinberg, Metabolism of native and of lactosylated human low density lipoprotein: Evidence for two pathways for catabolism of exogenous proteins in rat hepatocytes, Proc. Natl. Acad. Sci. U. S. A. 77:5923 (1980).

66. H. R. Slater, C. J. Packard, S. Bicker, and J. Shepherd,

Effects of cholestyramine on receptor-mediated plasma clearance and tissue uptake of human low density lipoproteins in the rabbit, J. Biol. Chem. 255:10210 (1980).

67. J. Shepherd, C. J. Packard, S. Bicker, T. D. V. Lawrie, and H. G. Morgan, Cholestyramine promotes receptor-mediated low-density-lipoprotein catabolism, N. Engl. J. Med. 302:1219 (1980).

68. R. S. Shulman, P. N. Herbert, K. Wehrly, and D. S. Fredrickson, The complete amino acid sequence of C-I (apolp-ser), an apolipoprotein from human very low density lipoproteins, J. Biol. Chem. 250:182 (1975).

69. R. L. Jackson, H. N. Baker, E. B. Gilliam, and A. M. Gotto, Jr., Primary structure of very low density apolipoprotein C-II of human plasma, Proc. Natl. Acad. Sci. U. S. A. 74:1942 (1977).

70. T. A. Musliner, P. N. Herbert, and E. C. Church, Activation of lipoprotein lipase by native and acylated peptides of apolipoprotein C-II, Biochim. Biophys. Acta 573:501 (1979).

71. H. B. Brewer, Jr., R. Shulman, P. Herbert, R. Ronan, and R. Wehrly, The complete amino acid sequence of alanine apolipoprotein (apoC-III), an apolipoprotein from human plasma very low density lipoproteins, J. Biol. Chem. 249:4975 (1974).

72. C. T. Lim, J. Chung, H. J. Kayden, and A. M. Scanu, Apoproteins of human serum high density lipoproteins. Isolation and characterization of the peptides of Sephadex fraction V from normal subjects and patients with abetalipoproteinemia, Biochim. Biophys. Acta 420:332 (1976).

73. J. D. Osborne, Jr., T. J. Bronzert, and H. B. Brewer, Jr., Self association of apoC-I from the human high density lipoprotein complex, J. Biol. Chem. 252:5756 (1977).

74. R. L. Jackson, J. D. Morrisett, J. T. Sparrow, J. P. Segrest, H. J. Pownall, L. C. Smith, H. F. Hoff, and A. M. Gotto, Jr., The interaction of apolipoprotein-serine with phosphatidyl-choline, J. Biol. Chem. 249:5314 (1974).

75. A. K. Soutar, C. W. Garner, H. N. Baker, J. T. Sparrow, R. L. Jackson, A. M. Gotto, and L. C. Smith, Effect of the human plasma apolipoproteins and phosphatidylcholine acyl donor on the activity of lecithin:cholesterol acyltransferase, Biochemistry 14:3057 (1975).

76. J. J. Albers, Lecithin:cholesterol acyltransferase, Artery 5:61 (1979).

77. P. E. Fielding and C. J. Fielding, A cholesteryl ester transfer complex in human plasma, Proc. Natl. Acad. Sci. U. S. A. 77:3327 (1980).

78. D. Ganesan, R. H. Bradford, P. Alaupovic and W. J. McConathy, Differential activation of lipoprotein lipase from human post-heparin plasma, milk and adipose tissue by polypeptides of human serum apolipoprotein C, FEBS Lett. 15:205 (1971).

79. M. L. Kashyap, L. S. Srivastava, C. Y. Chen, G. Perisutti, M.

Campbell, R. F. Lutmer, and C. J. Glueck, Radioimmunoassay of human apolipoprotein C-II. A study in normal and hypertri-glyceridemic subjects, J. Clin. Invest. 60:171 (1977).

80. R. J. Havel, L. Kotite, and J. P. Kane, Isoelectric hetero-geneity of the cofactor protein for lipoprotein lipase in human blood plasma, Biochem. Med. 21:121 (1979).

81. W. W. Mantulin, M. F. Rohde, A. M. Gotto, Jr., and H. Pownall, The conformational properties of human plasma apolipoprotein C-II, J. Biol. Chem. 255:8185 (1980).

82. A. L. Miller and L. C. Smith, Activation of lipoprotein lipase by apolipoprotein glutamic acid, J. Biol. Chem. 248:3359 (1973).

83. J. Chung, and A. M. Scanu, Isolation, molecular properties, and kinetic characterization of lipoprotein lipase from rat heart, J. Biol. Chem. 252:4202 (1977).

84. T. A. Musliner, E. C. Church, P. N. Herbert, M. J. Kingston, and R. S. Shulman, Lipoprotein lipase cofactor activity of a carboxyl-terminal peptide of apolipoprotein C-II, Proc. Natl. Acad. Sci. U. S. A. 74:5358 (1977).

85. T. A. Musliner, P. N. Herbert, and E. C. Church, Activation of lipoprotein lipase by native and acylated peptides of apo-lipoprotein C-II, Biochim. Biophys. Acta 573:501 (1979).

86. P. K. J. Kinnunen, R. L. Jackson, L. C. Smith, A. M. Gotto, Jr., and J. T. Sparrow, Activation of lipoprotein lipase by native and synthetic fragments of human plasma apolipoprotein C-II, Proc. Natl. Acad. Sci. U. S. A. 74:4848 (1977).

87. W. C. Breckenridge, J. A. Little, G. Steiner, A. Chow, and M. Poapst, Hypertriglyceridemia associated with deficiency of apolipoprotein C-II, N. Engl. J. Med. 298:1265 (1978).

88. E. J. Schaefer, D. M. Foster, L. L. Jenkins, F. T. Lindgren, M. Berman, R. I. Levy, and H. B. Brewer, Jr., The composition and metabolism of high density lipoprotein subfractions, Lipids 14:511 (1979).

89. R. S. Shulman, P. N. Herbert, D. S. Fredrickson, K. Wehrly, and H. B. Brewer, Jr., Isolation and alignment of the tryptic peptides of alanine apolipoprotein, an apolipoprotein from human plasma very low density lipoproteins, J. Biol. Chem. 249:4969 (1974).

90. W. V. Brown, R. I. Levy, and D. S. Fredrickson, Further charac-terization of apolipoproteins from the human plasma very low density lipoproteins, J. Biol. Chem. 245:6588 (1970).

91. J. J. Albers and A. M. Scanu, Isoelectric fractionation and characterization of polypeptides from human serum very low density lipoproteins, Biochim. Biophys. Acta 236:29 (1971).

92. J. D. Morrisett, J. S. K. David, H. J. Pownall, and A. M. Gotto, Jr., Interaction of an apolipoprotein (apolp-alanine) with phosphatidylcholine, Biochemistry 12:1290 (1973).

93. J. T. Sparrow, H. J. Pownall, F.-J. Hsu, L. E. Blumenthal, A. R. Culwell, and A. M. Gotto, Lipid binding by fragments of apolipoprotein C-III-1 obtained by thrombin cleavage,

Biochemistry 16:5427 (1977).

94. M. D. Curry, W. J. McConathy, J. D. Fesmire, and P. Alaupovic, Quantitative determination of human apolipoprotein C-III by electroimmunoassay, Biochim. Biophys. Acta 617:503 (1980).

95. A. M. Gotto, R. I. Levy, K. John, and D. S. Fredrickson, On the nature of the protein defect in abetalipoproteinemia, N. Engl. J. Med. 284:813 (1971).

96. L. A. Pottenger, L. E. Frazier, L. H. DuBien, G. S. Getz, and R. W. Wissler, Carbohydrate composition of lipoprotein apoproteins isolated from rat plasma and from the livers of rats fed orotic acid, Biochem. Biophys. Res. Commun. 54:770 (1973).

97. L. Henderson, P. Herbert, H. Windmueller, and R. Krauss, The C apolipoproteins of the orotic acid rat: A model for abetalipoproteinemia, Circulation 50:III-114 (1974).

98. W. V. Brown and M. L. Baginsky, Inhibition of lipoprotein lipase by an apoprotein of human very low density lipoprotein, Biochem. Biophys. Res. Commun. 46:375 (1972).

99. R. M. Krauss, P. N. Herbert, R. I. Levy, and D. S. Fredrickson, Further observations on the activation and inhibition of lipoprotein lipase by apolipoproteins, Circ. Res. 33:403 (1973).

100. W. J. McConathy and P. Alaupovic, Isolation and partial characterization of apolipoprotein D: A new protein moiety of the human plasma lipoprotein system, FEBS Lett. 37:178 (1973).

101. G. M. Kostner, Studies of the composition and structure of human serum lipoproteins: Isolation and partial characterization of apolipoprotein A-III, Biochim. Biophys. Acta 336:383 (1974).

102. J. J. Albers, M. C. Cheung, S. L. Ewens, and J. H. Tollefson, Characterization and immunoassay of apolipoprotein D, Atherosclerosis 39:395 (1981).

103. W. J. McConathy and P. Alaupovic, Studies on the isolation and partial characterization of apolipoprotein D and lipoprotein D of human plasma, Biochemistry 15:515 (1976).

104. T. Chajek and C. J. Fielding, Isolation and characterization of a human serum cholesteryl ester transfer protein, Proc. Natl. Acad. Sci. U. S. A. 75:3445 (1978).

105. M. D. Curry, W. J. McConathy, and P. Alaupovic, Quantitative determination of human apolipoprotein D by electroimmunoassay and radial immunodiffusion, Biochim. Biophys. Acta 491:232 (1977).

106. G. Kostner, Studies on the cofactor requirement for lecithin: cholesterol acyltransferase, Scand. J. Clin. Lab. Invest. 33, Suppl. 137:19 (1974).

107. J. J. Albers, Lecithin:cholesterol acyltransferase, Artery 5:61 (1979).

108. S. O. Olofsson and A. Gustafson, Degradation of high density lipoproteins (HDL) in vitro, Scand. J. Clin. Lab. Invest. 33, Suppl. 137:57 (1974).

109. P. E. Fielding and C. J. Fielding, A cholesteryl ester transfer
     complex in human plasma, Proc. Natl. Acad. Sci. U. S. A.
     77:3327 (1980).
110. R. E. Morton and D. B. Zilversmit, The separation of apolipo-
     protein D from cholesteryl ester transfer protein, Biochim.
     Biophys. Acta 663:350 (1981).
111. F. A. Shelburne and S. H. Quarfordt, A new apoprotein of
     human plasma very low density lipoproteins, J. Biol. Chem.
     249:1428 (1974).
112. V. I. Zannis and J. L. Breslow, Characterization of a unique
     human apolipoprotein E variant associated with type III
     hyperlipoproteinemia, J. Biol. Chem. 255:1759 (1980).
113. N. Tada, P. J. Nestel, N. Fidge, and G. Campbell, Abnormal
     apolipoprotein composition in alcoholic hepatitis, Biochim.
     Biophys. Acta 664:207 (1981).
114. N. Tada, N. Fidge, and P. Nestel, Identification and charac-
     terization of mixed disulphide complexes of E apoprotein
     in high density lipoprotein of subjects with acute alco-
     holic hepatitis, Biochem. Biophys. Res. Commun. 90:297
     (1979).
115. P. N. Herbert, R. J. Heinen, L. L. Bausserman, K. M. Lynch,
     L. O. Henderson, and T. A. Musliner, Abetalipoproteinemia
     and hypobetalipoproteinemia: Questions still exceed in-
     sights, in:"Atherosclerosis V. Proceedings of the Fifth
     International Symposium on Atherosclerosis," A. M. Gotto,
     Jr., L. C. Smith, and B. Allen, Eds., Springer-Verlag,
     New York (1980).
116. G. Utermann, Isolation and partial characterization of an
     arginine-rich apolipoprotein from human plasma very low
     density lipoproteins: apolipoprotein E, Hoppe-Seylers Z.
     Physiol. Chem. 356:1113 (1975).
117. K. H. Weisgraber, S. C. Rall, Jr., and R. W. Mahley, Human E
     apoprotein heterogeneity. Cysteine-arginine interchanges
     in the amino acid sequence of the apoE isoforms, J. Biol.
     Chem. 256:9077 (1981).
118. G. R. Warnick, C. Mayfield, J. J. Albers, and W. R. Hazzard,
     Gel isoelectric focusing method for specific diagnosis of
     familial hyperlipoproteinemia type 3, Clin. Chem. 25:279
     (1979).
119. G. Utermann, M. Hees, and A. Steinmetz, Polymorphism of apo-
     lipoprotein E and occurrence of dysbetalipoproteinaemia in
     man, Nature 269:604 (1977).
120. G. Utermann, G. Albrecht, and A. Steinmetz, Polymorphism of
     apolipoprotein E. I. Methodological aspects and diagnosis
     of hyperlipoproteinemia type III without ultracentrifuga-
     tion, Clin. Genet. 14:351 (1978).
121. R. J. Havel, L. Kotite, J.-L. Vigne, J. P. Kane, P. Tun,
     Nancy Phillips, and G. C. Chen, Radioimmunoassay of human
     arginine-rich apolipoprotein, apoprotein E, J. Clin. Invest.
     66:1351 (1980).

122. J. M. Falko, G. Schonfeld, J. L. Witztum, J. B. Kolar, S. W. Wiedman, and R. Steelman, Effects of diet on apoprotein E levels and on the apoprotein E subspecies in human plasma lipoproteins, J. Clin. Endocrinol. Metab. 50:521 (1980).

123. V. I. Zannis and J. L. Breslow, Human very low density lipoprotein apolipoprotein E isoprotein polymorphism is explained by genetic variation and posttranslational modification, Biochemistry 20:1033 (1981).

124. V. I. Zannis, P. W. Just, and J. L. Breslow, Human apolipoprotein E isoprotein subclasses are genetically determined, Am. J. Hum. Genet. 33:11 (1981).

125. T. L. Innerarity and R. W. Mahley, Enhanced binding by cultured human fibroblasts of apoE-containing lipoproteins as compared with low density lipoproteins, Biochemistry 17:1440 (1978).

126. Y. -s. Chao, E. E. Windler, G. C. Chen, and R. J. Havel, Hepatic catabolism of rat and human lipoproteins in rats treated with 17αethinyl estradiol, J. Biol. Chem. 254:11360 (1979).

127. R. J. Havel, Y. -s. Chao, E. E. Windler, L. Kotite, and L. S. S. Guo, Isoprotein specificity in the hepatic uptake of apolipoprotein E and the pathogenesis of familial dysbetalipoproteinemia. Proc. Natl. Acad. Sci. U. S. A. 77:4349 (1980).

128. R. E. Gregg, L. A. Zech, E. J. Schaefer, and H. B. Brewer, Jr., Type III hyperlipoproteinemia: Defective metabolism of an abnormal apolipoprotein E, Science 211:584 (1981).

129. C. B. Blum, L. Aron, and R. Sciacca, Radioimmunoassay studies of human apolipoprotein E, J. Clin. Invest. 66:1240 (1980).

130. R. S. Kushwaha, W. R. Hazzard, P. W. Wahl, and J. J. Hoover, Type III hyperlipoproteinemia: Diagnosis in whole plasma by apolipoprotein E immunoassay, Ann. Int. Med. 87:509 (1977).

131. J. D. Morrisett, R. L. Jackson, and A. M. Gotto, Jr., Lipid-protein interactions in the plasma lipoproteins, Biochim. Biophys. Acta 472:93 (1977).

132. R. I. Roth, R. L. Jackson, H. J. Pownall, and A. M. Gotto, Jr., Interaction of plasma "arginine-rich" apolipoprotein with dimyristoylphosphatidylcholine, Biochemistry 16:5030 (1977).

133. S. -O. Olofsson, W. J. McConathy, and P. Alaupovic, Isolation and partial characterization of a new acidic apolipoprotein (apolipoprotein F) from high density lipoproteins of human plasma, Biochemistry 17:1032 (1978).

134. M. Ayrault-Jarrier, J.-F. Alix, and J. Polonovski, Une nouvelle proteine des lipoproteines du serum humain: isolement et caracterisation partielle d'une apolipoproteine G, Biochimie 60:65 (1978).

135. Y. Nakaya, E. J. Schaefer, and H. B. Brewer, Jr., Activation of human post heparin lipoprotein lipase by apolipoprotein H (β_2-glycoprotein I), Biochem. Biophys. Res. Commun. 95:1168 (1980).

136. E. Polz and G. M. Kostner, The binding of β_2-glycoprotein-I

to human serum lipoproteins, FEBS Lett. 102:183 (1979).

137. H. E. Schultze, K. Heide, and H. Haupt, Über ein bisher unbe-
      kanntes niedermolekulares β2-Globulin des Humanserums,
      Naturwissenschaften 48:719 (1961).

138. E. Polz and G. M. Kostner, Binding of β2-glycoprotein-1 to
      intralipid: determination of the dissociation constant,
      Biochem. Biophys. Res. Commun. 90:1305 (1979).

139. E. Polz, G. M. Kostner, and A. Holasek, Studies on the protein
      composition of human serum very low density lipoproteins:
      demonstration of the β2-glycoprotein-1, Hoppe-Seyler's Z.
      Physiol. Chem. 360:1061 (1979).

140. T. Sata, R. J. Havel, L. Kotite, and J. P. Kane, New protein
      in human blood plasma, rich in proline, with lipid-binding
      properties, Proc. Natl. Acad. Sci. U. S. A. 73:1063 (1976).

141. E. P. Benditt and N. Eriksen, Amyloid protein SAA is associated
      with high density lipoprotein from human serum, Proc. Natl.
      Acad. Sci. U. S. A. 74:4025 (1977).

142. L. L. Bausserman, P. N. Herbert, and K. P. W. J. McAdam,
      Heterogeneity of human serum amyloid A proteins, J. Exp.
      Med. 152:641 (1980).

143. B. Shore and V. Shore, Isolation and characterization of poly-
      peptides of human serum lipoproteins, Biochemistry 8:4510
      (1969).

DETERMINANTS OF PLASMA HIGH DENSITY

LIPOPROTEIN CONCENTRATIONS

Peter N. Herbert, Paul D. Thompson, and Richard S. Shulman

Brown University Program in Medicine, Divisions of
Cardiology, and Nutrition and Metabolism, The Miriam
Hospital, Providence, Rhode Island, USA 02906

The inverse relationship between the plasma concentration of high density lipoproteins (HDL) and the prevalence and incidence of the complications of atherosclerosis is as well defined as any putative risk factor (see reference 1 for a recent review). Elsewhere in this volume, Dr. Kornitzer reviews criteria for inferring risk factor causality. When these are applied to assess the evidence linking low HDL levels to atherogenesis, a number of tentative conclusions are possible. The power of association of low HDL-cholesterol concentrations with coronary heart disease is as great or greater than any other lipid or lipoprotein factor,[2] and a dose-effect relationship has been suggested in two studies.[2,3] The observation has been repeatedly confirmed,[1-8] is independent of other "risk" factors,[2-4] and indeed appears to have predictive power.[6-8] Although an animal model has not yet been developed, logical pathogenetic mechanisms can readily be postulated. We first consider in this chapter the possible role of HDL in cholesterol homeostasis at the level of the arterial wall. The roles of genes, diet, activity, habits, drugs, and state of health as determinants of HDL levels are then reviewed.

HDL AND CHOLESTEROL BALANCE IN THE ARTERIAL WALL

The Problem

While the inverse statistical association between atherosclerosis risk and HDL levels is powerful, it must be appreciated that the task of direct demonstration of the role of HDL in cholesterol homeostasis at the arterial wall presents prodigous experimental problems. These problems are analogous to those previously encountered in attempts to demonstrate positive total-body cholesterol balance in hypercholesterolemia or atherosclerosis in general. Simply stated, the very small quantities of cholesterol that may accumulate in the arterial wall as a consequence of HDL deficiency are orders of magnitude smaller than the quantities of cholesterol that are cyclically coursing through various body compartments each day. Moreover, the accumulation of cholesterol as a consequence of imbalance in the concentrations of plasma lipoproteins is largely limited to the intimal and subintimal spaces. Even in familial hypercholesterolemia, most tissues in the body do not accumulate excess cholesterol.

Consider, for example, that the body of the typical 70kg man contains about 140g of cholesterol of which 75% is outside of the central nervous system. Blood contains about 10g of cholesterol (7% of the total) and half of this is in blood cells. Thus, only 5g of body cholesterol -- that present in the plasma compartment -- are directly relevant to the accretion of sterol in the arterial wall. Since the average plasma cholesterol difference between subjects at high or low risk for atheroscloerosis is only about 50 mg/dl, it can be calculated that the total quantity of plasma cholesterol accounting for this difference is of the order of 1g. When this "static" amount is contrasted with with the 3g of cholesterol normally entering and leaving the plasma compartment each day, or with the 12g to 40g of sterol moving through the enterohepatic circulation, it will be appreciated that the "background noise" of normal cholesterol traffic predictably will obscure the small daily imbalance in cholesterol transport that underlies atherogenesis. Studies relating HDL levels to total body cholesterol balance or even to plasma cholesterol and lipoprotein metabolism, therefore, are unlikely to reveal the link between HDL and arterial cholesterol deposition.

The Hypothesis and Supporting Evidence

As reviewed elsewhere in this volume, low density lipoproteins (LDL) are believed to be the source of the cholesterol which accumulates in atherosclerotic plaques.[9-11] HDL, in contrast, are thought to promote tissue cholesterol egress. HDL or their lipid-free proteins have been shown to promote cholesterol removal _in vitro_ from Landschütz ascites cells,[12-14] cultured human skin fibroblasts,[15-17] and mouse peritoneal macrophages.[18] The proteins of HDL alone appear minimally active or ineffective, but their cholesterol removing capacity is considerably enhanced after they are complexed with phospholipid.[13-15]

Interestingly, the smaller protein and phospholipid rich species of plasma HDL (HDL_3 and very high density lipoproteins) are able to decrease cell cholesterol content while the lipid rich HDL_2 fraction has the opposite effect.[17]

Questions naturally arise, therefore, concerning the possible existence of HDL subclasses that are particularly active in accepting tissue cholesterol and facilitating "reverse" cholesterol transport. It is possible that these are species enriched in protein and phospholipid. It should be recalled, however, that elevated HDL_2 concentrations are the hallmark of populations believed to be at low atherosclerosis risk; and HDL_2 is the subfraction correlating best with the total HDL-cholesterol concentration.[19] The population data are not necessarily at variance with the in vitro data since HDL_2 may be derived from HDL_3. But we must acknowledge that capacity to accept cellular cholesterol may not be the immediate or principle mechanism involved in the anti-atherogenic effect of HDL. HDL inhibition of LDL uptake by arterial wall cells, for example, may be more relevant in the decades over which atherosclerosis usually develops.[20]

HDL Origins and Fates

HDL contain more protein and less lipid (Fig. 1) than the other classes of plasma lipoproteins. They have α_1-electophoretic mobility and are often subdivided into ultracentrifugal fractions of density 1.063 to 1.120 (HDL_2) and 1.120 to 1.210 (HDL_3) g/ml. This subclassification of HDL has received considerable attention because, as noted above, variation in HDL_2 levels accounts for much of the interindividual differences in plasma HDL-cholesterol concentrations.[19] Relative to HDL_3, HDL_2 particles are larger and contain proportionately more unesterified cholesterol, triglyceride, and C-apoproteins. The relative proportions of the major HDL apoproteins also differ with an apo A-I/apo A-II weight ratio of about six in HDL_2, and of about three in HDL_3.

The intestine and liver can both synthesize the major HDL apolipoproteins, apo A-1 and apo A-II.[21-24] Newly secreted rat HDL of hepatic and intestinal origin (Fig. 2) are discoidal particles rich in phospholipid and cholesterol with little cholesteryl esters.[25,26] Such HDL from liver contain primarily apoE[25] and those from intestine mainly apo A-I.[26] Discoidal HDL cannot be visualized in normal human plasma suggesting a short life span. They are readily identified in the plasma of subjects with familial[27] or acquired[28] deficiencies of the enzyme lecithin cholesterol acyltransferase (LCAT), providing evidence that LCAT is involved in the generation of HDL of normal morphology (Fig. 2).

There is considerable circumstantial evidence that HDL modulate catabolism of the triglyceride rich lipoproteins. They serve as reservoirs for the C-apolipoproteins between tides of alimentary lipemia,[29] are preferred substrates for the LCAT reaction[30] which generates almost all the plasma cholesteryl esters, and they accept redundant surface material produced during chylomicron and very low density lipoprotein (VLDL) catabolism.[31-33] The latter phenomenon is

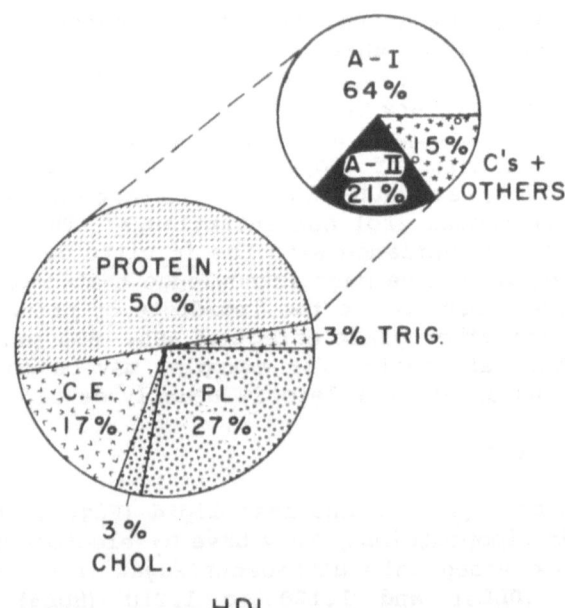

Fig.1. Chemical and protein composition of high density lipoproteins.
Phospholipid (PL) and cholesteryl esters (CE) are the major lipids
while the content of unesterified cholesterol (CHOL) and triglyceride
(TRIG) is quite low. Apolipoproteins A-I and A-II account for 85%
of the total protein; the three C-apolipoproteins, apo D, apo E, and
others comprise 15%.

thought to generate HDL directly in the blood stream (Fig. 2), and it
has been persuasively argued that plasma HDL levels are directly
related to tissue lipoprotein lipase activity and the efficiency of
chylomicron and VLDL triglyceride hydrolysis.[34] The validity of this
postulate is supported by the observation that subjects who either
lack lipoprotein lipase (type 1 hyperlipoproteinmia) or who elaborate
no chylomicrons and VLDL (abetalipoproteinemia) have HDL levels that
are typically half normal.

Our meager knowledge of tissue sites and mechanisms of HDL
catabolism raises more questions than are readily answered (Fig 3).
Lipoproteins, in general, pose special problems in this regard since
catabolism of each of the lipid classes and proteins comprising these
particles is probably under separate metabolic control. The phospholipids, unesterified cholesterol, cholesteryl esters, and triglycerides of HDL are in dynamic equilibrium with those in other lipo-

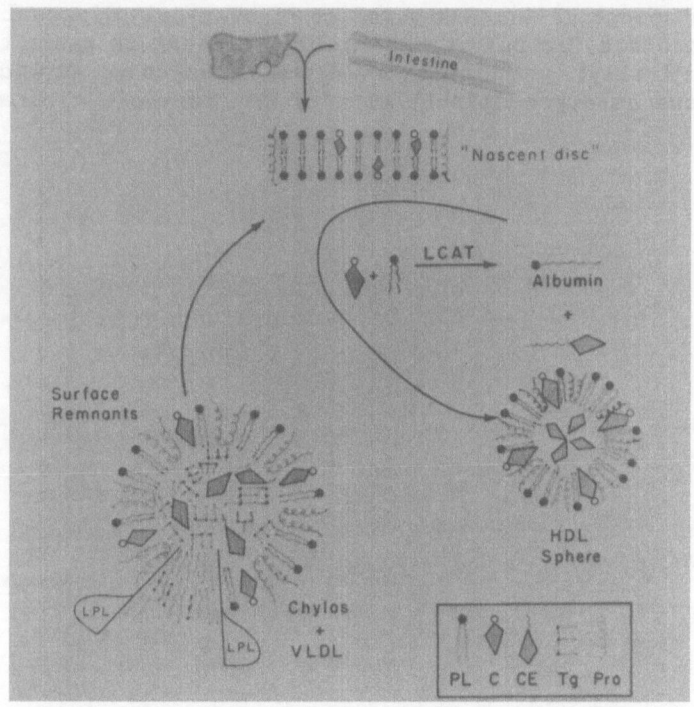

Fig. 2. Formation of normal HDL is completed in the plasma compartment. Discoidal particles, rich in unesterified cholesterol (C) and phospholipid (PL), are secreted by both liver and intestine. Similar "nascent" structures are derived from triglyceride-rich lipoprotein surface material, after triglyceride (Tg) hydrolysis by lipoprotein lipase (LPL) at the capillary endothelium. Cholesteryl esters (CE),which come to occupy the apolar core of spherical HDL, are produced when lecithin: cholesterol acyltransferase (LCAT) transfers a fatty acid from phosphatidyl choline to unesterified cholesterol. Albumin serves to accept lysolecithin which is produced as a byproduct of the LCAT reaction.

protein classes (or tissues) and function as components of larger metabolic pools. Since the A apoproteins are relatively unique to HDL, their synthesis and catabolism have been studied to probe effects specific to HDL. It is likely, however, that the biological fate of the HDL proteins is inextricably linked to that of the HDL lipids. Moreover, the HDL proteins can be viewed as vehicles whose cargo is in rapid flux, turning over at a much greater rate than the vehicles themselves. Knowledge of the eventual disposal of the vehicles, therefore, is only tangentially relevant to their transport function. Finally, available evidence does not implicate any specific tissue as a predominant site of HDL particle clearance from plasma.

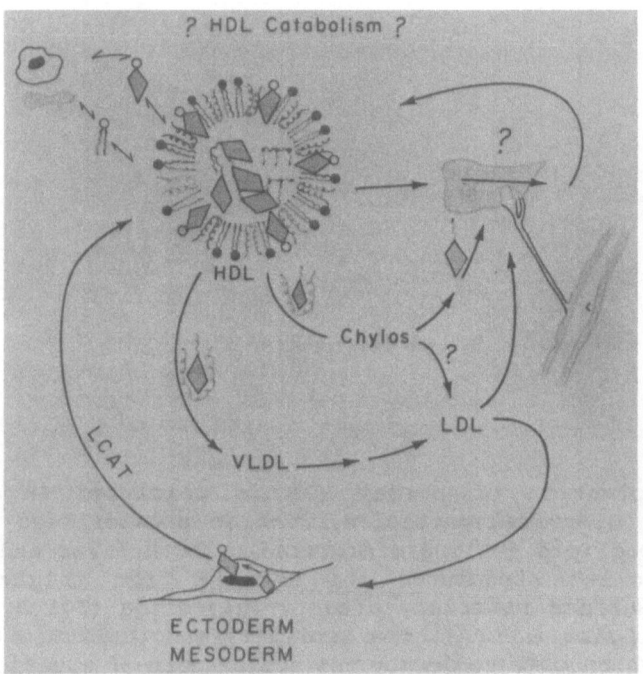

Fig. 3. Removal of intact HDL particles from the circulation may not be the major pathway for removal of HDL chemical components. Phospholipids and unesterified cholesterol from the HDL surface exchange with and transfer to lower density classes of lipoproteins and tissues. Net transfer of cholesteryl esters to both chylomicrons VLDL, and perhaps to the liver also occurs. A proportion of the cholesterol and cholesteryl esters participate in a futile cycle from HDL → VLDL → LDL → tissue → HDL. HDL apoproteins may be removed with intact particles or after they lose their lipoprotein moorings.

HDL-CHOLESTEROL LEVELS IN NORMALS AND SUBJECTS WITH CORONARY ARTERY DISEASE

The HDL-cholesterol level, estimated as the residual cholesterol in sera or plasma after precipitation of VLDL and LDL,[35] is the most widely employed measure of HDL concentration. Prepubertal boys and girls have very similar HDL-cholesterol levels while postpubertal women have levels 10-15 mg/dl greater than men (Table 1). Although estrogen levels fall dramatically in menopausal women, this change is not associated with alterations in HDL concentrations.

Typical differences in the HDL levels of controls and populations with clinically apparent coronary heart disease have been small and in the range of 3-4 mg/dl.[4,7,8] The magnitude of this difference has created considerable anxiety about the wisdom of applying the HDL-cholesterol test to the estimation of an individual's atherosclerotic risk. The anxiety relates to the poor precision and accuracy of the HDL-cholesterol measurement in many laboratories. Adequate quality control measures, however, can obviate the technical difficulties. It is also clear that the test is quite useful in the identification of individuals with profoundly low HDL levels, and in segregating subjects with hyperalphalipoproteinemia in whom mild elevations of the total cholesterol concentration do not connote atherosclerosis risk.

GENES AS DETERMINANTS OF HDL LEVELS

The largest study of familial interrelations of HDL levels reported to date showed a positive correlation only in pairs of first-degree relatives involving the mother, i.e., mother-son and mother-daughter; and in sib-sib pairs of the same sex where the correlation was quite striking.[38] As recognized by the investigators, "this pattern is not consistent either with sex-linked or with single-gene-dominant or recessive inheritance."

Similarly, in studies of familial aggregation of hyper-alpha-lipoproteinemia[39] the correlation between sibs of the same sex was impressive whereas brother-sister and parent-offspring correlations were weak or nonexistant. An analysis of 26 kindreds containing at least one subject with an HDL-cholesterol greater than 70 mg/dl suggested bimodality (and perhaps a major gene effect) in white but not black kindreds.[40] Only five of fifteen white families, however, demonstrated vertical transmission of the high HDL concentrations. Another study of 500 nuclear families failed to convincingly demonstrate a major gene effect in determining HDL levels.[41,42] Path analysis of the same data did suggest that genetic heritability accounted for about 30% of interindividual variance with cultural heritability accounting for 15%.[43]

Observations in small numbers of relatives of coronary heart

TABLE 1

Plasma High Density Lipoprotein Cholesterol Levels
Of White Males and Females in the United States*

Age	Males		Females	
		5-95th		5-95th
Years	Mean	Percentile	Mean	Percentile
>10	50	40-75	55	30-75
10-19	50	35-75	50	35-75
20-29	45	30-65	55	35-80
30-39	45	30-65	55	35-80
40-49	45	30-65	60	35-90
50-59	45	30-65	60	35-95
60-69	50	30-80	65	35-95
70+	50	30-80	60	35-95

Data from the North American Lipid Research Clinics[36,37]. The means and 5th and 95th percentiles have been rounded to the nearest 5 mg/dl. Recalculation of data by 10-year striata courtesy of Dr. Basil Rifkind, NHLBI, and adopted from reference 46.

disease victims have defined familial clustering of individuals with low HDL concentrations,[44,45] but environmental, cultural, and genetic effects could all have contributed. The best defined example of familial deficiency of HDL is Tangier disease.[46] The disorder is inherited as an autosomal trait. Heterozygotes have HDL levels that are about 50% of controls and homozygotes have no detectable normal HDL. Only 26 homozygotes with this condition have been recognized indicating that the trait does not account for a significant fraction of hypoalphalipoproteinemic subjects in a general population.

Racial differences in HDL levels have been defined but there is no compelling evidence that these have a genetic basis. Black men and women have higher HDL-cholesterols than whites,[47] and HDL levels are relatively high in the Japanese compared with those reported for Western populations.[48] In contrast, white men and women in London, Naples, Uppsala, and Genoa have different total cholesterol and triglyceride distributions but quite similar HDL-cholesterol concentrations.[49]

DIET AS A DETERMINANT OF HDL LEVELS

Total Fat and Carbohydrate

Vegetarians ingest as many calories as subjects on unrestricted diets but derive 25% fewer calories from fat while consuming proportionately more carbohydrate. Their HDL levels are about 10 mg/dl less than age and sex matched controls.[50] School children in developing countries in Africa and Asia have not only lower total cholesterol levels but HDL-cholesterol concentrations that are at least 10 mg/dl less than children in Europe and the USA.[51] Tarahumara Indians of northwestern Mexico, famous as endurance runners, consume only 10% of total calories as fat and have HDL-cholesterol levels of 25 mg/dl.[52] Finally, substitution of carbohydrate for fat in the diets of five hyperlipoproteinemics and two normal subjects increased fasting triglycerides and lowered the HDL-cholesterol.[53]

These observations do not distinguish between independent effects of high carbohydrate or low fat diets. But subjects such as endurance athletes, who consume large quantities of carbohydrate and relatively normal amounts of fat, have high rather than low HDL levels.[54] It seems probable, therefore, that habitually low fat rather than high carbohydrate diets result in lower HDL concentrations. Moreover, any dietary stimulus that increases serum triglycerides and reduces the efficiency of chylomicron and VLDL catabolism may decrease HDL levels by reducing the amount of lipoprotein surface material available for incorporation into HDL (Fig. 3).

Cholesterol

One diet survey demonstrated a positive correlation between reported egg consumption and the HDL-cholesterol level[54] and certain studies cited above relating fat (triglyceride) consumption and HDL levels might be alternatively interpreted in terms of dietary cholesterol. Cholesterol feeding in animals may induce formation of an abnormal lipoprotein of α-mobility[55] which is also present in small quantities in humans consuming high cholesterol diets.[56]

Conversely, other population surveys have not linked dietary cholesterol intake and plasma HDL-cholesterol.[57] It is also possible that HDL-cholesterol increases in subjects receiving supplements such as egg yolk may well be attributable to the fat rather than cholesterol content of eggs.[58] Our personal experience suggests that the contribution of dietary cholesterol to the total HDL-cholesterol is small and indeed may be transient.

Saturated and Polyunsaturated Fat

Maintaining total dietary fat content constant while substituting polyunsaturated fat for saturated fat produces a fall in both plasma total and HDL cholesterol concentrations (Table 2). The effect may be greater in men than women,[63] and in one study was associated with reduced synthesis as opposed to increased catabolism of apoprotein A-I.[61] It is not known if the lowering of HDL is caused by the addition of polyunsaturated fat or the isocaloric removal of

TABLE 2

Alteration of Dietary P:S Ratio
And Plasma HDL-Cholesterol Concentrations

Number Subjects	Δ P:S	Change in Cholesterol Total	HDL	Reference
23	. 2 →2.4	−16%	0%	59
5	. 1 →1.0	− 9%	+1	60
4	.25 →4.0	−24%	−33%	61
9	? →2.0	−23%	−15%	62
30	. 3 →2.0	−10 to 20%	−10 to 36%	63

saturated fat. These alternatives should be distinguished experimentally and the information applied in the design of hypocholesterolemic diets. It is the experience of many clinicians that the HDL and LDL lowering effects of P:S altered diets are separable in outpatients consuming diest of P:S~1,and anecdotal testimony supporting this observation has been published.[64]

Total Calories

HDL-cholesterol levels vary inversely with body mass.[65,66] In the Lipid Research Clinics prevalence study, mean HDL-cholesterol levels for individuals at the Quetelet (weight/height^2) tenth percentile were 3 mg/dl higher than those at the fiftieth percentile; and the latter, in turn, were 3 to 4 mg/dl higher than those at the ninetieth percentile.[65] Short-term caloric restriction in obese subjects usually produces a fall in HDL levels[67,68] that may be related to both decreases in chylomicron and VLDL production (Fig. 2) and reduced lipoprotein lipase activity.[68] Obese subjects who are able to maintain long-term weight reductions, however, have demonstrated HDL cholesterol increases of more than 50%.[69] Our laboratory's experience with modest weight losses (5 kg) in obese women suggests that smaller increases (3-4 mg/dl) in HDL-cholesterol are more typical.

HABITUAL EXERCISE AS A DETERMINANT OF HDL LEVELS

Populations that by virtue of life style,[70] work,[71] or leisure-time activity[72-74] engage in habitual strenuous physical activity have greater than average HDL concentrations. Endurance training of sedentary individuals, moreover, in some[75-78] but not all[79-82] trials has led to an increase in plasma HDL concentrations. In general, studies employing less intensive exercise regimens induced little or no change in HDL levels, and minimal changes are observed when exercise and caloric restriction are combined. Diet changes during training are probably common and have not been excluded as important variables in most studies of the effects of exercise.

It is unlikely that higher HDL levels are an acute effect of exercise. We have not observed changes in HDL levels after single intensive exercise sessions in trained or untrained subjects; nor did a 42 km footrace increase the HDL concentrations of twelve marathoners.[84] Similarly, a ten day walk of 50 km a day without food produced no increase in HDL cholesterol.[85] A 70 km cross-country ski race was reported to increase HDL-cholesterol levels by 17%[86]; but samples were analyzed three years after the race and this may have introduced artifacts since the reported HDL levels were quite low. Most available evidence, therefore, suggests that increases in HDL levels are an effect of regular rather than sporadic exercise. Indeed, cessation of exercise in trained subjects does not appear to produce any immediate lowering of HDL concentrations.[87]

Muscle does not secrete lipoproteins so regular endurance exercise must mediate its effects through changes in hepatic and intestinal lipoprotein production, or in peripheral lipoprotein catabolism. We have found that runners consume about 23% more calories than their sedentary counterparts, and these additional calories are primarily carbohydrate. Thus VLDL turnover may exceed that in normals. In addition, lipoprotein lipase activity is greater in adipose tissue of trained men and women[88] and enzyme activity increases when previously sedentary subjects engage in regular vigorous physical activity.[78] Since endurance athletes character- istically have low plasma triglycerides,[89] it is likely that their catabolism of chylomicrons and VLDL is highly efficient.[34] This could directly provide more surface lipids for HDL formation (Fig. 2).

DRUGS AS DETERMINANTS OF HDL LEVELS

Alcohol

Three surveys of large populations in the USA,[90,91] Hawaii,[92] and Great Britain[93] have demonstrated a graded direct relationship between alcohol consumption and HDL-cholesterol levels. Differences between teetotalers and moderately heavy imbibers of ethanol exceeded 10 mg/dl. Even in physician marathoners, alcohol consumption contributes to the variation in HDL-cholesterol concentrations.[94]

After recent drinking bouts, 87% of chronic alcoholics admitted to an alcohol clinic had increased HDL levels that normalized within two weeks.[95] Nine healthy young men who consumed 75g of ethanol each day for five weeks increased their alphalipoprotein concentrations by almost 30%, with a very gradual return to baseline values in the four weeks after alcohol cessation.[96] No correlation between indices of liver damage and alphalipoprotein concentrations was found in the chronic alcoholics, although 87% had γ-glutamyltransferase levels in the abnormal range.[95] The student drinkers increased their serum and hepatic levels of γ-glutamyltransferase, and serum and liver trigly-ceride levels also rose transiently.[96] Other serum enzymes reflecting liver function did not change in a consistent pattern but these observations raise the obvious possibility that mild hepatic damage may occur paripassu when ethanol ingestion raises HDL levels.

The effects of ethanol on either lipoprotein synthesis or lipoprotein lipase activity may account for the elevation of HDL concentrations. Alcohol consumption leads to increased hepatic secretion of VLDL[97-99] which in turn may provide precursors of HDL lipids (Fig. 2). Alcohol is known to induce smooth endoplasmic reticulum hyperplasia[96] and may directly or indirectly "induce" apolipoprotein synthesis. A third possible mechanism involves stimulation of adipose tissue lipoprotein lipase activity which was observed in one prospective study.[96]

Drugs Affecting Lipoprotein Metabolism

Most of the drugs prescribed to lower plasma cholesterol or triglycerides also affect the concentration or distribution of HDL. Bile acid sequestrants (cholestyramine and colestipol) do not consis-tently alter HDL-cholesterol levels.[100-102] These drugs have been reported to cause slight increases in apo A-I[102-103] and in the relative amount of HDL_2,[103] and reductions of apo A-II.[103,104] D-thyroxine also has little or no effect on HDL levels.[105]

Treatment with clofibrate is accompanied in some but not all cases by an increase in various indices of HDL mass. Mean HDL-cholesterol rose from 41 to 49 mg/dl, apo A-I from 126 to 137 mg/dl, and apo A-II from 34 to 43 mg/dl when 14 mild hyperlipidemics were treated with clofibrate.[102] Conversely, discontinuation of clofibrate therapy in ten hyperlipidemic subjects produced a fall of 7 mg/dl in HDL-cholesterol and 13 mg/dl in apo A-I.[106] The most dramatic changes are seen in type 3 hyperlipoproteinemia where increases of 10 to 15 mg/dl in HDL-cholesterol are not unusual.[107] The effect of clofibrate on HDL levels may relate to stimulation of lipoprotein lipase activity[108] (Fig. 2). It is not known if lipase stimulation invariably accompanies clofibrate administration, and whether the many subjects with low HDL levels unaffected by clofibrate[109] can be segregated by their lipoprotein lipase response.

Nicotinic acid also increases HDL levels in many but not all patients with hypoalphalipoproteinemia. Normal subjects increase their HDL-cholesterol levels by 7 to 19 mg/dl with dramatic increases in their HDL_2:HDL_3 mass ratios while receiving 3g of nicotinic acid each day.[110,111] These changes are accompanied by a fall in serum triglycerides and in the catabolic rates of the proteins of HDL.[110,111] In most hypertriglyceridemic subjects much less striking effects are seen despite considerable falls in serum triglycerides.[112] Inefficient catabolism of triglyceride rich lipoproteins, unaffected by nicotinic acid, may account for the different response in the latter patients.

Probucol is the only lipid-lowering drug that consistently lowers HDL levels,[113] probably by substantially reducing synthesis of apo A-I.[114] In a group of nine subjects demonstrating a 20% reduction of HDL-cholesterol there was a 6% fall in plasma apo A-I concentrations. HDL-cholesterol fell an average of 30% in ten other familial hypercholesterolemics, and there was a 34% reduction of apo A-I in these subjects.[115] The mechanism involved is not known but it may involve reduction of apo A-I synthesis in the intestine.[114]

Other Drugs

Subjects exposed to chlorinated hydrocarbon pesticides, i.e., lindane and DDT, have elevated HDL cholesterol concentrations[116] which fall when exposure is terminated.[117] Use of the antiepileptic drug phenytoin, another inducer of hepatic microsomal enzymes, is also associated with above average HDL-cholesterol levels.[118] Mono- and bicyclic terpenes, prescribed for the dissolution of gall stones, have variable effects but in general increase HDL-cholesterol concentrations.[119]

Two population studies in the USA[120,121] showed an inverse relationship between cigarette smoking and HDL-cholesterols while a third in Scandinavia failed to find an association.[122] In the Lipid Research Clinics Program Prevalence Study, cigarette smokers had lower HDL-cholesterol levels than nonsmokers, and the difference was greater in women (9 mg/dl) than in men (5 mg/dl). The effect correlated with the number of cigarettes smoked and was independent of other variables such as age, obesity, alcohol consumption, and regular exercise.[120] Apo A-I and apo A-II levels are also lower in smokers.[123] HDL-cholesterol concentrations have been lowered by the administration of propranolol[124] and chlorthalidone[125] to hypertensive patients. The reductions with these drugs have averaged 5 to 7 mg/dl.

SEX HORMONES AS DETERMINANTS OF HDL LEVELS

Use of estrogenic hormones is associated with higher HDL-cholesterol levels while use of progestins has the opposite effect. Changes in HDL levels with use of mixed formulations for oral contraception depend on the relative amounts of estrogens and progestins.[126] The relationship between endogenous estrogens and HDL levels, however, is not as well defined. Natural menopause is not associated with a fall in HDL in women since increasing age is positively associated with HDL-cholesterol concentrations.[1,126] Plasma estradiol levels correlate only weakly (r = 0.23), whereas plasma sex hormone binding globulin (SHBG) levels correlate strongly (r = 0.53) with HDL-cholesterol concentrations.[127] The latter relationship suggests common determinants rather than cause and effect.

Testosterone administration appears to reduce HDL levels[128-130] and HDL-cholesterol falls in males after puberty.[1] Conversely, in a small group of healthy young men, a positive association between HDL-cholesterol and serum testosterone was observed,[131] whereas no association could be documented in another study.[132] It appears that while pharmacologic doses of exogenous testosterone reproducibly lower HDL levels, there is no direct relationship between endogenously produced hormone and HDL concentrations. This paradox is not dissimilar to that already noted for estrogens and HDL.

DISEASES AS DETERMINANTS OF HDL LEVELS

Any illness with deleterious effects on the nutritional status, activity patterns, hepatic and gastrointestinal function, or endocrine balance of man can potentially alter the concentration, composition, or particle distribution of HDL. A few illustrative examples are cited here but an exhaustive treatment of this subject is outside the scope of this review.

Liver Disease

The liver synthesizes both HDL apolipoproteins and the plasma enzyme lecithin: cholesterol acyltransferase (LCAT). LCAT is necessary to produce normal HDL in the plasma compartment (Fig. 2). Severe parenchymal liver disease with cirrhosis may be associated with low concentrations of HDL and other plasma lipoproteins. HDL may actually be absent from the plasma of subjects with certain viral illnesses or lymphomatous infiltration of the liver; and with spontaneous or induced regression of disease the HDL concentrations can return to normal.

Alcoholic hepatitis with intrahepatic cholestasis, primary biliary cirrhosis, and extrahepatic biliary obstruction may produce HDL changes like those in familial LCAT deficiency.[28] During resolution of alcoholic hepatitis or treatment of primary bilary cirrhosis with anionic exchange resins the HDL levels may transiently reach very high values before normalizing. This latter phenomenon may relate to LCAT mediated clearance of the phospholipid and cholesterol enriched Lp-X lipoprotein which often accumulates in plasma in cholestasis.[133]

Mild or clinically silent liver disease may be associated with greater than average HDL concentrations. In the Lipid Research Clinics Program Prevalence Study, subjects with high serum bilirubin or serum aspartate aminotransferase (AST, SGOT) values had higher HDL cholesterol levels.[134] History of gall bladder disease, interestingly is associated with a reduced concentration of HDL-cholesterol.[135]

Diabetes Mellitus

Profound insulin deficiency with hyperlipidemia and ketoacidosis is regularly associated with striking transient depression of HDL levels. This is likely due to the lipoprotein lipase deficiency (Fig. 2) which characterizes this disorder.

An inverse relationship between diabetic control and HDL levels was suggested in a study correlating HDL-cholesterol and glycosylated hemoglobin concentrations,[136] a result that was shortly challenged.[137] Moreover, insulin and HDL-cholesterol levels were found to be inversely correlated in Samoans.[138] In the latter study it is probable that obesity was common to both above average insulins and lower than normal HDL-cholesterols.

Treatment of patients having type 1 diabetes mellitus with continuous subcutaneous insulin infusions has led to an 8 mg/dl increase in mean HDL-cholesterol over 26 weeks.[139] Therapy with oral hypoglycemics, in contrast, was associated with lower HDL-cholesterols than found in controls, or patients receiving insulin or diet alone. It is not known if the salubrious effect of insulin in these patients is mediated through lipoprotein lipase or another aspect of lipoprotein metabolism.

Other Disorders

Subjects hospitalized for a wide variety of maladies usually show a fall in HDL levels that is proportional to the severity of their illness. Patients with myocardial infarction or major surgery, for example, demonstrate HDL-cholesterol decreases of 10 mg/dl that reach a nadir seven to ten days after infarction or surgery. This effect may have multiple causes that include intravenous overhydration, radical diet changes, medications, and marked restriction of activity.

Other disease related influences on HDL concentrations will undoubtedly surface. Increased HDL-cholesterol in obstructive pulmonary disease has recently been described and attributed to the work of breathing in these patients.[140] An alternative possibility, not excluded, is that drugs such as theophyllines, almost universally used, may affect lipoprotein metabolism.

Acknowledgements:

Work described herein that was performed in the author's laboratory was supported in part by a grant from Reynold's Industries, The Miriam Hospital Cardiology and Atherosclerosis Research Trust, and N.I.H. Grants HL23789, HL28467 and HLO1003.

REFERENCES

1.   G. Heiss, N.J. Johnson, S. Reiland, C.E. Davis, H.A. Tyroler,The epidemiology of plasma high-density lipoprotein cholesterol levels, **Circulation** 62(IV):116-136 (1980).

2.   W.B. Kannel, W.P. Castelli, T. Gordon, Cholesterol in the prediction of atherosclerotic disease, **Ann Intern Med** 90:85-91 (1979).

3.   G.G. Rhoads, C.L. Gulbrandsen, A. Kagan, Serum lipoproteins and coronary heart disease in a population study of hawaii japanese men, **N Engl J Med** 294:293-298 (1976).

4.   W.P. Castelli, J.T. Doyle, T. Gordon, C.G. Hames, M.C. Hjortland, S.B. Hulley, A. Kagan, W.J. Zukel, HDL cholesterol and other lipids in coronary heart disease, **Circulation** 55:767- 772 (1977).

5.   K. Berg, A. Borresen, G. Dahlen, Serum high density lipoprotein and atherosclerotic heart disease, **Lancet** i:499-501 (1976).

6.   T. Gordon, W.P. Castelli, M.C. Hjortland, W.B. Kannel, T.R. Dawber, High density lipoprotein as a protective factor against coronary heart disease, **Am J Med** 62:707-714 (1977)

7.   N.E. Miller, D.S. Thelle, O.H. Forde, O.D. Mjos, The Tromoso heart study, **Lancet** i:965-968 (1977).

8.   U. Goldbourt, J.H. Medalie, High density lipoprotein cholesterol and incidence of coronary heart disease -- the Israeli ischemic heart disease study, **Am J Epidemiol** 109:296-308 (1979).

9.   D.M. Kramsch, W. Hollander, The interaction of serum and arterial lipoproteins with elastin of the arterial intima and its role in the lipid accumulation in atherosclerotic plaques, **J Clin Invest** 52:236-247 (1973).

10. E.B. Smith, R.S. Slater, J.A. Hunter, Quantitative studies on
     fibrinogen and low-density lipoprotein in human aortic
     intima, **Atherosclerosis** 18:479-487 (1973).

11. H.F. Hoff, R.L. Jackson, S.J. Mao, A. M. Gotto, Jr.,
     Localization of low-density lipoproteins in athero-
     sclerotic lesions from human normolipemics employing a
     purified florescent-labeled antibody, **Biochim Biophys Acta**
     351:407-415 (1974).

12. O. Stein, Y. Stein, The removal of cholesterol from Landschutz
     ascites cells by high-density apolipoprotein, **Biochim
     Biophys Acta** 326:232-244 (1973).

13. Y. Stein, M.C. Glandeaud, M. Fainaru, O. Stein, The removal of
     cholesterol from aortic smooth muscle cells in culture and
     Landschutz ascites cells by fractions of human high-density
     apolipoprotein, **Biochim Biophys Acta** 380:106-118 (1975).

14. R. L. Jackson, A. M. Gotto, O. Stein, Y. Stein, A comparative
     study on the removal of cellular lipids from Landschutz
     ascites cells by human plasma apolipoproteins, **J Biol Chem**
     250:7204-7209 (1975).

15. O. Stein, M. Fainaru, Y. Stein, The role of lysophospha-
     tidylcholine and apolipoprotein a_1 in the cholesterol-
     removing capacity of lipoprotein-deficient serum in tissue
     culture, **Biochim Biophys Acta** 574:495-504 (1979).

16. R.J. Daniels, L.S. Guertler, T.S. Parker, D. Steinberg, Studies
     on the rate of efflux of cholesterol from cultured human
     skin fibroblasts, **J Biol Chem** 256:4978-4983 (1981).

17. J.F. Oram, J.J. Albers, M.C. Cheung, E.L. Bierman, The effects
     of subfractions of high density lipoprotein on cholesterol
     efflux from cultured fibroblasts, **J Biol Chem** 256:8348-8356
     (1981).

18. Y.K. Ho, M.S. Brown, J.L. Goldstein, Hydrolysis and excretion of
     cytoplasmic cholesteryl esters by macrophages: stimulation
     by high density lipoprotein and other agents, **J Lipid Res**
     21:391-398 (1980).

19. D.W. Anderson, A.V. Nichols, S.S. Pan, F.T. Lindgren, High
     density lipoprotein distribution, **Atherosclerosis** 29:161-
     179 (1978).

20. T.E. Carew, S.B. Hayes, T. Koschinsky, D. Steinberg, A mechanism by which high-density lipoproteins may slow the atherogenic process, **Lancet** i:1315:1317 (1976).

21. H.G. Windmueller, P.N. Herbert, R.I Levy, Biosynthesis of lymph and plasma lipoprotein apoproteins by isolated perfused rat liver and intestine, **J Lipid Res** 14:215-223 (1973).

22. T.E. Felker, M. Fainaru, R.L. Hamilton, R.J. Havel, Secretion of the arginine-rich and a-i apolipoproteins by the isolated perfused rate liver, **J Lipid Res** 18:465-472 (1977).

23. G. Assmann, A. Capurso, E. Smootz, U. Wellner, Apoprotein A metabolism in Tangier disease, **Atherosclerosis** 30:321-332 (1978).

24. R.M. Glickman, A. Kilgore, J. Khorana, Chylomicron apoprotein localization within rat intestinal epithelium: studies of normal and impaired lipid absorption, **J Lipid Res** 19:260-268 (1978).

25. R.L. Hamilton, M.C. Williams, C.J. Fielding, R.J. Havel, Discoidal bilayer structure of nascent high density lipoproteins from perfused rat liver, **J Clin Invest** 58:667-680 (1976).

26. P.H. Green, A.R. Tall, R.M. Glickman, Rat intestine secretes discoid high density lipoprotein, **J Clin Invest** 61:528-534 (1978).

27. C.D. Mitchell, W.C. King, K.R. Applegate, T. Forte, J.A. Glomset, K.R. Norum, E. Gjone, Characterization of apolipoprotein E-rich high density lipoproteins in familial lecithin: cholesterol acyltransferase deficiency, **J Lipid Res** 21:625-634 (1980).

28. S.M. Sabesin, H.L. Hawkins, L. Kuiken, J.B. Ragland, Abnormal plasma lipoproteins and lecithin-cholesterol acyltransferase deficiency in alcoholic liver disease, **Gastroenterology** 72:510-518 (1977).

29. R.J. Havel, J.P. Kane, E.O. Balasse, N. Segel, L.V. Basso, Splanchnic metabolism of free fatty acids and production of triglycerides of very low density lipoproteins in normotriglyceridemic and hypertriglyceridemic humans, **J Clin Invest** 49:2017 (1970).

30. C.J. Fielding, P.E. Fielding, Purification and substrate specificity of lecithin-cholesterol acyltransferase from

human plasma, **FEBS Lett** 15:335-358 (1971).

31. T.G. Redgrave, D.M. Small, Quantitation of the transfer of surface phospholipid of chylomicrons to the high density lipoprotein fraction during the catabolism of chylomicrons in the rat, **J Clin Invest** 64:162 (1979).

32. A.R. Tall, P.H. Green, R.M. Glickman, J.W. Riley, Metabolic fat of chylomicron phospholipids and apoproteins in the rat, **J Clin Invest** 64:977-989 (1979).

33. J.R. Patsch, A.M. Gotto,Jr., T. Olivecrona, S. Eisenberg, Formation of high density lipoprotein$_2$-like particles during lipolysis of very low density lipoproteins in vitro, **Proc Natl Acad Sci** 75:4519-4523 (1978).

34. M. Kekki, Lipoprotein-lipase action determining plasma high density lipoprotein cholesterol level in adult normolipaemics, **Atherosclerosis** 37:143-150 (1980).

35. J.J. Albers, G.R. Warnick, M.C. Chenng, Quantitation of high density lipoproteins, **Lipids** 13:926-932 (1978).

36. G. Heiss, I. Tamir, C.E. Davis, H.A. Tyroler, B.M. Rifkind, G. Schnofeld, D. Jacobs, I.D. Frantz, Jr., Lipoprotein-cholesterol distributions in selected North American populations: The Lipid Research Clinics Program Prevalence Study, **Circulation** 61:302-315 (1980).

37. R. Beaglehole, D.C. Trost, I. Tamir, P. Kwiterovich, C.J. Glueck, W. Insull, B. Christensen, Plasma high-density lipoprotein cholesterol in children and young adults, **Circulation** 62(IV):83-92 (1980).

38. O.D. Mjos, D.S. Thelle, O.H. Forde, H. Vik-Mo, Family study of high density lipoprotein cholesterol and the relation to age and sex, **Acta Med Scand** 201:323-329 (1977).

39. C.J. Glueck, R.W. Fallat, F. Millett, P. Gartside, R.C. Elston, R.C. Go, Familial hyper-alpha-lipoproteinemia: studies in eighteen kindreds, **Metabolism** 24:1243-1265 (1975).

40. R.M. Siervogel, J.A. Morrison, K. Kelly, M. Mellies, P. Gartside, C.J. Glueck, Familial hyper-alpha-lipoproteinemia in 26 kindreds, **Clin Genet** 17:13-25 (1980).

41. M.E. Morton, C.J. MacLean, A. Kagan, C.L. Gulbrandsen, G.G. Rhoads, S. Yee, R. Lew, Commingling in distributions of

lipids and related variables, **Amer J. Hum Genet** 29:52-59
(1977).

42. N.E. Morton, C.L. Gulbrandsen, G.G. Rhoads, A. Kagan, R. Lew,
     Major loci for lipoprotein concentrations, **Amer J. Hum
     Genet** 30:583-589 (1978).

43. D.C. Rao, N.E. Morton, C.L. Gulbrandsen, G.G. Rhoads, A. Kagan,
     S. Yee, Cultural and biological determinants of lipoprotein
     concentrations, **Ann Hum Genet** 42:467-477 (1979).

44. M.S. Nupuf, W.H. Sutherland, High density lipoprotein levels in
     children of young men with ischaemic heart disease,
     Atherosclerosis 33:365-370 (1979).

45. H. Micheli, D. Pometta, C. Jornot, J.R. Scherrer, High density
     lipoprotein cholesterol in male relatives of patients with
     coronary heart disease, **Atherosclerosis** 32:269-276 (1979).

46. P.N. Herbert, G. Assmann, A.M. Gotto,Jr., D.S. Fredrickson,
     Familial lipoprotein deficiency, in "The Metabolic Basis of
     Inherited Disease," J.B. Stanbury, et al, McGraw-Hill Book
     Co., New York (1982).

47. H.A. Tyroler, C.J. Glueck, B. Christensen, P.O. Kwiterovich,
     Jr., Plasma high-density lipoprotein cholesterol
     comparisons in black and white populations, **Circulation**
     62(IV):99-107 (1980).

48. Y. Yano, N. Irie, Y. Homma, M. Tsushima, I. Takeuchi, N. Nakaya,
     Y. Goto, High density lipoprotein cholesterol levels in the
     Japanese, **Atherosclerosis** 36:173-181 (1980).

49. B. Lewis, A. Chait, G. Sigurdsson, M. Mancini, E. Farinaro, P.
     Oriente, L.A. Carlson, M. Ericsson, H. Micheli, D. Pometta,
     Serum lipoproteins in four European communities: a
     quantitative comparison, **Eur J Clin Invest** 8:165-173
     (1978).

50. J. Burslem, G. Schonfeld, M.A. Howald, S.W. Weidman, J.P.
     Miller, Plasma apoprotein and lipoprotein lipid levels in
     vegetarians, **Metabolism** 27:711-719 (1978).

51. J.T. Knuiman, R.J. Hermus, J.G. Hautvast, Serum total and high
     density lipoprotein (HDL) cholesterol concentrations in
     rural and urban boys from 16 countries, **Atherosclerosis**
     36:529-537 (1980).

52. W.E. Connor, M.T. Cerqueira, R.W. Connor, R.B. Wallace, M.R. Malinow, H.R. Casdorph, The plasma lipids, lipoproteins, and diet of the Tarahumara Indians of Mexico, **Am J Clin Nutr** 31:1131-1142 (1978).

53. D.E. Wilson, R.S. Lees, Metabolic relationships among the plasma lipoproteins, **J Clin Invest** 51:1051-1056 (1972).

54. G.H. Hartung, J.P. Foreyt, R.E. Mitchell, I. Vlasek, A.M. Gotto,Jr., Relation of diet to high-density lipoprotein cholesterol in middle-aged marathon runners, joggers, and inactive men, **N Engl J Med** 302:357-361 (1980).

55. R.W. Mahley, K.H. Weisgraber, T. Innerarity, H.B. Brewer,Jr., G. Assmann, Swine lipoproteins and atherosclerosis, **Biochemistry** 14:2817-2823 (1975).

56. R.W. Mahley, R.P. Bersot, T.L. Innerarity, A. Lipson, S. Margolis, Alterations in human high-density lipoproteins, with or without increased plasma-cholesterol, induced by diets high in cholesterol, **Lancet** ii:807-809 (1978).

57. N. Ernst, M. Fisher, W. Smith, T. Gordon, B.M. Rifkind, J.A. Little, M.A. Mishkel, O.D. Williams, The association of plasma high-density lipoprotein cholesterol with dietary intake and alcohol consumption, **Circulation** 62(IV):41-52 (1980).

58. D. Applebaum-Bowden, W.R. Hazzard, J. Cain, M.C. Cheung, R.S. Kushwaha, J.J. Albers, Short-term egg yolk feeding in humans, **Atherosclerosis** 33:385-396 (1979).

59. A. Chait, A. Onitiri, A. Nicoll, E. Rabaya, J. Davies, B. Lewis, Reduction of serum triglyceride levels by polyunsaturated fat, **Atherosclerosis** 20:347-364 (1974).

60. P.J. Nestel, N. Havenstein, Y. Homma, T.W. Scott, L.J. Cook, Increased sterol excretion with polyunsaturated-fat high-cholesterol diets, **Metabolism** 24:189-198 (1975).

61. J. Shepherd, C.J. Packard, J.R. Patsch, A.M. Gotto,Jr, O.D. Taunton, Effects of dietary polyunsaturated and saturated fat on the properties of high density lipoproteins and the metabolism of apolipoprotein A-I, **J Clin Invest** 61:1582-1592 (1978).

62. B. Vessby, J. Boberg, I.B. Gustafsson, B. Karlstrom, H. Lithell, A.M. Ostlund-Lindqvist, Reduction of high density lipoprotein cholesterol and apolipoprotein A-I

63. N. Ernst, P. Bowen, M. Fisher, E.J. Schaefer, R.I. Levy, Changes
     in plasma lipids and lipoproteins after a modifed fat diet,
     Lancet ii:111-112 (1980).

64. I. Hjermann, S. C. Enger, A. Helgeland, I. Holme, P. Leren, K.
     Trygg, The effect of dietary changes on high density
     lipoprotein cholesterol, **Am J Med** 66:105-109 (1979).

65. C.J. Glueck, H.L. Taylor, D. Jacobs, J.A. Morrison, R.
     Beaglehole, O.D. Williams, Plasma high-density lipoprotein
     cholesterol: association with measurements of body mass,
     Circulation 62(IV):62-69 (1980).

66. N.R. Phillips, R.J. Havel, J.P. Kane, Levels and
     interrelationships of serum and lipoprotein cholesterol and
     triglycerides, **Arterioclerosis** 1:13-24 (1981).

67. P.D. Thompson, R.W. Jeffery, R.R. Wing, P.D. Wood, Unexpected
     decrease in plasma high density lipoprotein cholesterol
     with weight loss, **Am J Clin Nutr** 32:2016-2021 (1979).

68. J.R. Taskinen, E.A. Nikkila, Effects of caloric restriction on
     lipid metabolism in man, **Atherosclerosis** 32:289-299 (1979).

69. F. Contaldo, P. Strazzullo, A. Postiglione, G. Riccardi, L.
     Patti, G. Di Biase, M. Mancini, Plasma high density
     lipoprotein in severe obesity after stable weight loss,
     Atherosclerosis 37:163-167 (1980).

70. H.O. Bang, J. Dyerberg, A.B. Nielsen, Plasma lipid and
     lipoprotein pattern in Greenlandic west-coast Eskimos,
     Lancet i:1143-1146 (1971).

71. A. Lehtonen, J. Viikari, The effect of vigorous physical
     activity at work on serum lipids with a special reference
     to serum high-density lipoprotein cholesterol, **Acta Physiol
     Scand** 104:117-121 (1978).

72. P.D. Wood, w. Haskell, H. Klein, S. Lewis, M.P. Stern, J.W.
     Farquhar, The distribution of plasma lipoproteins in
     middle-aged male runners, **Metabolism** 11:1249-1257 (1976).

73. A. Lehtonen, J. Viikari, Serum triglycerides and cholesterol and
     serum high-density lipoprotein cholesterol in highly
     physically active men, **Acta Med Scand** 204:111-114 (1978).
     concentrations by a lipid-lowering diet, **Atherosclerosis**
     35:21-27 (1980).

74. S.C. Enger, K. Herbjornsen, J. Serikssen, A. Fretland, High
     density lipoproteins (HDL) and physical activity: the
     influence of physical exercise, age and smoking on HDL-
     cholesterol and the HDL-total cholesterol ratio, **Scand J
     Clin Lab Invest** 37:251-255 (1977).

75. A. Lopez, R. Vial, L. Balart, G. Arroyave, Effect of exercise and
     physical fitness on serum lipids and lipoproteins,
     Atherosclerosis 20:1-9 (1974).

76. J.K. Huttunen, E. Lansimies, E. Voutilainen, C. Ehnholm, E.
     Heitanen, I. Penttila, O. Siitonen, R. Rauramaa, Effect of
     moderate physical exercise on serum lipoproteins,
     Circulation 60:1220-1229 (1979).

77. P.A. Farrell, J. Barboriak, The time course of alterations in
     plasma lipid and lipoprotein concentrations during eight
     weeks of endurance training, **Atherosclerosis** 37:231-238
     (1980).

78. P. Peltonen, J. Marniemi, E. Hietanen, I. Vuolri, C. Ehnholm,
     Changes in serum lipids, lipoproteins, and heparin
     releasable lipolytic enzymes during moderate physical
     training in man: a longitudinal study, **Metabolism** 30:518-
     526 (1981).

79. M.E. Moll, R.S. Williams, R.M. Lester, S.H. Quarfordt, A.G.
     Wallace, Cholesterol metabolism in non-obese women,
     Atherosclerosis 34:159-166 (1979).

80. R.J. Shephard, P.E. Youldon, M. Cox, C. West, Effects of a 6-
     momth industrial fitness programme on serum lipid
     concentrations, **Atherosclerosis** 35:277-286 (1980).

81. E.R. Nye, K. Carlson, P. Kirstein, S. Rossner, Changes in high
     density lipoprotein subfractions and other lipoproteins
     induced by exercise, **Clin Chim Acta** 113:51-57 (1981).

82. T.G. Allison, R.M. Iammarino, K.F. Metz, G.S. Skrinar, L.H.
     Kuller, R.J. Robertson, Failure of exercise to increase
     high density lipoprotein cholesterol, **J Card Rehab** 1:257-
     265 (1981).

83. L.C. Lipson, R.O. Bonow, E.J. Schaefer, H.B. Brewer, F.T.
     Lindgren, Effect of exercise conditioning on plasma high
     density lipoproteins and other lipoproteins,
     Atherosclerosis 37:529-538 (1980).

84. P.D. Thompson, E. Cullinane, L.O. Henderson, P.N. Herbert, Acute
     effects of prolonged exercise on serum lipids, **Metabolism**
     29:662-665 (1980).

85. L.A. Carlson, S.O. Froberg, Blood lipid and glucose levels
     during a ten-day period of low-calorie intake and exercise
     in man, **Metabolism** 16:624-634 (1967).

86. W.H. Sutherland, S.P. Woodhouse, S. Williamson, B. Smith,
     Decreased and continued physical activity and plasma
     lipoprotein lipids in previously trained men,
     Atherosclerosis 39:307-311 (1981).

87. S.C. Enger, S.B. Stromme, H.E. Refsum, High density lipoprotein
     cholesterol, total cholesterol and triglycerides in serum
     after a single exposure to prolonged heavy exercise, **Scand
     J Clin Lab Invest** 40:1-5 (1980).

88. E. A. Nikkila, J.R. Taskinen, S. Rehunen, M. Harkonen,
     Lipoprotein lipase activity in adipose tissue and skeletal
     muscle of runners: relation to serum lipoproteins,
     Metabolism 27:1661-1671 (1978).

89. P.D. Wood, W.L. Haskell, The effect of exercise on plasma high
     density lipoproteins, **Lipids** 14:417-427 (1979).

90. W.P. Castelli, T. Gordon, M.C. Hjortland, A. Kagan, J.T. Doyle,
     C.G. Hames, S.B. Hulley, W.J. Zukel, Alcohol and blood
     lipids, **Lancet** i:153-155 (1977).

91. N. Ernst, M. Fisher, W. Smith, T. Gordon, B.M. Rifkind, J.A.
     Little, M.A. Mishkel, O.D. Williams, The association of
     plasma high-density lipoprotein cholesterol with dietary
     intake and alcohol consumption, **Circulation** 62(IV):41-52
     (1980).

92. K. Yano, G.G. Rhoads, A. Kagan, Coffee, alcohol and risk of
     coronary heart disease among Japanese men living in Hawaii,
     N Engl J Med 297:405-409 (1977).

93. P. Williams, D. Robinson, A. Bailey, High-density lipoprotein
     and coronary risk factors in normal men, **Lancet** i:72-75
     (1979).

94. W. Willett, C.H. Hennekens, A.J. Siegel, M.M. Adner, W.P.
     Castelli, Alcohol consumption and high-density lipoprotein
     cholesterol in marathon runners, **N Engl J Med** 303:1159-1161
     (1980).

95. B.G. Johansson, A. Medhus, Increase in plasma alpha-lipoproteins in chronic alcoholics after acute abuse, **Acta Med Scand** 195:273-277 (1974).

96. P. Belfrage, B. Berg, I. Hagerstrand, P. Nilsson-Ehle, H. Tornqvist, T. Wiebe, Alterations of lipid metabolism in healthy volunteers during long-term ethanol intake, **Eur J Clin Invest** 7:127-131 (1977).

97. R.H. Schapiro, R.L. Scheig, G.D. Drummey, J.H. Mendelson, K.J. Isselbacher, Effect of prolonged ethanol ingestion on the transport and metabolism of lipids in man, **N Engl J Med** 272:610-615 (1965).

98. A. Chait, A.W. February, M. Mancini, B. Lewis, Clinical and metabolic study of alcoholic hyperlipidaemia, **Lancet** ii:62-64 (1972).

99. E. Baraona, C.S. Lieber, Effects of ethanol on lipid metabolism, **J Lipid Res** 20:289-315 (1979).

100. R.I. Levy, D.S. Fredrickson, N.J. Stone, D.W. Bilheimer, W.V. Brown, C.J. Glueck, A.M. Gotto, P.N. Herbert, P.O. Kwiterovich, T. Langer, J. LaRosa, S.E. Lux, A.K. Rider, R.S. Shulman, H.R. Sloan, Cholestyramine in Type II hyperlipoproteinemia, **Ann Intern Med**, 79:51-58 (1973).

101. P.T. Kuo, K. Hayase, J.B. Kostis, A.E. Moreyra, Use of combined diet and colestipol in long-term (7-7½ years) treatment of patients with Type II hyperlipoproteinemia, **Circulation** 59:199-211 (1979).

102. M.C. Cheung, J.J. Albers, P.W. Wahl, W.R. Hazzard, High density lipoproteins during hypolipidemic therapy, **Atherosclerosis** 35:215-228 (1980).

103. J. Shepherd, C.J. Packard, H.G. Morgan, J.L. Third, J.M. Stewart, T.D. Lawrie, The effects of cholestyramine on high density lipoprotein metabolism, **Atherosclerosis** 33:433-444 (1979).

104. J.L. Witztum, G. Schonfeld, S.W. Weidman, W.E. Giese, M.A. Dilingham, Bile sequestrant therapy alters the compositions of low-density and high-density lipoproteins, **Metabolism** 28:221-229 (1979).

105. P. Schwandt, P. Weisweiler, The effect of D-thyroxine on lipoprotein lipids and apolipoproteins in primary Type IIa hyperlipoproteinemia, **Atherosclerosis** 35:301-306 (1980).

106. P.J. Nestel, D. Hunt, M.L. Wahlqvist, Clofibrate raises plasma
     apoprotein A-I and HDL-cholesterol concentrations,
     Atherosclerosis 37:625-629 (1980).

107. J.M. Falko, J.L. Witztum, G. Schonfeld, S.W. Weidman, J.B.
     Kolar, Type III hyperlipoproteinemia, **Am J Med** 66:303-310
     (1979).

108. Y. Maruhama, A. Yanbe, R. Abe, A. Ohneda, S. Yamagata, Effect of
     clofibrate administration on plasma post-heparin lipolytic
     activity in man, **Tohoku J Exp Med** 113:343-349 (1974).

109. S.C. Enger, J. Erikssen, V. Johnsen, A. Samuelsen, K.
     Herbjornsen, E.A. Laws, The effect of clofibrate on high
     density lipoprotein and total cholesterol in patients with
     coronary heart disease, **Artery** 4:28-35 (1978).

110. C.B. Blum, R.I. Levy, S. Eisenberg, M. Hall, R.H. Goebel, M.
     Berman, High density lipoprotein metabolism in man, **J Clin
     Invest** 60:795-807 (1977).

111. J. Shepherd, C.J. Packard, J.R. Patsch, A.M. Gotto,Jr., O.D.
     Taunton, Effects of nicotinic acid therapy on plasma high
     density lipoprotein subfraction distribution and
     composition and on apolipoprotein A metabolism, **J Clin
     Invest** 63:858-867 (1979).

112. C.J. Packard, J.M. Stewart, J.L. Third, H.G. Morgan, T.D.
     Lawrie, J. Shepherd, Effects of nicotinic acid therapy on
     high-density lipoprotein metabolism in Type II and Type IV
     hyperlipoproteinaemia, **Biochim Biophys Acta** 618:53-62
     (1980).

113. J. LeLorier, S. DuBreuil-Quidoz, S. Lussier-Cacan, Y.S. Huang,
     J. Davignon, Diet and probucol in lowering cholesterol
     concentrations, **Arch Intern Med** 137:1429-1434 (1977).

114. P.J. Nestel, T. Billington, Effects of probucol on low density
     lipoprotein removal and high density lipoprotein synthesis,
     Atherosclerosis 38:203-209 (1981).

115. M.J. Mellies, P.S. Gartside, L. Glatfelter, P. Vink, G. Guy, G.
     Schonfeld, C.J. Glueck, Effects of probucol on plasma
     cholesterol, high and low density lipoprotein cholesterol,
     and apolipoproteins A1 and A2 in adults with primary
     familial hypercholesterolemia, **Metabolism** 29:956-964
     (1980).

116. L.A. Carlson, B. Kolmodin-Hedman, Hyper-alpha-lipoproteinemia

in men exposed to chlorinated hydrocarbon pesticides, **Acta Med Scand**, 192:29-32 (1972).

117. L.A. Carlson, B. Kolmodin-Hedman, Decrease in alpha-lipoprotein cholesterol in men after cessation of exposure to chlorinated hydrocarbon pesticides, **Acta Med Scand** 201:375-376 (1977).

118. E.A. Nikkila, M. Kaste, C. Ehnholm, J. Viikari, Increase of serum high-density lipoprotein in phenytoin users, **Br Med J** 2:99 (1978).

119. G.D. Bell, J.P. Bradshaw, A. Burgess, W. Ellis, J. Hatton, A. Middleton, B. Middleton, T. Orchard, D.A. White, Elevation of serum high density lipoprotein cholesterol by rowachol, a proprietary mixture of six pure monoterpenes, **Athersclerosis** 36:47-54 (1980).

120. M.H. Crique, R.B. Wallace, G. Heiss, M. Mishkel, G. Schonfeld, G.T. Jones, Cigarette smoking and plasma high-density lipoprotein cholesterol, **Circulation** 62(IV):70-76 (1980).

121. R.J. Garrison, W.B. Kannel, M. Feinleib, W.P. Castelli, P.M. McNamara, S.J. Padgett, Cigarette smoking and HDL cholesterol, **Atherosclerosis** 30:17-25 (1978).

122. J. Erikssen, S.C. Enger, The effect of smoking on selected coronary heart disease risk factors in middle-aged men, **Acta Med Scand** 203:27-30 (1978).

123. K. Berg, A.L. Borresen, G. Dahlen, Effect of smoking on serum levels of HDL apoproteins, **Atherosclerosis** 34:339-343 (1979).

124. P. Leren, A. Helgeland, I. Holme, P.O. Foss, I. Hjermann, P.G. Lund-Larsen, Effect of propranolol and prazosin on blood lipids, **Lancet** ii:4-6 (1980).

125. T. Rosenthal, E. Holtzman, P. Segal, The effect of chlorthalidone on serum lipids and lipoproteins, **Athersclerosis** 36:111-115 (1980).

126. D.D. Bradley, J. Wingerd, D.B. Petitti, R.M. Krauss, S. Ramcharan, Serum high-density-lipoprotein cholesterol in women using oral contraceptives, estrogens and progestins, **N Engl J Med** 299:17-20 (1978).

127. J.R. Masarei, B.K. Armstrong, M.W. Skinner, T. Ratajczak, R. Hahnel, D. Crooke, H.T. Clarke, HDL-cholesterol and sex-hormone status, **Lancet** i:208 (1980).

128. A. Solyom, Effects of androgens on serum lipids and
     lipoproteins, **Lipids** 7:100-105 (1971).

129. R.H. Furman, P. Alaupovic, R.P. Howard, Effects of androgens and
     estrogens on serum lipids and the composition and
     concentration of serum lipoproteins in normolipemic and
     hyperlipidemic states, **Prog Biochem Pharmacol** 2:215-249
     (1967).

130. W. Insull,Jr., R.T. Kirkland, J.L. Probstfield, B.S. Keenan,
     G.W. Clayton, Control of HDL-cholesterol plasma levels by
     testosterone in pubertal males, **Circulation** 64(IV):113
     (1981).

131. A. Nordoy, A. Aakvaag, D. Thelle, Sex hormones and high density
     lipoproteins in healthy males, **Atherosclerosis** 34:431-436
     (1979).

132. J.A. Morrison, J. Gutal, T.J. Orchard, P.R. Khoury, W. Dai, R.E.
     LaPorte, C.J. Glueck, Plasma testosterone and high density
     lipoprotein cholesterol in adolescence: a marked absence of
     association, **Circulation** 64(IV):113 (1981).

133. E. Manzato, R. Fellin, G. Baggio, S. Walch, W. Neubeck, D.
     Seidel, Formation of lipoprotein-X, **J Clin Invest** 57:1248-
     1260 (1976).

134. R.L. Patten, D. Hewitt, G.T. Waldman, G. Jones, J.A. Little,
     Associations of plasma high-density lipoprotein
     cholesterol with clinical chemistry data, **Circulation**
     62(IV):31-41 (1980).

135. D.B. Petitti, G.D. Friedman, A.L. Klatsky, Association of a
     history of gallbladder disease with a reduced concentration
     of high-density-lipoprotein cholesterol, **N Engl J Med**
     304:1396-1398 (1981).

136. G.D. Calvert, T. Mannik, J.J. Graham, P.H. Wise, R.A. Yeates,
     Effects of therapy on plasma-high-density-lipoprotein-
     cholesterol concentration in diabetes mellitus, **Lancet**
     2:66-68 (1978).

137. R.S. Elkeles, J. Wu, J. Hambley, Haemoglobin A_1, blood glucose,
     and high-density lipoprotein cholesterol in insulin-
     requiring diabetics, **Lancet** ii:547-548 (1978).

138. C.A. Hornick, B.D. Fellmeth, High density lipoprotein
     cholesterol, insulin, and obesity in Samoans,
     Atherosclerosis 39:321-328 (1981).

139. F.L. Dunn, A. Pietri, P. Raskin, Plasma lipid and lipoprotein
     levels with continuous subcutaneous insulin infusion in
     Type I diabetes mellitus, **Ann Intern Med** 95:426-431 (1981).

140. G.M. Tisi, A. Conrique, E. Barrett-Connor, S.M. Grundy,
     Increased high density lipoprotein cholesterol in
     obstructive pulmonary disease (predominant emphysematous
     type), **Metabolism** 30:340-346 (1981).

APOLIPOPROTEIN DISORDERS

G. Assmann and H.-J. Menzel

Zentrallaboratorium der Medizinischen Einrichtungen
der Westfälischen Wilhelms-Universität
Domagkstrasse 3, 4400 Münster/Westf.
WEST GERMANY

Apolipoprotein disorders encompass a range of diseases
attributable to a defect in the structure or metabolism (biosynthesis, secretion, catabolism) of apolipoproteins. Section I of
this study deals with the biochemistry of apolipoproteins while
the pathophysiology and clinical aspects of apolipoprotein disorders are discussed in Section II.

I. APOLIPOPROTEINS

Among the individual serum lipoproteins (chylomicrons,
very low density lipoproteins (VLDL), low density lipoproteins
(LDL) and high density lipoproteins (HDL)) there are a number of
apolipoproteins varying in chemical structure (Table 1) whose amino
acid sequences and functional properties are known to some degree
|1|. Table 2 provides an orientation to the distribution of
apolipoproteins in serum lipoproteins (Table 3).

Insight has been gained into the pathophysiology of the
structure and metabolism of various lipoproteins on the basis of
knowledge regarding the primary structure of apolipoproteins
(e.g. lipid affinity of apolar regions, genetically determined
presence of isoproteins, biological activity of synthetic pep-
tides) |2, 3|. Several diseases of lipid metabolism may be classi-
fied today as apolipoprotein disorders.

Apolipoprotein A-I and A-II

The amino acid sequences of Apo A-I and Apo A-II have been
described |4, 5, 6|. Apo A-I, the major apolipoprotein of HDL, has
a molecular weight of 28,331 (245 amino acids) and is characterized

213

G. ASSMAN AND H.-J. MENZEL

Table 1. : Apolipoproteins

Apolipo-protein	Molecular Weight x 10^{-3}	Site of synthesis	Serum concentration (mg/dl)	Function
A-I	28.3	intestine, liver	100-150	Cofactor of lecithin:cholesterol transferase; structural protein of HDL
A-II	17.0	intestine, ? liver	30-150	Phospholipoid-binding properties; structural protein of HDL
A-IV	46.0	intestine	15	unknown
B-100	549.0	liver	80-100	Intracellular construction or transport of VLDL; receptor interaction (LDL) with apoprotein B-E-receptor cells
B-48	265.0	intestine + liver	?	Intracellular construction or transcellular transport of chylomicrons and VLDL; receptor interaction with apoprotein B receptor?
C-I	6.5	liver	10	Cofactor of adipose tissue lipoprotein lipase (particularly saturated fatty acids)
C-II	8.8	liver	3- 8	Cofactor of adipose tissue lipoprotein lipase
$C-III_{0,1,2}$	8.9	liver	8- 15	unknown
D	20.0	?	10	unknown; question of role in LCAT reaction and cholesteryl ester metabolism
E	39.0	liver	3- 5	Receptor interaction with Apo B, E-receptor cells and with hepatic Apo E-receptor; inhibitor of adipose tissue lipoprotein lipase?

Table 2. : Apolipoprotein composition of serum lipoproteins
(data according to Herbert, P.N., this symposium)

	Chylomicrons %	VLDL %	LDL %	HDL$_2$ %	HDL$_3$ %
A-I	33	trace	trace	65	62
A-II	trace	trace	trace	10	23
A-IV	14	-	-	?	trace
B	5	25	95	3	-
C	32	55	2	13	5
D	?	?	?	2	4
E	10	15	3	3	1
other	6	5	5	4	5

Table 3. : Apolipoprotein disorders

```
-------------------------------------------------------------
Apolipoprotein    Defect
-------------------------------------------------------------
A-I               Tangier disease

                  Apo A-I Milano Variant
                  Apo A-I Marburg Variant
                  Apo A-I Münster Variants 1-3
-------------------------------------------------------------
B                 Recessive abetalipoproteinemia

                  Homozygotic hypobetalipoproteinemia

                  Normotriglyceridemic abetalipoproteinemia
-------------------------------------------------------------
C                 Apolipoprotein C-II deficiency
-------------------------------------------------------------
E                 Apolipoprotein E-2 homozygosity

                  a) Dysbetalipoproteinemia
                  b) Familial type III hyperlipoproteinemia
-------------------------------------------------------------
```

by a high frequency of helical regions in the secondary structure.
A substantial proportion of the HDL Apo A-I is synthesized in the
intestine and first enters the plasma as a component of chylomicrons. Upon entry into the circulation the chylomicrons are
subjected to rapid breakdown. This leads to the formation of Apo
A-I-containing lamellar particles rich in phospholipids as "surface
remnants" of the chylomicrons, which are considered the precursors
of plasma HDL.

    Apo A-I is an activator apolipoprotein for lecithin:choleste-
rol acyltransferase |8, 9, 10|. This enzyme transfers the beta-
carbon fatty acid residue (usually linoleic acid) from phosphatidyl
choline to the 3-β-hydroxy group of cholesterol |11|. The cataly-
tic activity of this enzyme enables the lamellar surface structures
of the chylomicrons, via de novo synthesis of cholesteryl esters
(arranged in the center of the macromolecule) and lysolecithin
(bound to albumin), to be transformed into pseudomicellar spherical
HDL. The enzyme LCAT is also involved in the biosynthesis of HDL-1
and HDL-2 subfractions from HDL-3 |12, 13|.

    Apolipoprotein A-I is present even in normal serum in various
polymorphic forms |14|. Structural variants of Apo A-I have been
described (Apo A-I Milano |15, 16|; Apo A-I Marburg |17|; Apo A-I
Münster |18|) (see below). Apo A-I is present in extremely low
plasma concentrations (< 1% of the normal value) in Tangier
disease |19, 20|.

    Apo A-II, also a structural protein in HDL, consists of two
identical protein chains of 77 amino acids each, joined by a
disulfide bridge. The dimeric molecule has a molecular weight of
approx. 17,000 and is comprised of the two identical polypeptide
chains of 77 amino acid residues each |4|.

    Both A-apolipoproteins characteristically bind phospholipids
(phosphatidyl choline, sphingomyelin) to form protein-phospholipid
complexes, whereby the proportion of α-helical regions is increased
|21, 22, 23|. The apolipoprotein-phospholipid complexes
can be isolated by ultracentrifugation in the density range from
1.063 to 1.21 g/ml and are capable of binding cellular cholesterol. Apo A-II exhibits a higher degree of interaction with phospholipids than does Apo A-I. In addition to these properties both
apolipoproteins show a strong tendency to form associations (pro-
tein-protein interaction). No structural variants of Apo A-II have
been identified to date.

Apo A-III (Apo D)

    Apolipoprotein A-III has a molecular weight of approx. 20,000
and occurs particularly in the HDL density range (< 5% of HDL
apolipoproteins) |24, 25|. It was originally thought that this

apolipoprotein activates the enzyme LCAT |26|, though this finding
could not be confirmed in follow-up investigations. According to
studies by Fielding et al. apolipoprotein D together with apolipoprotein A-I and the enzyme LCAT form a component of the "cholesteryl ester transfer complex", which transfers newly synthesized
cholesteryl ester to other lipoproteins |27, 28, 29|. The involve-
ment of the cholesteryl ester transfer complex in the transport of
cholesterol from peripheral somatic cells is still hypothetical,
though at least some aspects have been confirmed experimentally.

Apo A-IV

Apolipoprotein A-IV is synthesized in the intestine, has a
molecular weight of 46,000 and occurs as a component of chylomi-
crons and the lipoprotein-free plasma fraction |30, 31, 32|. A
funtion has not yet been reported for this apolipoprotein.

Apolipoprotein B

Apo B is a structural protein of chylomicrons, VLDL, LDL and
Lp(a). It is synthesized in the intestine and the liver and is
important in the secretion and transport of these lipoproteins. In
the case of abetalipoproteinemia the apolipoprotein B-containing
lipoproteins are not detectable in serum.

As a result of its insolubility in water following delipida-
tion this apolipoprotein is difficult to analyze chemically. There
are as yet no precise data for the molecular weight or structure of
Apo B. According to studies by Kane et al. at least two subtypes
can be distinguished, designated Apo B-100 (M.W. 549,000) and Apo
B-48 (M.W. 265,000) |33|. Apo B-48 is a structural protein of
chylomicrons although it cannot be detected in LDL. On the other
hand, Apo B-100 is a structural apolipoprotein of VLDL, IDL and LDL
|34|. As a structural component of LDL Apo B-100 interacts with
so-called Apo B,E-receptors (i.e. LDL receptors), peripheral somatic
cells (e.g. dermal fibroblasts, intimal endothelial cells, smooth
muscle cells of the arterial wall) and with corresponding hepatocy-
tic receptors, with the LDL being taken up into the cells and
catabolized |35|. Chemical modification of the arginine residues
in Apo B using cyclohexanedione increases the half-life of circula-
ting LDL |36, 37|. This finding may be considered an important
indication of the significance of apolipoprotein B in the catabolism of LDL.

In the case of normotriglyceridemic abetalipoproteinemia
neither VLDL, IDl nor LDL can be detected in plasma |38|. However,
in contrast to recessive abetalipoproteinemia and homozygotic
hypobetalipoproteinemia lipids contained in the diet can be transported via chylomicrons. This indicates that a number of genes are
involved in the regulation of Apo B biosynthesis.

In a normal case as well as in the case of isolated hypercholesterolemia more than 90% of the total apolipoprotein B is located
in the LDL.   In hypertriglyceridemia 20-50% of the total apolipopro-
tein B may occur in VLDL or chylomicrons |39, 40|.   Lipoprotein (a)
(Lp(a)), which also contains apolipoprotein B, may be markedly
elevated in concentration and contribute significantly to the
plasma concentration of apolipoprotein B |41, 42, 43|.

C Apolipoproteins

The C apolipoproteins are of relatively low molecular weight
and can be separated by means of ion exchange chromatography and
polyacrylamide gel electrophoresis into C-I, C-II, C-III-0, C-III-1
and C-III-2 fractions.   Apo C-III-0, Apo C-III-1 and Apo C-III-2
are distinguished by differing content of N-acetyl neuraminic
acid.   The C apolipoproteins, just as the apolipoproteins, are
capable of forming protein-phospholipid complexes with phospholipids.   The primary structure of C apolipoproteins has been descri-
bed |44, 45, 46, 47|.

Apo C-I

Approximately 10% of the total protein of VLDL and roughly 2%
of the total protein of HDL consist of Apo C-I.   This apolipopro-
tein has been synthesized entirely |48|.   A synthetic peptide
(amino acids 32-57) binds phospholipids.   Native and synthetic Apo
C-I activate the enzyme LCAT with artificial substrates. The
physiological significance of LCAT activation in comparison to Apo
A-I is unknown at present.

Apo C-II

Approximately 10% of the total protein of VLDL, 1-2% of the
total protein of HDL-2 and less than 1% of the total protein of
HDL-3 consists of Apo C-II |49|.   This apoprotein is a specific
cofactor of lipoprotein lipase |50, 51| and is transferred during
lipolysis from HDL-2 to triglyceride-rich lipoproteins, in order to
accelerate catabolism.   The phospholipid-binding and lipoprotein
lipase activating properties of this apolipoprotein are, in contrast to apo A-I, arranged in different segments of the primary
structure |52, 53, 54|.   A genetic lack of Apo C-II results in
hypertriglyceridemia (hyperchylomicronemia) |55|.   A structural
variant of Apo C-II has been discovered only recently |56|.

Apo C-III

Apo C-III comprises approximately 40% of the total protein of
VLDL and roughly 2% of the total protein of HDL |57|.   In the case
of hypertriglyceridemia often more than 50% of the total Apo C-III

is found in the VLDL |58|. Under certain experimental conditions
Apo C-III may inhibit lipoprotein lipase |59, 60|, though the
physiological significance of this observation is disputed.

Apolipoprotein E

Approximately 10-20% of the total protein of VLDL consists of
Apo E. This apolipoprotein is also present in all other lipoprotein fractions, though in low concentrations. The molecular weight
is stated to be 33,000 or 38,000 |61, 62|. A portion of the
apolipoprotein E exists in the form of a complex with apolipopro-
tein A-II |63, 64|. Apolipoprotein E is synthesized in the liver
|65| and its serum concentration corresponds to that of triglyceri-
des |66|. The highest concentrations of Apo E in serum are measu-
red in Type III hyperlipoproteinemia |67, 68|.

After removal of neuraminic acid from the VLDL, apolipoprotein
E can be separated by isoelectric focusing in 6 M urea into several
genetically determined isomeric forms, designated Apo E-2, E-3 and
E-4 |69, 79| (Fig.1) (Table 4). The primary sequences of the
isomeric forms of Apo E are known; they differ in content of
cysteine and arginine |71|. Apo E is of importance in receptor
interaction and in the metabolism of various lipoproteins (chylomi-
cron remnants, VLDL remnants, HDL-1) |71, 72, 73, 74, 75|.

II APOLIPOPROTEIN DISORDERS

Apolipoprotein disorders are defined here as diseases in which
the etiology and pathophysiology are directly related to a structural defect, a defect in biosynthesis or secretion, or to a defect
in cell recognition and catabolism of an apolipoprotein. The
precise biochemical defect has not yet been determined for each
individual case discussed below.

1. Tangier Disease

Tangier disease |76, 77, 78, 79, 80| was first described by
Fredrickson in 1961 and is named for Tangier Island, Virginia,
where the patients first known to have the disease lived. The most
striking clinical symptom in Tangier disease is substantial enlargement and yellow-orange discoloration of the tonsils. In addition, splenomegaly is seen in most patients as is peripheral
neuropathy.

The disease is characterized by the following laboratory
findings :
1. Low plasma cholesterol concentrations (< 100 mg/dl) and
   normal or elevated plasma triglycerides.

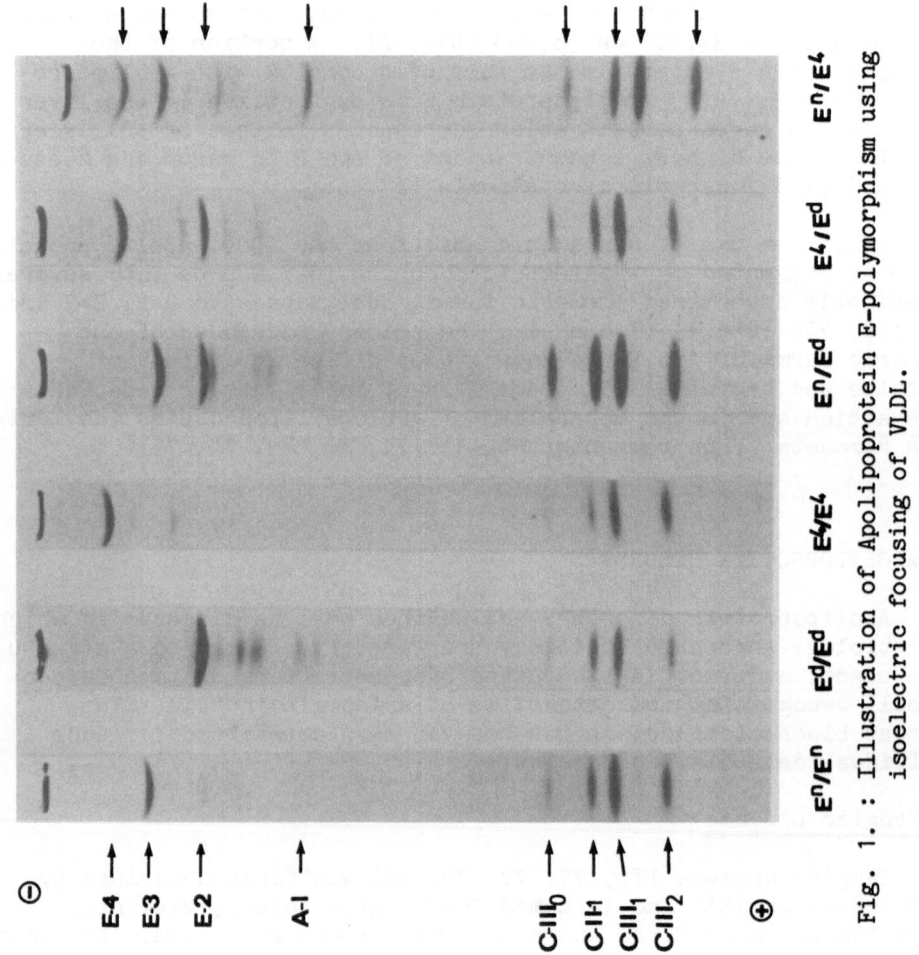

Fig. 1. : Illustration of Apolipoprotein E-polymorphism using isoelectric focusing of VLDL.

Table 4. : Apolipoprotein E polymorphism

GENOTYPE	E^D/E^D	E^N/E^D	E^4/E^D	E^N/E^N	E^N/E^4	E^4/E^4
PHENOTYPE	E-2	E-3 / E-2	E-4 / E-2	E-3	E-4 / E-3	E-4
LIPOPROTEIN PATTERN	VLDL Chol	?	?	normal	normal	normal
	LDL Chol					
	− VLDL +					
FREQUENCY IN POPULATION	1%	13%	3%	59%	22%	2%

2. Nearly total absence of high density lipoproteins (HDL) in plasma in conjunction with altered chemical composition of other plasma lipoproteins.

3. Concentration of cholesteryl esters in numerous organs |81, 82|, primarily in the macrophages of tonsils, lymph nodes, thymus, bone marrow, liver, spleen and rectal mucosa. In addition to the storage of cholesteryl esters there is accumulation of lipid in Schwann cells and intestinal smooth muscle cells. Arterial smooth muscle cells or other cells of the arterial wall are not affected. Arteriosclerosis is not a clinical symptom of this disease. The combination of low plasma cholesterol and enlarged, yellow-orange tonsils is characteristically indicative of Tangier disease.

The biochemical cause of analphalipoproteinemia is probably a structural defect in apolipoprotein A-I. This apolipoprotein is present in the serum of Tangier patients at a concentration of 1% of the normal concentration |19, 20|. In contrast to normal apolipoprotein A-I, which is detected as a component of HDL falling almost exclusively in the density range of 1.063-1.21 g/ml KBr, Tangier apolipoprotein A-I is found in the fraction ⟩1.21 g/ml in density. Isolated Tangier Apo A-I shows loss of the ability to reassociate with normal HDL. Storage of cholesteryl esters in the macrophages must be considered a direct consequence of the analphalipoproteinemia. As yet no definitive statement can be made regarding why, in spite of the complete absence of normal HDL, arteriosclerosis is not seen as a complication in Tangier disease.

2. Hypoalphalipoproteinemias

The familial hypoalphalipoproteinemias are a biochemically heterogeneous group of disorders with their origin in the reduced biosynthesis or accelerated catabolism of HDL |80|. It is probable that the defective metabolism of HDL is not due to an apolipoprotein defect in every case, and thus the classification chosen here may require modification.

The criteria for diagnosis are as follows :

1. HDL cholesterol ⟨ 25 mg/dl.
2. Exclusion of secondary causes (e.g. obesity, hypertriglyceridemia, diabetes mellitus).
3. Confirmation of hypoalphalipoproteinemia in family members.
4. Possible determination of a structural variant of apolipoprotein A-I.

In view of the fact that to date only a few cases of primary hypoalphalipoproteinemia (e.g. heterozygous patients with Tangier disease) have been observed, it is not yet possible to address potential clinical complications or the risk of arteriosclerosis.

3. Structural Variants of Apolipoprotein A-I

Structural variants of Apo A-I can be identified in native serum by isoelectric focusing (Fig. 2). In our own studies of 700 patients subjected to coronary angiography three different familial apolipoprotein A-I structural variants were discovered (Apo A-I Münster 1-3 |18|). Normal Apo A-I in the probands in these families was reduced to approx. 50% of the normal serum concentration, though there was no indication of hypoalphalipoproteinemia. Apparently, despite the defective structure of the apolipoprotein A-I Münster 1-3, the physicochemical properties (protein-protein interaction, protein-lipid interaction) are intact, such that functional deficiencies in terms of altered HDL concentration are nonexistent.

4. Abetalipoproteinemia

The disease described in a Jewish girl by Bassen and Kornzweig in 1950 is, analogous to Friedreich's ataxia and fat malabsorption syndrome, characterized by retinitis pigmentosa, acanthocytosis and neurological symptoms |80, 83, 84|. The diagnosis is confirmed by extremely low levels of cholesterol ($<$ 100 mg/dl) and triglycerides ($<$ 30 mg/dl) and the total absence of apolipoprotein B-containing lipoproteins (chylomicrons, VLDL, LDL, Lp(a)).

For reasons heretofore unknown not only is there no apolipoprotein B but also no apolipoprotein C-III-1 present in plasma. On the basis of family studies two forms of abetalipoproteinemia can be distinguished, on the one hand, recessive abetalipoproteinemia (autosomal recessive inheritance) and, on the other hand, the homozygous form of hypobetalipoproteinemia. In the case of recessive abetalipoproteinemia the parents of the probands exhibit normal concentrations of apolipoprotein B and LDL, while in the other case both parents have extremely low apolipoprotein B levels (Table 5).

The precise biochemical defect responsible for the apolipoprotein B deficiency is not yet known. Apolipoprotein B cannot be detected immunologically either in plasma or the intestinal mucosa (site of synthesis of chylomicrons).

Regardless of the precise genetic diagnosis fat in the diet should be avoided in treating abetalipoproteinemia on account of the absence of a resorption mechanism and fat-soluble vitamins should be added to the diet. In particular, it is of the utmost

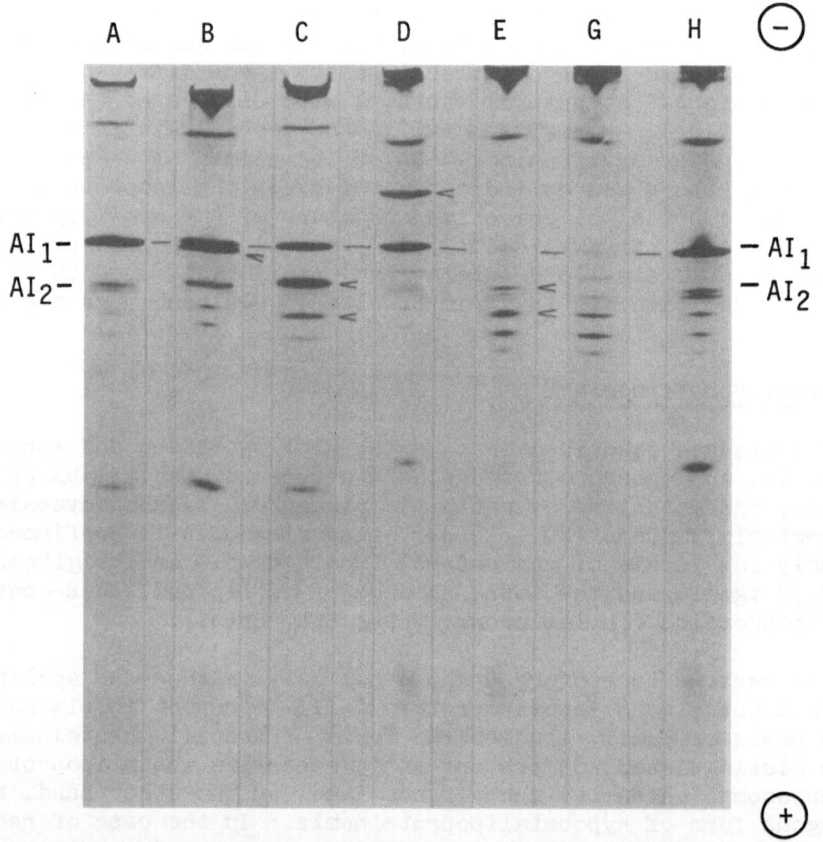

Fig. 2. : Illustration of Apolipoprotein A-I structural
          variants (using isoelectric focusing of nati-
          ve serum).

    Gel A + H : normal serum
    Gel B   : Apolipoprotein A-I Münster-1 variant
    Gel C   : Apolipoprotein A-I Münster-2 variant
    Gel D   : Apolipoprotein A-I Münster-3 variant
    Gel E   : Apolipoprotein A-I Milano variant
    Gel F   : Tangier disease

Table 5. : Apolipoprotein B mutants

Classification	Genetic type	LDL cholesterol	Remarks Apo B-100	Apo B-48
I. Abetalipoproteinemia	autosomal recessive	0 mg/dl	not detectable	not detectable
II. Hypobetalipoproteinemia	autosomal dominant			
- heterozygous form		10-40 mg/dl	?	?
- homozygous form		0 mg/dl	not detectable	not detectable
III. Hypobetalipoproteinemia variants				
a) normotriglyceridemic abetalipoproteinemia	?	0 mg/dl	not detectable	not detectable
b) asymptomatic hypobeta lipoproteinemia with fasting chylomicronemia (homozygous)	autosomal dominant	4- 8 mg/dl	?	?

importance to add Vitamin E (100 mg/kg/day), since it is thus
possible to favorably influence the progression of the retinitis
pigmentosa and neuromuscular symptoms.

5. Normotriglyceridemic Abetalipoproteinemia

In this variant, in contrast to the classical form of abetalipoproteinemia, triglycerides are resorbed in the intestine and
chylomicrons formed and secreted |38|. The intestinal synthesis of
apolipoprotein B-48 is evidently not affected (Table 5). However,
as a consequence of selective inhibition of hepatic synthesis of
apolipoprotein B-100, neither VLDL nor LDL is present in plasma.
This metabolic defect, although reported only once to date, is, in
the case of further confirmation, an indication of the fact that
apolipoprotein B-100 and apolipoprotein B-48 are under separate
genetic control. Furthermore, it may be assumed that chylomicron
apolipoprotein B (B-48) is not a precursor of LDL apolipoprotein B
(B-100).

6. Hyperbetalipoproteinemia

The disease is inherited as autosomal dominant. Homozygous
patients cannot be distinguished either in clinical appearance or
in laboratory results from patients with recessive abetalipopro-
teinemia |80, 84|. Since hypobetalipoproteinemia is generally
asymptomatic, little is known about its frequency in the population. Due to the extremely low cholesterol level the risk of
arteriosclerosis is small and the life expectancy is consequently
increased (longevity syndrome).

The criteria for diagnosis are as follows :

1. Abnormally low, but nevertheless immunochemically detectable
   LDL, concentration of HDL normal.
2. Exclusion of secondary causes of hyperbetalipoproteinemia
   (e.g. malnutrition, liver or intestinal disease).
3. Identical findings in family members.

As a rule, a simultaneous reduction in cholesterol and triglycerides (< 100 mg/dl) is observed, with LDL cholesterol reduced to
10-50% of the normal concentration. Clinical findings such as fat
intolerance or neurological complications of abetalipoproteinemia
are not observed.

Analogous to hypoalphalipoproteinemia, it is probable that a
number of biochemical defects can cause hypobetalipoproteinemia.
In this regard, a new system of classification will be necessary
here as well.

7. Apolipoprotein C-II Deficiency

In the case of hyperchylomicronemia it is imperative that a check be made to see whether the serum apolipoprotein C-II concentration is normal. Clear semi-quantitative results are generally available by urea-polyacrylamide gel electrophoresis or isolelectric focusing of lipoproteins < 1.006 g/ml in density; immunochemical tests (radioimmunoassay, immunoelectrophoresis) with monospecific antibodies confirm the diagnosis. To date, an apoliprotein C-II deficiency as the cause of reduced lipoprotein lipase activity with consecutive hyperchylomicronemia has been described in only a very few cases |55, 85, 86, 87, 88, 89|.

Just as in familial lipoprotein lipase deficiency, hyperchylomicronemia is seen as early as the childhood years and leads to similar clinical complications, particularly acute pancreatitis. In contrast to familial lipoprotein lipase deficiency, neither xanthomatosis nor hepatomegaly has been observed to date in patients with apolipoprotein C-II deficiency. The few cases described up to now do not permit generalizations with reference to clinical complications of this disease.

8. Apolipoprotein E-2 Homozygosity

In the case of apolipoprotein E-2 homozygosity (approx. 1% of population (Fig. 1, Table 4) there is resultant dysbetalipoproteinemia as consequence of disturbed catabolism of chylomicron remnants and IDL |90, 91|. In the lipoprotein electrophoresis β-VLDL is found in the d < 1.006 g/ml supernatant (i.e. dysbetalipoproteinemia), VLDL cholesterol is elevated, LDL cholesterol and total cholesterol are reduced. The abnormal β-VLDL have the following properties :

- spherical particles 250 A in diameter on average (normal VLDL : approx. 400 A)
- float in S_f-range 20-60 (normal VLDL : S_f 20-400)
- rich in cholesterol (normal VLDL : triglyceride rich)
- high apolipoprotein E concentration
- no normal apoliporotein E (i.e. Apo E-3 or Apo E-4), only defective apolipoprotein E (Apo E-2) present

It is assumed that the β-VLDL are metabolic products of the chylomicrons (i.e. chylomicron remnants) or normal VLDL (i.e. VLDL remnants) |92, 93|. Evidently, as a result of a structural mutation of apolipoprotein E-3 yielding apolipoprotein E-2 (arginine-cystein exchange at position 116) the remnants of the triglyceride-rich molecules are not properly recognized by the hepatic apoprotein E receptor and thus accumulate in the plasma.

Table 6. : Apolipoprotein E polymorphism and coronary heart disease

Frequency of Apoprotein E Genotypes

	E^N/E^N	E^D/E^D	E^4/E^4	E^N/E^D	E^N/E^4	E^D/E^4
Coronary sclerosis + (coronary angiography on 214 patients)	59.8	2.8	3.3	9.8	23.4	0.9
Coronary sclerosis − (coronary angiography on 322 patients)	59.3	0.9	2.2	14.0	22.0	1.1
Company employees (From periodic check-ups)	62.5	0.7	2.5	11.0	20.0	3.7

It has not been possible to date to determine whether this dys-betalipoproteinemia is associated with an increased coronary risk. In our own studies of a group of patients who underwent coronary angiography apolipoprotein E-2 homozygosity occurred with greater frequency among those with coronary heart disease than among unaffected patients or in the general population (Table 6). The low number of cases does not permit any conclusion as to whether apolipoprotein E-2 may be considered a biochemical indicator of increased coronary risk. Apolipoprotein homozygosity (phenotype E-2/E-3 or E-2/E-4) is represented in the group with approximately equal frequency (Table 6). One to two percent of the patients with apolipoprotein E-2 homozygosity progress to a condition characterized by severe early coronary arteriosclerosis, peripheral arteriosclerosis and xanthomatosis : Type III hyperlipoproteinemia.

9. Familial Type III Hyperlipoproteinemia

Familial Type III hyperlipoproteinemia was described initially in 1967 by Frederickson et al. |94|. Employing a combination of ultracentrifugation and lipoprotein electrophoresis these authors discovered abnormal VLDL in the plasma of patients of this type, which did not exhibit the usual pre- β mobility, but rather β mobility. These abnormal lipoproteins were designated " β-VLDL" or "floating β-lipoproteins", which yield a broad β-band in the electrophoresis of native serum '"broad β disease"). Later studies by Havel and Kane showed a high concentration of apolipoprotein E in the β-VLDL. In 1975 Utermann described the genetic defect of Type III hyperlipoproteinemia as an increase in Apo E-2 with simultaneous absence of Apo E-3 and Apo E-4 |66|. Zanis and Breslow in 1979 introduced a triallelic model for Apo E (E-N, E-D and E-4), corresponding to six different genotypes and phenotypes in the population (Table 4) |69, 70|. Consequently, apolipoprotein E-2 homozygosity corresponds to the genotype E-D/E-D. In 1981 Weisgraber et al identified a structural mutation of apolipoprotein E-3 as a biochemical defect of Type III hyperlipoproteinemia |71|.

Only 2% of all patients with the apolipoprotein genotype E-D/E-D (homozygous for Apo E-2) developed clinical signs of Type III hyperlipoproteinemia |96|. Type III hyperlipoproteinemia becomes manifested when, in addition to Apo E-2 homozygosity, there is either a further inborn error of lipid metabolism present (e.g. familial hypercholesterolemia, familial hypertriglyceridemia, familial combined hyperlipidemia, polygenetic hypercholesterolemia) or there is a concomitant secondary hyperlipoproteinemia (e.g. in hyperthyroidism) present |90, 96, 97, 98| (Table 7). Obviously, under these circumstances, that is, apolipoprotein E-2 homozygosity combined with increased biosynthesis of VLDL or reduced catabolism of LDL, the condition in question is extreme dysbetalipoproteinemia, causally related to atherosclerosis and xanthomatosis.

Table 7. : Apoprotein E-2 homozygosity (E^D/E^D) : biochemical and clinical findings.

- Frequency in population : approx. 1%

- VLDL cholesterol concentration elevated

- Total serum cholesterol reduced, LDL cholesterol reduced

- Simultaneous inheritance of additional lipoprotein metabolic defect causes Type III hyperlipoproteinemia

- Hypothyroidism, obesity, estrogen deficiency or glucose intolerance may also result in expression of Type III hyperlipoproteinemia

- 1 in 50 people develop a Type III hyperlipoproteinemia

- 1 in 5000 people in the general population exhibit clinical signs of Type III hyperlipoproteinemia

The diagnosis of familial Type III hyperlipoproteinemia (frequency approx. 1:5000) can be confirmed on the basis of the clinical findings (xanthomas of the hand lines, tuberous xanthomas, intermittent claudication, coronary heart disease) and the biochemical findings (Apo E-2 homozygosity, β-VLDL, hyperlipidemia with elevated cholesterol and triglycerides) |96|. The early occurrence of coronary heart disease and/or peripheral vascular occlusion (often before age 40) are frequent complications of this disorder of lipid metabolism. Type III hyperlipoproteinemia must be implicated in the case of combined hyperlipidemia and peripheral vascular occlusion. Particularly characteristic of Type III hyperlipoproteinemia are planar xanthomas of the hand lines, not occurring in any other genetic hyperlipidemia. Furthermore, tuberous and tuberoeruptive xanthomas are observed on the elbow, occasionally periosteal tendinous xanthomas in the region of the Achille's tendon and the extensor tendons of the hands. Xanthelasmas and arcus corneae are somewhat rare. In addition to arteriosclerosis and xanthomatosis patients with familial Type III hyperlipoproteinemia frequently exhibit hyperuricemia and reduced glucose tolerance as metabolic anomalies |99, 100|.

As a consequence of the marked dependence of the lipid level on the caloric supply in Type III hyperlipoproteinemia, the cholesterol and triglyceride values are extremely variable and are generally measured between 300 and 1000 mg/dl. The majority of

cholesterol is not transported in the LDL, but in the VLDL. HDL
cholesterol values are usually reduced.

It has been demonstrated in family studies of patients with
Type III hyperlipoproteinemia that heterozygous family members
(genotype E-N/E-D or E-4/E-D) have clearly higher VLDL cholesterol
and VLDL apolipoprotein E concentrations than family members with the
normal apolipoprotein E genotype (E-N/E-N, E-4/E-4, E-N/E-4) |64|.
The risk of arteriosclerosis for heterozygous patients in families
with Type III hyperlipoproteinemia has not been determined to date.

The diagnostic possibilities for detecting Type III hyperlipoproteinemia are evaluated as follows :

1. Lipoprotein electrophoresis |94, 101, 102|

   Not reliable, since, on the one hand, a broad β band is seen
   in only half of all patients with Type III hyperlipoproteinemia and, on the other hand, it may occur in patients with
   other familial metabolic defects.

2. Quotients | 103, 104, 105|

   E.g. VLDL cholesterol/serum triglycerides ⟩ 0.3 or VLDL
   cholesterol/VLDL triglycerides ⟩ 0.42 : a good indicator, but
   not conclusive proof, since it is dependent on the individual
   metabolic situation and the applicable β -VLDL concentration,
   which may also fall below limit values.

3. Apolipoprotein E Polymorphism |66, 97, 98, 106, 107, 108|

   Best criterion : Genotype E-D/E-D; phenotype E-2 homozygous;
   offers conclusive proof in conjunction with corresponding
   clinical findings (hyperlipidemia, xanthomas of the hand
   lines, arteriosclerosis).

The differentiation of apolipoprotein E-2 homozygosity from
Type III hyperlipoproteinemia is at present possible only on the
basis of clinical observations. Of particular clinical interest is
the question of which patients, if any, with apolipoprotein E-2
homozygosity have an increased coronary risk. In any case, apolipoprotein E-2 homozygosity occurs in the population with a frequency
of 1% and is characterized by dysbetalipoproteinemia, which, at
least in a number of patients, is accompanied by the early onset of
coronary sclerosis. Between Type III hyperlipoproteinemia with
extreme elevation of β-VLDL and apoprotein E-2 homozygosity with
low serum lipid levels and slight elevation of β -VLDL and apolipoprotein E-2 is an entire spectrum of metabolic anomalies whose
relationship to coronary sclerosis is in need of explanation.

The authors would like to express their gratitude to Mr. Glenn Whitted for preparing the English text.

REFERENCES

1. Morrisett, J.D., Jackson, R.L., Gotto, A.M., Jr., Lipoproteins : structure and function, Ann. Rev. Biochem., 44 : 183 (1975), J. Biol. Chem., 249 : 5314 (1974).
2. Jackson, R.L., Morrisett, J.D., Gotto A.M., Jr., Segrest, J.P., The mechanism of lipid-binding by plasma lipoproteins, Mol. Cell Biochem., 6 : 43 (1975).
3. Jackson R.L., Morrisett, J.D., Gotto, A.M., Jr., Lipoproteins and lipid transport : Structural and functional concepts, in : Hyperlipidemia, Diagnosis and Therapy, Levy, R.I., Rifkind, B.M., eds., p.1, Grune and Stratton, New York (1977).
4. Brewer, H.B., Jr., Lux, S.E., Ronan, R., John, K.M., Amino acid sequence of human apo Lp-Gln-II (apo A-II), an apolipoprotein isolated from the high density lipoprotein complex, Proc. Natl. Acad. Sci., USA,, 69 : 1304 (1972).
5. Baker, H.N., Delahunty, T., Gotto, A.M., Jr., Jackson, R.L., The primary structure of high density apolipoprotein-glutamine-I, Proc. Natl. Acad. Sci., USA,, 71 : 3631 (1974).
6. Brewer, H.B., Jr., Fairwell, T., Larne, A., Ronan, R., Houser, A., Bronzert, T.J., The amino acid sequence of human apo A-I, an apolipoprotein isolated from high density lipoproteins, Biochem. Biophys. Res. Comm., 80 : 623 (1978).
7. Nicols, A., Miller, N.E., Lewis, B., High-density lipoprotein metabolism, Adv. Lipid Res., 17 : 53 (1980).
8. Fielding, C.J., Shore, V.G., Fielding, P.E., A protein cofactor of lecithin : cholesterol acyltransferase, Biochem. Biophys. Res. Comm., 46 : 1493 (1972).
9. Albers, J.J., Lecithin : cholesterol acyltransferase, Artery, 5 : 61 (1979).
10. Soutar, A.K., Garner, C.W., Baker, H.N., Sparrow, J.T., Jackson, R.L., Gotto, A.M., Smith, L.C., Effect of the human plasma apolipoproteins and phosphatidylcholine acyl donor on the activity of lecithin : cholesterol acyltransferase, Biochemistry, 14 : 3057 (1975).
11. Glomset, J.A., The plasma lecithin : cholesterol acyltransferase reaction, J. Lipid Res., 9 : 155 (1968).
12. Schmitz, G., Assmann, G., Melnik, B., The role of lecithin : cholesterol acyltransferase in high density lipoprotein-3/high density lipoprotein-2 interconversion in man, Clin. Chim. Acta, in press (1981).
13. Schmitz, G., Assmann, G., Isolation of human serum HDL-1 by zonal ultracentrifugation, J. Lipid. Res., submitted (1981).
14. Nestruck, A.C., Suzue, G., Marcel, Y.L., Studies on the polymorphism of human apolipoprotein A-I, Biochim. Biophys. Acta, 617 : 110 (1980).

15. Franceschini, G., Sirtori, C.R., Capurso, A., Weisgraber, K.H., Mahley, R.W., A-I-Milano Apoprotein. Decreased high density lipoprotein cholesterol levels with significant lipoprotein modifications and without clinical atherosclerosis in an Italian family, J. Clin. Invest., 66 : 892 (1980).

16. Weisgraber, K.H., Bersot, T.P., Mahley, R.W., Franceschini, G., Sirtori, C.R., A-I-Milano Apoprotein. Isolation and characterization of a cystein-containing variant of the A-I apoprotein from human high density lipoprotein, J. Clin. Invest., 66 : 901 (1980).

17. Utermann, G., Steinmetz, A., Haas, J., Feusner, G., Franceschini, G., Apolipoproteinopathies : rapid method for screening and characterization of genetic apolipoprotein A variants, J. Biol. Chem., in press (1981).

18. Menzel, H.-J., Dittmar, K., Assmann, G., One step screening method for the polymorphism of apolipoproteins A-I, A-II and A-IV, J. Lipid. Res., submitted (1981).

19. Assmann, G., Smootz, E., Adler, K., Capurso, A., Oette, K., The lipoprotein abnormality in Tangier disease, quantification of A-apoproteins, J. Clin. Invest., 59 : 565 (1977).

20. Assmann, G., Simantke, O., Schaefer, H.-E., Smooth, E., Characterization of high density lipoproteins in patients heterozygous for Tangier disease, J. Clin. Invest., 60 : 1025 (1977).

21. Mao, S.J.T., Sparrow, J.T., Gilliam, E.B., Gotto, A.M., Jr., Jackson, R.L., Mechanism of lipid-protein interaction in the plasma lipoproteins : the lipid-binding properties of synthetic fragments of apolipoprotein A-II, Biochemistry, 16 : 4150 (1977).

22. Segrest, J.P., Jackson, R.L., Morrisett, J.D., Gotto, A.M., Jr., A molecular theory of lipid protein interactions in the plasma lipoproteins, FEBS Let., 38 : 247 (1974).

23. Mao, S.J.T., Jackson, R.L., Gotto, A.M., Sparrow, J.T., Mechanism of lipid-protein interaction in the plasma lipoproteins : Identification of a lipid binding site in apolipoprotein A-II, Biochemistry, 20 : 1676 (1981).

24. Kostner, G.M., Studies of the composition and structure of human serum lipoproteins : Isolation and partial characterization of apolipoprotein A-III, Biochim. Biophys. Acta, 336 : 383 (1974).

25. McConathy, W.J., Alaupovic, P., Isolation and partial charaterization of apolipoprotein D : A new protein moiety of the human plasma lipoprotein system, FEBS Let., 37 : 178 (1973).

26. Kostner, G., Studies on the cofactor requirement for lecithin : Cholesterol acyltransferase, Scand. J. Clin. Lab. Invest., 33 suppl. 137 : 19 (1974).

27. Chajek, T., Fielding, C.J., Isolation and characterization of a human serum cholesteryl ester transfer protein, Proc. Natl. Acad. Sci., USA, 75 : 3445 (1978).

28. Fielding, P.E., Fielding, C.J., A cholesteryl ester trans-
    fer complex in human plasma, Proc. Natl. Acad. Sci., USA, 77 :
    3327 (1980).
29. Fielding, C.J., Fielding, P.E., Regulation of human plasma
    lecithin cholesterol acyltransferase activity by lipoprotein
    acceptor cholesteryl ester content, J. Biol. Chem., 256 : 2102
    (1981).
30. Green, P.H.R., Glickman, R.M., Riley, J.W., Quinet, E.,
    Human apolipoprotein A-IV. Intestinal origin and distribution
    in plasma, J. Clin. Invest., 65 : 911 (1980).
31. Weisgraber, K.H., Bersot, T.P., Mahley, R.W., Isolation and
    characterization of an apoprotein from the d ⟨ 1.006 lipopro-
    teins of human and canine lymph homologous with the rat A-IV
    apoprotein, Biochem. Biophys. Res. Commun., 85 : 287 (1978).
32. Utermann, G., Beisiegel, U., Apolipoprotein A-IV : A
    protein occuring in human mesenteric lymph chylomicrons and
    free in plasma, Europ. J. Biochem., 99 : 33 (1979).
33. Kane, J.P., Hardman, D.A., Paulus, H.E., Heterogeneity of
    apolipoprotein B : Isolation of a new species from human
    chylomicrons, Proc. Natl. Acad. Sci., USA, 77 : 2465 (1980).
34. Havel, R.J., International Congress for Clinical Chemistry,
    Wien (1981).
35. Brown, M.S., Kovanen, P.T., Goldstein, J.L., Regulation of
    plasma cholesterol by lipoprotein receptors, Science, 212 :
    628 (1981).
36. Shepherd, J., Bicker, S, Lorimer, A.R., Packard, C.J.,
    Receptor-mediated low density lipoprotein catabolism in man,
    J. Lipid. Res., 20 : 999 (1979).
37. Shepherd, J., Packard, C.J., Bicker, S., Lawrie, T.D.V.,
    Morgan, H.G., Cholesterylamine promotes receptor-mediated
    low-density-lipoprotein catabolism, N. Engl. J. Med., 302 :
    1219 (1980).
38. Malloy, M.J., Kane, J.P., Harmann, D.A., Hamilton, R.L.,
    Dalal, K.B., Normotriglyceridemic Abetalipoproteinemia.
    Absence of the B-100 apolipoprotein, J. Clin. Invest., 67 :
    1441 (1981).
39. Schonfeld, G., Lees, R.S., George, P.K., Pfleger, B., Assay
    of total plasma apolipoprotein B concentration in human
    subjects, J. Clin. Invest., 53 : 1458 (1974).
40. Albers, J.J., Cabana, V.G., Hazzard, W.R., Immunoassay of
    human plasma apolipoprotein B, Metabolism, 24 : 1339 (1975).
41. Utermann, G., Lipp, K., Wiegandt, H., Studies on the
    Lp(a)-lipoprotein of human serum, IV. The disaggregation
    of the Lp(a)-lipoprotein, Humangenetik, 14 : 142 (1972).
42. Albers, J.J., Adolphons, J.L., Hazzard, W.R., Radioimmuno-
    assay of human plasma Lp(a) lipoprotein, J. Lipid. Res., 18 :
    331 (1977).

43. Kostner, G.M., Avogardo, P., Cazzolato, G., Marth, E., Bittolo-Bon, G., Quinci, G.B., Lipoprotein Lp(a) and the risk for myocardial infarction, Atherosclerosis, 38 : 51 (1981).

44. Shulman, R.S., Herbert, P.N., Wehrly, K., Fredrickson, D.S., The complete amino acid sequence of C-I (Apo Lp-Ser), an apolipoprotein from human very low density lipoproteins, J. Biol. Chem.,250 : 182 (1975).

45. Jackson, R.L., Sparrow, J.T., Baker, H.N., Morrisett, J., Taunton, O.D., Gotto, A.M., Jr.,The primary structure of apolipoprotein-serine, J. Biol. Chem., 249 : 5308, (1974).

46. Jackson, R.L., Baker, H.N., Gilliam, E.B., Gotto, A.M., Jr., Primary structure of very low density apolipoprotein C-II of human plasma, Proc. Natl. Acad. Sci., USA, 74 : 1942 (1977).

47. Brewer, H.B., Shulman, R., Herbert, P., Ronan, R., Wehrly, K., The complete amino acid sequence of alanine apolipoprotein (apo C-III), an apolipoprotein from human plasma very low density lipoproteins, J. Biol. Chem., 249 : 4975 (1974).

48. Jackson, R.L., Morrisett, J.D., Sparrow, J.R., Segrest, J.P., Pownall, H.J., Smith, L.C., Hoff, H.F., Gotto, A.M., Jr., The interaction of apolipoprotein-serine with phosphatidylcholine, J. Biol. Chem., 249 : 5314 (1974).

49. Kashyap, M.L., Srivastava, L.S., Chen, C.Y., Perisutti, G., Campbell, M., Lutmer, R.J.F., Glueck, C.J., Radioimmunoassay of human apolipoprotein C-II. A study in normal and hypertriglyceridemic subjects, J. Clin. Invest., 60 : 171 (1977).

50. Havel, R.J., Shore, V.G., Shore, B., Biou, D.M., Role of the specific glycopeptides of human serum lipoproteins in the activation of lipoprotein lipase, Circ. Res., 27 : 595 (1970).

51. LaRosa, J.C., Levy, R.I., Herbert, P.N., Lux, S.E., Fredrickson, D.S., A specific apoprotein activator for lipoprotein lipase, Biochem. Biophys. Res. Commun., 41 : 57 (1970).

52. Smith, L.C., Voyta, J.C., Catapano, A.L., Kinnunen, P.K.J., Gotto, A.M., Jr., Sparrow, J.T., Activation of lipoprotein lipase by synthetic fragments of apo C-II, in : Atherosclerosis V, Gotto, A.M., Jr., Smith, L.C., Allen, B., eds., p. 397, Springer-Verlag, New York (1980).

53. Musliner, T.A., Herbert, P.N., Church, E.C., Activation of lipoprotein lipase by native and acylated peptides of apolipoprotein C-II, Biochim. Biophys. Acta, 573 : 501 (1979).

54. Kinnunen, P.K.J., Jackson, R.L., Smith, L.C., Gotto, A.M., Sparrow, J.T., Activation of lipoprotein lipase by native and synthetic fragments of human plasma apolipoprotein C-II, Proc. Natl. Acad. Sci., USA, 74 : 4848 (1977).

55. Breckenridge, W.C., Little, J.A., Steiner, G., Chow, A., Poapst, M., Hypertriglyceridemia associated with deficiency of apolipoprotein C-II, N. Engl. J. Med., 298 : 1265 (1978).

56. Havel, R., Kotite, L., Kane, J., Isoelectric heterogeneity of the cofactor protein for lipoprotein lipase and human blood plasma, Biochem. Med., 21 : 121 (1979).

57. Catapano, A.L., The distribution of apo C-II and apo C-III in very low density lipoproteins of normal and type IV subjects, Atherosclerosis, 35 : 419 (1980).

58. Curry, M.D., McConathy, W.J., Fesmire, J.D., Alaupovic, P., Quantitative determination of human apolipoprotein C-III by electro-immunoassay, Biochim. Biochphys. Acta, 617 : 503 (1980).

59. Brown, W.V., Baginsky, M.L., Inhibition of lipoprotein lipase by an apoprotein of human very low density lipoprotein, Biochem. Biophys. Res. Commun., 46 : 375 (1972).

60. Kraus, R.M., Herbert, P.N., Levy, R.I., Fredrickson, D.S., Further observations on the activation and inhibition of lipoprotein lipase by apolipoproteins, Circ. Res., 33 : 403 (1973).

61. Zannis, V.I., Breslow, J.L., Characterization of a unique human apolipoprotein E variant associated with type III hyperlipoproteinemia, J. Biol. Chem., 255 : 1759 (1980).

62. Shelburne, F.A., Quarfordt, S.H., A new apoprotein of human plasma very low density lipoproteins, J. Biol. Chem., 249 : 1428 (1974).

63. Weisgraber, K.H., Mahley, R.W., Apoprotein (E-A-II) complex of human plasma lipoproteins, J. Biol. Chem., 253 : 6281 (1978).

64. Innerarity, T.L., Mahley, R.W., Weisgraber, K.H., Bersot, T.P., Apoprotein (E-A-II) complex of human plasma lipoprotein. II. Receptor binding activity of a high density lipoprotein subfraction modulated by apo (E-A-II) complex, J. Biol. Chem., 253 : 6289 (1978).

65. Wu, A.-L., Windmüller, H.G., Relative contributions by liver and intestine to individual plasma apolipoproteins in the rat, J. Biol. Chem., 254 : 7316 (1979).

66. Uterman, G.N., Jaeschke, M., Menzel, J., Familial hyperlipoproteinemia Type III : Deficiency of a specific apolipoprotein (apo E-III) in the very low density lipoproteins, FEBS Let., 56 : 352 (1975).

67. Havel R.J., Kotite, L., Vigne, J.-L., Kane, J.P., Tun, P., Phillips, N., Chen, G.C., Radioimmunoassay of human arginine-rich apolipoprotein, apoprotein E. Concentration in blood and lipoproteins as affected by apoprotein E-3 deficiency, J. Clin. Invest., 66 : 1351 (1980).

68. Kushwaha, R.S., Hazzard, W.R., Wahl, P.W., Hoover, J.J., Type III hyperlipoproteinemia : Diagnosis in whole plasma by apolipoprotein-E immunoassay, Ann. Intern. Med., 87 : 509 (1977).

69. Zannis, V.I., Breslow, J.L., Human very low density lipoprotein apolipoprotein E isoprotein polymorphism is explained by genetic variation and posttranslational modification, Biochemistry, 20 : 1033 (1981).

70. Zannis, V.J., Just, P.W., Breslow, J.L., Human apolipopro-

tein E isoprotein subclasses are genetically determined, Amer.
J. Hum. Genet., 33 : 11 (1981).

71. Weisgraber, K.H., Rall, S.C., Jr., Mahley, R.W., Human E
    apoprotein heterogeneity : Cystein-arginine interchanges in
    the amino acid sequence of the apo-E isoforms, J. Biol. Chem.,
    in press (1981).

72. Chao, Y.-S., Windler, E.E., Chen, G.C., Havel, R.J., Hepatic
    catabolism of rat and human lipoproteins in rats treated with
    17 alpha-ethinyl estradiol, J. Biol. Chem., 254 : 11360
    (1979).

73. Pitas, R.E., Innerarity, T.L., Mahley, R.W., Cell surface
    receptor binding of phospholipid protein complexes containing
    different ratios of receptor-active and -inactive E apopro-
    tein, J. Biol. Chem., 255 : 5454 (1980).

74. Innerarity, T.L., Pitas, R.E., Mahley, R.W., Receptor
    binding of cholesterol-induced high-density lipoproteins
    containing predominantly apoprotein E to cultured fibroblasts
    with mutations at the low-density lipoprotein receptor locus,
    Biochemistry, 19 : 4359 (1974).

75. Havel, R.J., Chao, Y.-S., Windler, E.E., Kolite, L., Guo,
    L.S.S., Isoprotein specificity in the hepatic uptake of
    apolipoprotein E and the pathogenesis of familial dysbetalipo-
    proteinemia, Proc. Natl. Acad. Sci., USA, 77 : 4349 (1980).

76. Assmann, G., Tangier-Krankheit, in : Stoffwelchselkrankhei-
    ten, Schettler, G., Greten, H., Schlierf, G., Seidel, D.,
    eds., Springer-Verlag, Berlin Heidelberg New York (Handbuch
    der Inneren Medizin, 5, Aufl. Bd. VII Teil 4, S. 461) (1976).

77. Assmann, G., Die Tangier-Krankheit - Klinik und Pathophysio-
    logie, Klin. Wschr., 57 : 53 (1979).

78. Herbert, P.N., Gotto, A.M., Fredrickson, D.S., Familial
    lipoprotein deficiency (abetalipoproteinemia, hypobetalipopro-
    teinemia and Tangier disease), in : The metabolic basis of
    inherited disease, Stanbury, J.B., Wyngaarden, J.B., Fredrick-
    son, D.S., eds., p. 544 (Ch. 28), McGraw-Hill, New York
    (1978).

79. Assmann G., Tangier disease and the possible role of high
    density lipoproteins in atherosclerosis, Atherosclerosis Rev.,
    6 : 1 (1979).

80. Herbert, P.N., Assman, G., Gotto, A.M., Fredrickson,
    D.S., Familial lipoprotein deficiency (abetalipoproteinemia,
    hypobetalipoproteinemia and Tangier disease), in : The metabo-
    lic basis of inherited disease, Stanbury, M.S., Wyngaarden,
    J.B., Fredrickson, D.S., Goldstein, J.L., Brown, M.S., eds.,
    Ch. 29, McGraw-Hill, in press (1982).

81. Ferrans, V.I., Fredrickson, D.S., The pathology of Tangier
    disease. A light and electron microscopic study, Am. J.
    Pathol., 78 : 101 (1975).

82. Katz, S.S., Small, D.M., Brook, I.G., Lees, R.W., The
    storage lipids in Tangier disease. A physical chemical study,

J. Clin. Invest., 59 : 1045 (1977).

83. Herbert, P.N., Heinen, R.J., Bausserman, L.L., Henderson,
    L.O., Musliner, T.A., Abetalipoproteinemia and hypobetalipo-
    proteinemia : question still exceed insights, in : Atheroscle-
    rosis V. Proceedings of the fifth international symposium on
    atherosclerosis, Gotto, A.M., Jr., Smith, L.C., Allem, B.,
    eds., p. 684-688, Springer Verlag, New York (1980).

84. Herbert, P.N., Fredrickson, D.S., The hypobetalipoprotein-
    emias, in : Handbüch der Inneren Medizin, VII/4, Fettstoff-
    wechsel, Schettler, G., Greten, H., Schlierf, G., Seidel, D.,
    eds., p. 485, Springer Verlag, Heidelberg (1976).

85. Cox, D.W., Breckenridge, W.C., Little, J.A., Inheritance of
    apolipoprotein C-II deficiency with hypertriglyceridemia and
    pancreatitis, N. Engl. J. Med., 299 : 1421 (1978).

86. Yamamura, T., Sudo, H., Ishikawa, K., Yamamoto, A., Familial
    type I hyperlipoproteinemia caused by apolipoprotein C-II
    deficiency, Atherosclerosis, 34 : 53 (1979).

87. Capurso, A., Pace, L., Bonomo, L., Catapano, A., Schiliro,
    G., LaRosa, M., Assmann, G., New case of apoprotein C-II
    deficiency, Lancet 1, 268 (1980).

88. Crepaldi, G., Fellin, R., Baggio, G., Augustin, J., Greten,
    H., Lipoprotein and apoprotein, adipose tissue and hepatic
    lipoprotein lipase levels in patients with familial hyperchy-
    lomicronemia and their immediate family members, in : Athero-
    sclerosis V, Gotto, A.M., Jr., Smith, L.C., Allen, B., eds.,
    p. 250, Springer-Verlag, New York (1980).

89. Miller, N.E., Rao, S.N., Alaupovic, P., Noble, N., Slack,
    J., Brunzell, J.D., Lewis, B., Familial apolipoprotein C-II
    deficiency, plasma lipoproteins and apolipoprotein in hetero-
    zygous and homozygous subjects and the effects of plasma
    infusion, Eur. J. Clin. Invest., 11 : 69 (1981).

90. Utermann, G., Hees, M., Steinmetz, A., Polymorphism of
    apolipoprotein E and occurrence of dysbetalipoproteinemia in
    men, Nature, 269 : 604 (1977).

91. Utermann, G., Pruin, N., Steinmetz, A., Effect of a single
    polymorphic gene locus on plasma lipid levels in man, Clin.
    Genet., 15 : 63 (1979).

92. Havel, R.J., Goldstein, J.L., Brown, M.S., Lipoproteins and
    lipid transport, in : Metabolic control and disease, 8th ed.,
    Bondy, P.K., Rosenberg, L.E., eds., p. 393 (Ch. 7), Saunders,
    W.B. Co, Philadelphia (1980).

93. Gregg, R.E., Zech, L.A., Schaefer, E.J., Brewer, H.B., Jr.,
    Type III hyperlipoproteinemia : Defective metabolism of an
    abnormal apolipoprotein E, Science, 211 : 584 (1981).

94. Fredrickson, D.S., Levy, R.I., Lees, R.S., Fat transport in
    lipoproteins - an integrated approach to mechanisms and
    disorders, N. Engl. J. Med., 276 : 32, 94 : 148, 215 : 273
    (1967).

95. Havel, R.J., Kane, J.P., Primary dysbetalipoproteinemia :
    Predominance of a specific apolipoprotein species in triglyce-
    ride-rich lipoproteins, Proc. Natl. Acad. Sci., USA, 70 : 2015
    (1973).
96. Brown, M.S., Goldstein, J.L., Fredrickson, D.S., Familial
    type 3 hyperlipoproteinemia, in : The metabolic basis of
    inherited disease, Stanbury, J.B., Wyngaarden, J.B., Fredrick-
    son, D.S., Goldstein, J.L., Brown, M.S., eds., Ch. 32, McGraw-
    Hill, New York, in press (1982).
97. Utermann, G., Langenbeck, U., Beisiegel, U., Weber, W.,
    Genetics of the Apo-E-system in man, Am. J. Hum. Genet., 32 :
    339 (1980).
98. Utermann, G., Vogelberg, K.H., Steinmetz, A., Schoenborn,
    W., Pruin, N., Jaeschke, M., Hees, M., Canzler, H., Polimor-
    phism of apolipoprotein E, Clin. Genet., 15 : 37 (1979).
99. Morganroth, J., Levy, R.I., Fredrickson, D.S., The biochemi-
    cal, clinical and genetic features of type III hyperlipopro-
    teinemia, Ann. Intern. Med., 82 : 158 (1975).
100. Levy, R.I., Assmann, G., Type III - Hyperlipoproteinemia, in :
    Stoffwechselkrankheiten, Schettler, G., Greten, H., Schlierf,
    G., Seidel, D., eds., Springer-Verlag, Berlin Heidelberg New
    York (Handbuch der Inneren Medizin, 5, Aufl. Bd. VII Teil 4,
    S. 301) (1976).
101. Masket, B.H., Levy, R.I., Fredrickson, D.S., The use of
    polyacrylamide electrophoresis in differentiating type III
    hyperlipoproteinemia, J. Lab. Clin. Med., 82 : 794 (1973).
102. Schneider, J., Maurer, M., Kaffarnik, H., Häufigkeit der
    Hyperlipoproteinämie Typ III bei elektrophoretisch nachweis-
    barer breiter -Bande, Klin. Wschr., 52 : 941 (1974).
103. Fredrickson, D.S., Morganroth, J., Levy, R.I., Type III
    hyperlipoproteinemia : An analysis of two contemporary defini-
    tions, Ann. Intern. Med., 82 : 150 (1975).
104. Mishkel, M., Nazir, D.J., Crother, S., A longitudinal
    assessment of lipid ratios in the diagnosis of type III
    hyperlipoproteinemia, Clin. Chim. Acta, 58 : 121 (1975).
105. Hazzard, W.R., Porte, D., Bierman, E.L., Abnormal lipid
    composition of very low density lipoproteins in diagnosis of
    broad beta disease (type III hyperlipoproteinemia), Metabo-
    lism, 21 : 1009 (1972).
106. Utermann, G., Albrecht, G., Steinmetz, A., Polymorphism of
    Apolipoprotein E. I. Methodological aspects and diagnosis of
    hyperlipoproteinemia type III without ultracentrifugation,
    Clin. Genet., 14 : 351 (1978).
107. Warnick, G.R., Mayfield, C., Albers, J.J., Hazzard, R.W.,
    Gel isoelectric focussing method for specific diagnosis of
    familial hyperlipoproteinemia type III, Clin. Chem., 25 : 279
    (1979).

108. Weidman, S.W., Suarez, B., Falko, J.M., Witzum, J.L., Kolar, J., Raben, M., Schonfeld, G., Type III hyperlipoproteinemia : Development of a VLDL Apo E gel isoelectric focusing technique and application in family studies, J. Lab. Clin. Med., 93 : 549 (1979).

HEMOSTASIS AND ATHEROSCLEROSIS

Fedor Bachmann

Hematology Division and Thrombosis Research Laboratory
University of Lausanne, Medical School, CHUV
CH-1011 Lausanne, Switzerland

INTRODUCTION

This review, although not intending to call into question the important role of hyperlipidemia and especially of LDL-cholesterol in the pathogenesis of atherosclerosis, aims to familiarize the reader with other etiologic factors of atherosclerosis. Recent experimental work clearly shows that under certain conditions, the development of atherosclerotic plaques can be inhibited despite hypercholesteremia. Kramsch et al. fed rabbits an atherogenic diet with and without increasing doses of lanthanum chloride, a potent calcium antagonist. Whereas all animals exhibited severe cholesteremia of 20 to 25 g/l, extensive atherosclerotic lesions comprising 64% of the aortic surface area developed only in those given the atherogenic diet without lanthanum [1]. There was a progressive reduction of aortic surface area involvement with increasing dosage of lanthanum to 16% (20 mg $LaCl_3$/kg/d) and to less than 3% (40 mg $LaCl_3$/kg/d). Fuster et al. observed that the aortas of pigs afflicted with homozygous von Willebrand's disease did not exhibit multiple atheromatous plaques whereas those of normal pigs did [2]. These authors undertook a prospective trial on the role of von Willebrand factor (the multimeric blood coagulation Factor VIII complex) in the pathogenesis of atherosclerosis. They fed a 2% cholesterol diet to 11 control pigs and to 7 pigs with von Willebrand's disease. All of the controls developed atherosclerotic plaques in the aorta and in 9, at least 13% of the entire surface was involved. In contrast, 4 of the

---

Abbreviations: G, (giga) = 10^9; PDGF, platelet derived grow factor; PF4, platelet factor 4; SMC, smooth muscle cells.

pigs with von Willebrand's disease did not develop such lesions, 2
had lesions affecting 6 and 7% of the aortic surface and only one
had 13% of the aortic surface involved. In pigs with von Willebrand
disease, the extent of endothelial damage was equally severe as in
the controls, and there was extensive nonproliferative, nonathero-
sclerotic intimal fat infiltration.

These experiments demonstrate that hypercholesteremia resulted
in increased permeability of the endothelium to lipids but did not
suffice per se to produce atherosclerotic plaques. The presence of
von Willebrand factor is necessary for platelets to adhere to subendothelium and thus to initiate the repair mechanisms in the event
of endothelial damage. Patients and animals with homozygous von
Willebrand disease are functionally thrombocytopenic and have severe hemorrhagic manifestations. Several lines of evidence point to
the important role of platelet-vessel wall interactions consecutive
to endothelial damage in the pathogenesis of atherosclerosis.

THE RESPONSE TO INJURY HYPOTHESIS OF ATHEROSCLEROSIS

The hypothesis that arterial endothelial lesions, which induce
the formation of a thrombotic process and involve the participation
of platelets are the substrate for the formation of atherosclerotic
plaques, dates book to the work of Rokitansky and of Virchow[3-4].
The response-to-injury hypothesis has been extended by Duguid,
French, Mustard and Packham, Stemerman, Ross and other[5-9] and has
been well reviewed by Ross and Glomset[10].

A number of factors, such as increased shear stress in hypertension, hyperlipidemia, congenital homocysteinemia, diabetes,
smoking, hormone dysfunction and perhaps even constituants released
from hyperactive platelets may injure the endothelium and lead to
platelet-vessel wall interaction. Platelets attach to the exposed
subendothelium, aggregate and release from their α-granules fibrinogen, β-thromboglobulin, platelet factor 4 (PF4) and platelet-
derived growth factor (PDGF) into the surroundings. PDGF is a potent
mitogenic factor and induces smooth muscle cell (SMC) proliferation.
Steuerman demonstrated that PF4 does indeed enter the vessel wall
after mechanical removal of the aortic endothelium by a balloon
catheter[11]. Using a fluorescin-labeled antibody to PF4, he showed
that, 10 minutes after endothelial desquamation, PF4 was present in
one third of the vessel wall. Thirty minutes after ballooning the
entire vessel wall was permeated by PF4. Infusion of prostacycline
at the start of deendothelialization greatly reduced platelet adhesion to the exposed subendothelium and release of PF4 into the vessel wall. Stemerman also measured growth of SMC's by ^{3}H-thymidine
incorporation into SMC-DNA, and found that reballooning of the abdominal aorta caused a proliferative spurt of thoracic aortic SMC's,
thus demonstrating that a humoral signal can initiate SMC proliferation. He believes that mitogenic factors released from platelets

may indeed find their way through more permeable endothelium without the need for close platelet-vessel wall interaction and proposes that the response-to-injury hypothesis of atherosclerosis be
broadened to the response-to-signal concept. This new concept sig-
nifies that any alteration of platelet reactivity resulting in an
increased release of PDGF from α-granules is per se atherogenic in
the presence of increased endothelial permeability.

PREVENTION OF ATHEROSCLEROSIS BY REDUCTION OF PLATELET REACTIVITY

Four well conducted experimental studies underline the important etiologic role of platelets in the formation of atherosclerotic
lesions. I have already discussed the study of Fuster et al., who
showed that pigs with a congenital deficiency of von Willebrand
factor, a condition which prevents platelets from adhering in a
normal fashion to subendothelium, are protected against atherosclerosis[2].

Moore and collaborators placed PE60 polyethylene catheters in
the aortas of 35 rabbits fed standard rabbit chow[12]. The animals
were randomly divided into 2 groups. The experimental group of 17
rabbits received injections of antiplatelet serum preoperatively
and for 13 additional days. Mean platelet counts on days 4 and 14
were 6, respectively 7 G/l. The control group of 18 rabbits received no anti-platelet serum. Mean platelet counts on days 4 and 14
were 434 and 436 G/l respectively. The animals were killed after
14 days. The extent of lesions was estimated by photographing the
opened aortas, projecting the photographs on cardboard, cutting the
areas occupied by the different lesions and weighing the cardboard.
In the control group, the mean weight of raised lesions was 6 to 7
times greater than in the experimental group (p < 0.001). In animals
with platelet counts < 1 G/l, raised lesions were completely prevented. Raised lesions were defined as having a thickened intima
in which lipid containing cells, sometimes recognizable as SMC,
were present. Many lesions showed in addition a central lipid pool
and calcifications. They were distinctly elevated above the intimal
surface and had a covering layer of thrombus.

Friedman et al. pursued a similar but more elaborate approach[13].
They produced aortic de-endothelialization by the intra-arterial
balloon catheter technique in over 200 rabbits. In the experimental
groups thrombocytopenia was induced and maintained (mean platelet
count 5.6 G/l) for up to 31 days by daily injections of highly specific sheep anti-rabbit platelet sera. Control animals received
identically treated normal sheep sera, and had mean daily platelet
counts of 363 G/l. Prior to killing, animals were given Evans blue
intravenously to study the degree of re-endothelialization. Intimal
thickness of the aortas was assessed by counting cell layers in se-
mithin sections. There was no difference in endothelial regrowth in
controls and in the thrombocytopenic animals; re-endothelialization

was progressive over the 28 day experimental period and reached 20%
of the aortic surface after 7 days, 40% after 14 days and 60% after
28 days. In the controls, there was marked and progressive neointimal proliferation. 14 days after endothelial denudation, Evans blue-
negative areas showed an endothelial cell covering layer overlying
a mean SMC neointimal proliferation of 6.3 cell layers. Blue regions
exhibited a mean neointimal SMC proliferation of 9.5 cell layers. 28
days after ballooning, non-blue areas and blue areas showed a SMC
proliferation of 13.1 and 18.2 cell layers respectively ($p < 0.001$),
whereas mean neointimal SMC proliferation in thrombopenic animals
was less than 1 SMC cell layer over denuded and re-endothelialized
aorta. These results clearly demonstrate that platelet play an important role in SMC proliferative response (which probably is an
obligatory event in atherogenesis) following endothelial injury.

The fourth study was designed to clarify the mechanism responsible for the markedly accelerated atherosclerosis in patients with
chronic homocystinemia, an inborn deficiency of cystathionine syntha-
se. This condition typically leads to death before the 3rd decade of
life due to atherosclerotic occlusion of cerebral, myocardial, renal
and pulmonary arteries[14] . Harker and collaborators infused into baboons throughout a 3 month period a solution of 1-homocysteine (26
animals) or a control solution (8 animals). The infusions produced
plasma homocystine levels of 0.1 to 0.2 mM due to the endogenous
transformation of homocysteine to homocystine. 11 of the 26 experimental animals received orally dipyridamole, a phosphodiesterase inhibitor, 10 mg/kg t.i.d. In the 8 control animals, endothelial cell
coverage was entirely intact as evidenced by pressure-perfusion fi-
xation in vivo, using either 0.3% AgNO staining or scanning elec-
tronmicroscopy. Patchy endothelial cell loss comprised 7 to 10% of
the aortic surface observed in both experimental groups. The administration of dipyridamole, therefore, did not significantly reduce
the extent of endothelial damage. Platelet survival was 5.4 days in
the controls. It was markedly shortened to 2.8 days ($p < 0.001$) in
the 15 animals receiving chronic homocysteine infusions alone and
only slightly shortened to 4.8 days (n.s.) in 11 baboons receiving
both homocysteine infusions and dipyridamole. Likewise dipyridamole
administration normalized the excessive platelet turnover of 183 G/l
per day to 76 G/l per day (controls 63 G/l per day). All of the ho-
mocystinemic animals developed lesions similar to the fibromuscular
elastic lesions in man. These contained numerous SMC's surrounded by
large amounts of small collagen fibers and elastic fibers rich in
microfibrils, suggesting that the elastic fibers were relatively immature. The lesion score in the animals receiving no dipyridamole
correlated directly with the overall mean homocystine concentration
(r:0.96). It was four times lower in the baboons who were given dipyridamole ($p < 0.001$). These experiments strongly suggest that homo-
cystine-induced endothelial cell injury resulted in atherosclerosis
through platelet-mediated intimal proliferation of SMC's that can
be partially prevented by drug-induced platelet dysfunction.

THE PLATELET-DERIVED GROWTH FACTOR (PDGF)

Most in vitro cell cultures require the presence of serum for
growth. In 1973, Balk et al. discovered that plasma lacks this
growth promoting activity and that cultures of chicken fibroblasts
were arrested in the G_0/G_1 phase of the cell cycle in the absence of serum[15]. Ross et al. subsequently reported that platelets
release a potent mitogenic factor during the coagulation of blood[16].
PDGF is identical to the growth factor in human serum that stimulates
proliferation of mouse 3T3 cells [17]. It is also mitogenic for other
mesenchymal cells, such as SMC's[16]), glial cells[18], primate dermal
fibroblasts[19] and synovial cells[20]. PDGF is stored in the α-gra-
nules of platelets [21] and released into the surrounding medium upon
activation of platelets by thrombin, ADP, collagen, epinephrine or
arachidonate [21-23]. Apparently, the release of PDGF involves the
activation of the prostaglandin pathway since arachidonate mediated
release was suppressed by indomethacin, an inhibitor of cyclooxygenase[23]. Patients with the gray platelet syndrome, a hereditary selective deficiency of platelet α-granules release no or little PDGF
from their stimulated platelets[22].

Human PDGF has been purified to homogeneity by two groups of investigators, but different molecular weights are reported. This may
be due to the extremely small yield of approximately 25 to 50 µg of
PDGF per 100 liters of blood, which hampers extensive biochemical
analysis of the purified polypeptide. Antoniades et al. reported a
molecular weight of 13'000 to 16'000 daltons and an isoelectric point
of 9.8 [24]. Heldin et al. found a molecular weight of 33'000 daltons. In the presence of reducing agents, PDGF was converted into
two distinct components of 17'000 and 14'000 daltons respectively.
These authors conclude, therefore, that PDGF is a two-chain polypeptide, linked by disulphide bridges.

Pure PDGF is active at 10^{-10}M, i.e. at concentrations at which
known polypeptide hormones are characteristically active [24]. PDGF is
necessary, but not sufficient for the movement of quiescent BALB/c
3T3 fibroblasts in the G_0/G_1 phase of the cell cycle into the S
phase[26]. Apparently quiescent 3T3 cells are rendered competent by
PDGF to initiate DNA synthesis in the presence of somatomedin-C and
of at least one other unknown progression factor [27]. Heldin et al.
demonstrated specific receptors for PDGF on skin fibroblasts, normal
and malignant glial cells, SMC's and 3T3 cells, but not on epithelial-
derived cells, neuroblastoma cells, endothelial cells or peripheral
lymphocytes[28]. In human foreskin fibroblast cultures, Scatchard analysis of binding indicated a single class of receptors with a K_d of
10^{-9} M. The number of PDGF-binding sites was approximately $3x10^5$ per
cell and there was no competition for PDGF-binding by epidermal
growth factor, fibroblast growth factor or insulin. The observation
that only the receptor-positive cells - i.e. the connective tissue-
and glia-derived cells - were responsive to stimulation with PDGF,

implies that the PDGF-receptor has functional significance[28].

Mammalian cells require cholesterol as a structural component of their membranes. Fibroblasts, arterial SMC's and a number of other mesenchymal cells take up cholesterol from LDL via LDL-receptors, followed by endocytotic incorporation of cholesterol into the cell[29]. When cells are grown in the absence of cholesterol, LDL-receptor activity becomes greatly increased. Witte and Cornicelli[30] have shown, that PDGF stimulates LDL-receptor activity in cultured human fibroblasts and leads to a dose-related increase in ^{125}I-LDL binding to a maximum of approximately 300%. In the presence of added LDL, this increase in LDL binding was not observed. Cholesterol esterification was also stimulated by PDGF as well as after a conditioning of fibroblasts in LDL- and PDGF-depleted medium followed by the addition of LDL. Fibroblasts from a patient with homozygous familial hypercholesterolemia, which lack the LDL-receptor also showed a significant increase in cholesterol esterification with PDGF alone, whereas LDL had no effect[30].

SMC's attach to different types of collagen by different mechanisms. They are stimulated to attach to types I and III collagens by serum and by purified fibronectin but appear to attach directly to type V collagen via a component of the SMC surface[31]. Grotendorst et al. coated nucleopore filters with type I or type V collagen. Using a modified Boyden chamber assay for chemotaxis, they then added freshly trypsinized SMC's to the upper chamber and the supernatant of a suspension of platelets having undergone thrombin-induced aggregation to the lower chamber[31]. The material released from platelets as well as purified PDGF were chemotactic for SMC's, but fibroblast growth factor and epidermal growth factor were not. When PDGF was present on both sides of the filter, no migration occurred from the upper to the lower chamber. Since PDGF is also chemotactic for fibroblasts, these authors suggest, that PDGF may be a regulator of wound-healing. It appears to act by attracting connective tissue cells to sites of injury and activating them for the proliferative response needed to repair the damage.

This short review on some properties of PDGF underlines the many roles PDGF may play in the pathogenesis of atherosclerosis. It is able to: (i) stimulate the proliferation of SMC's and of fibroblasts [16-19], to which it attaches via PDGF-receptors [28], (ii) stimulate LDL-receptor activity and cholesterol esterification in human fibroblasts [30],(iii) act as a chemotactic factor for SMC's and for fibroblasts [31], and (iv) appears to be able to penetrate into the arterial wall through a damaged and more permeable endothelium[11].

EFFECT OF LIPIDS AND LIPOPROTEINS ON PLATELETS AND THE BLOOD
COAGULATION SYSTEM

Over the last two decades, many investigators have been concerned with the effect of lipids on blood coagulation, platelet
function and fibrinolytic activity of the blood.

By means of the simplest coagulation test, the plasma recalcification time in siliconized glass tubes, Botti and Ratnoff
found that the addition of small amounts of C 16 and of C 18 unsaturated fatty acids to whole plasma resulted in a significant
shortening of the clotting time[32]. No such shortening of global
plasma coagulability occurred when C 12 to C 14 saturated or C 18
non-saturated fatty acids were added to plasma. Hoak et al. observed
that palmitic and stearic acid, when added to platelet rich plasma,
furthermore increased the platelet aggregation response induced by
ADP [33]. Enhancement of platelet aggregability was not observed,
however, after the addition of linoleic acid. Farbiszewski et al.
found a correlation between the amount of β-lipoprotein added to
platelet rich plasma and platelet adhesiveness and aggregation response to ADP and thrombin[34]. Nordøy studied the effect of a 72
hours fasting period on free fatty acid (FFA) mobilization in 10
healthy volunteers[35]. There was a 3-fold increase of FFA, the most
marked increase being observed for oleic acid, the main component
of adipose tissue triglyceride fatty acids. After 48 hours of fasting, there was a drop of the platelet count and an increase in the
number of circulating platelet aggregates and of PF 4, indicating
that platelets had been stimulated and that a release reaction had
taken place.

Numerous studies reveal an association of platelet hyperreactivity and arterial disease. Platelet function abnormalities found
include : spontaneous aggregation of platelets,decreased threshold
to aggregation induced by ADP, collagen, epinephrine and arachidonic
acid, increased retention of platelets on glass beads, increased
thromboxane production, decreased platelet survival and increased
platelet turnover, and the presence of circulating platelet aggregates in blood. Clinical conditions in which platelet hyperreactivity was found comprise diabetes mellitus[36,37], peripheral vascular
disease [38], coronary heart disease [39,40] cerebrovascular disease[41-45],
and hyperbetalipoproteinemia [46]. The mere association of platelet
hyperfunction and arterial disease generally due to atherosclerosis
does by no means prove a causal relationship. It is conceivable that
the contact of platelets with endothelial raised lesions in the vasculature or the presence of thrombin and activated clotting factors
in intravascular thrombi lead to their activation. Indeed, Daugherty
et al. have shown that platelet hyperreactivity exists only in the
acute phase of cerebral ischemia and returns spontaneously to normal
within 6 weeks [47], and Mettinger et al. did not find increased platelet reactivity in 52 patients with ischemic cerebrovascular disease
6 to 16 weeks after the acute disease event[48].

Platelets of patients with Type II hyperlipoproteinemia show
marked hyperreactivity, Carvalho et al. examined 17 such patients
(mean LDL-cholesterol 290 mg/100 ml) and found that their platelets
aggregated in response to 1/25 the mean concentration of epinephrine and to one third the concentration of collagen or ADP. Total nucleotide release was increased from 4 to 6 fold with all aggregating
agents[46]. It is interesting to note that normal platelets, when
incubated up to 60 minutes with Type II hyperlipoproteinemic plasma,
did not develop hyperreactivity. Thus, it appears that the mere presence of high concentrations of LDL-cholesterol in the plasma is not
the principal factor inducing hyperreactivity. The same authors
found that the platelets of patients with Type IV hyperlipoproteinemia show normal sensitivity to aggregating agents. However, in the
latter syndrome, Rosing et al. found an impairment of the diurnal
fibrinolytic pattern[49].

Let us now consider a heretical hypothesis for the pathogenesis
of atherosclerosis. According to this view, an inordinate intake of
saturated long-chain fatty acids and/or of cholesterol resulting in
higher VLDL- and LDL-cholesterol has two major consequences : (i) it
increases endothelial permeability and, (ii) it renders platelets
hyperactive. Since hypercholesteremia alone does not suffice to produce atherosclerotic lesions [1,2], platelet hyperreactivity appears to
be the cardinal etiologic factor for atherosclerosis. Stimulated hyperactive platelets undergoing the platelet release reaction will
liberate from their α-granules PDGF. The mitogenic, circulating PDGF
penetrates through a damaged endothelium and induces SMC proliferation (Stemerman's response-to-signal hypothesis[11]). In order for
this hypothesis to be taken seriously we would have to demonstrate
that the intake of a diet high in saturated fat by healthy volunteers
produces platelet hyperreactivity. Conversely we would expect that
the ingestion of polyunsaturated fats, which lowers serum triglycerides and cholesterol, will result in decreased platelet activity.
Several studies have investigated the effect of diet on platelet
function. In a first study,O'Brien et al. demonstrated that platelet
reactivity increased after a large meal of saturated fats[50]. In a
subsequent large study, 39 apparently fit working men aged 23 to 53
were studied three times at weekly intervals while on their normal
diet[51]. 19 were then put on a diet in which the normal saturated
fats were replaced as far as convenient by sunflower-oil based products such as margarine, cooking oil, cakes, etc., containing up to
65% linoleic acid. The other 20 maintained their normal diet. In
the group receiving the diet rich in polyunsaturated fat, most tests
changed in a direction opposite to that found in vascular disease
(see above) and the following parameters were significantly different when study period results were compared to baseline results :
lowering of serum cholesterol, lengthening of the heparine thrombin
clotting time and of the Stypven time, lowering of the platelet retention on glass-beads, and of circulating platelet aggregates, as
measured by the spinning loose method. Renaud et al. studied 2

groups of farmers in the Var and in the Moselle region of France [52].
Official statistics reveal that the incidence of coronary heart disease is considerably higher in the Moselle than in the Var region.
Farmers were selected for these studies because more than any other
social class, they have a comparable way of life and a similar degree of physical activity. In a given area their habits, and particularly the dietary habits are quite similar, do not change much
from day to day and can be easily evaluated since they take all
their meals at home. Among over 400 subjects tested, there were no
differences between Var and Moselle farmers in : total serum and
HDL-cholesterol, serum triglycerides, body weight, systolic and diastolic blood pressure. Moselle farmers, however, smoked more and
had a significantly higher intake in lipids, mostly in saturated
fats than Var farmers. Total protein, carbohydrate, polyunsaturated
fat, cellulose and alcohol intake were comparable in the two groups.
Platelet function studies revealed that the recalcification time of
platelet rich plasma and the platelet factor 3 clotting time (both
tests measure platelet factor 3 availability) were significantly
shorter, and platelet aggregation responses induced by thrombin, ADP,
epinephrine and collagen were greater in the Moselle farmers. Smokers and non-smokers exhibited no difference in platelet function.
In order to determine if platelet hyperactivity in Moselle farmers
was due to the higher intake of saturated fats, rather than to a genetic factor, a group of 53 men and 22 women were persuaded to replace the intake of butter and cream by soft margarine and vegetable
oil. Another group of 50 men and 22 women kept their dietory habits.
One year after the change of diet there were striking differences
in platelet reactivity, the plasma recalcification time of platelet
rich plasma and the PF 3 clotting time being significantly longer,
whereas the cephalin-clotting time of platelet poor plasma remained
unchanged. Thrombin and collagen induced platelet-aggregation normalized completely.

Acute or chronic changes in the intake of saturated and polyunsaturated fats profoundly effect platelet reactivity. These changes occur already after a short time period and, as far as the short
term studies are concerned, cannot possibly be secondary to the development, or, on the contrary to the improvement of atherosclerotic
lesions during this short a time period. It thus appears that hyperactive platelets may play a major role in the pathogenesis of atherosclerosis.

ARTERIAL DISEASE, INCREASED COAGULATION FACTORS AND DECREASED
FIBRINOLYTIC ACTIVITY

The Northwick Park heart study attempts to identify components
of the hemostatic system which may be involved in the pathogenesis
of clinically manifest arterial disease, especially ischemic heart
disease. A recent report of Meade et al. presents early results on
mortality and on hemostasis tests in a study group of 1510 white

men aged 40-64 years at the time of recruitment[53].

By the end of 1979, 49 men had died; in 27 the cause of death was cardiovascular. The mean interval between recruitment and death was 33 months. Compared with the survivors, mean factor VII, factor VIII:C and fibrinogen at recruitment were significantly higher in men who subsequently died of cardiovascular causes. The associations of factor VII and fibrinogen with cardiovascular death appeared to be at least as strong as the association between cholesterol and cardiovascular death. Fibrinolytic activity was lowest in the cardiovascular group, but the difference compared with the value for the survivors was not significant. The findings in the Northwick Park heart study are consistant with the presence of a hypercoagulable state in patients predisposed to develop cardiovascular disease. However, the study sheds no light on the crucial question, if a hypercoagulable state is a causal factor for or a secondary manifestation of arterial disease.

No simple relationship appears to exist between abnormal lipoprotein patterns and the blood fibrinolytic activity as measured by the euglobulin lysis time determined early in the morning[54,55]. However, there are numerous reports on the association between arterial disease and decreased fibrinolytic activity[44,48,55-59]. In this context it is noteworthy that a decreased fibrinolytic activity is the most frequently observed abnormality of hemostasis tests in patients with idiopathic recurrent deep vein thrombosis. In a study conducted by Isacson and Nilsson, fibrinolytic activity of the euglobulins and of vein biopsies was deficient in over half of the patients with this condition[60]. At the present time the methodologies to measure fibrinolytic activity of blood are still rather crude, but several plasminogen activators contributing to global fibrinolytic activity are in the process of being identified. Undoubtedly, future studies, using more refined methods will attempt to clarify the possible relations between atherosclerosis and defects of one or several plasminogen activators.

On the basis of the reported studies it is reasonable to assume that alterations of the hemostatic system, particularly a hypercoagulable state, increased platelet reactivity and a decreased fibrinolytic activity play an important role in the pathogenesis of atherosclerosis.

REFERENCES

1.   D. M. Kramsch, A. J. Aspen and C. S. Apstein, Suppression of experimental atherosclerosis by the Ca^{++}-antagonist lanthanum, J. Clin. Invest., 65:967-981 (1980).

2. V. Fuster, E. J. W. Bowie, J. C. Lewis, D. N. Fass, Ch. A. Owen
    and A. L. Brown, Resistance to arteriosclerosis in pigs with
    von Willebrand's disease, J. Clin. Invest., 61:722-730 (1978).
3. K. von Rokitansky, A manual of pathological anatomy, Sydenham
    Society, London, Vol. 4, (1852), 261-272.
4. R. Virchow, Phlogose und Thrombose im Gefässystem, Gesammelte
    Abhandlungen zur wissenschaftlichen Medizin, Meidinger Sohn
    und Companie, (1856), 458.
5. J. B. Duguid, Pathogenesis of arteriosclerosis, Lancet, 2:925-
    927 (1949).
6. J. E. French, Atherosclerosis in relation to the structure and
    function of the arterial intima, with special reference to the
    endothelium, Int. Rev. Exp. Pathol., 5:253-353 (1966).
7. J. F. Mustard and M. A. Packham, The role of blood and plate-
    lets in atherosclerosis and the complication of atherosclerosis,
    Thromb. Diath. Haemorrh., 33:444-456 (1975).
8. M. B. Stemerman and R. Ross, Experimental Arteriosclerosis. I.
    Fibrous plaque formation in primates; an electron microscope
    study, J. Exp. Med., 136:769-789 (1972).
9. R. Ross and J. A. Glomset, Atherosclerosis and the arterial
    smooth muscle cell, Science, 180:1332-1339 (1973).
10. R. Ross and J. A. Glomset, The pathogenesis of atherosclerosis
    New Eng. J. Med., 295:369-377 and 420-425 (1976).
11. M. B. Stemerman, Platelet and smooth muscle cell responses
    after endothelial desquamation, Thrombos. Haemostas., 46:248
    (1981).
12. S. Moore, R. J. Friedman, D. P. Singal, J. Gauldie, M.A. Blajch-
    man and R. S. Roberts, Inhibition of injury induced thrombo-
    atherosclerotic lesions by anti-platelet serum in rabbits,
    Thrombos. Haemostas., 35:70-81 (1976).
13. R. J. Friedman, M. B. Stemerman, B. Wenz, S. Moore, J. Gauldie,
    M. Gent, M. L. Tiell and T. S. Spaet, The effect of thrombo-
    cytopenia on experimental arteriosclerotic lesion formation in
    rabbits, J. Clin. Invest., 60:1191-1201 (1977).
14. L. A. Harker, R. Ross, S. J. Slichter and C. R. Scott, Homo-
    cystine-induced arteriosclerosis. The role of endothelial cell
    injury and platelet response in its genesis, J. Clin. Invest.,
    58:731-741 (1976).
15. S. D. Balk, J. F. Whitfield, T. Yondale and A. Braun, Roles of
    calcium, serum, plasma and folic acid in the control of proli-
    feration of normal and Rous sarcoma virus-infected chicken fi-
    broblasts, Proc. Nat. Acad. Sci. USA, 70:675-679 (1973).
16. R. Ross, J. Glomset, B. Kariya and L. Harker, A platelet-depen-
    dent serum factor that stimulates the proliferation of arteri-
    al smooth muscle cells in vitro, Proc. Nat. Acad. Sci. USA, 71:
    1207-1210 (1974).

17. N. H. Antoniades, D. Stathakos and C. D. Scher, Isolation of
    a cationic polypeptide from human serum that stimulates proli-
    feration of 3T3 cells, Proc. Nat. Acad. Sci. USA, 72:2635-2639
    (1975).
18. B. Westermark and A. Wasteson, A platelet factor stimulating
    human normal glial cells, Exp. Cell Res., 98:170-174 (1976).
19. R. B. Rutherford and R. Ross, Platelet factors stimulate fibro-
    blasts and smooth muscle cells quiescent in plasma serum to
    proliferate, J. Cell Biol., 69:196-203 (1976)
20. C. W. Castor, J. C. Ritchie, M. E. Scott and S. L. Whitney,
    Connective tissue activation:XI. Stimulation of glycosamino-
    glycan and DNA formation by a platelet factor, Arthritis Rheum.,
    20:859-868 (1977).
21. D. R. Kaplan, F. C. Chao, Ch. D. Stiles, H. N. Antoniades and
    Ch. D. Scher, Platelet α-granules contain a growth factor for
    fibroblasts, Blood, 53:1043-1052 (1979).
22. J. M. Gerrard, D. R. Phillips, G. H. R. Rao, E. F. Plow,
    D. A. Walz, R. Ross, L. A. Harker and J. G. White, Biochemical
    studies of two patients with the gray platelet syndrome. Select-
    ive deficiency of platelet alpha granules, J. Clin. Invest., 66:
    102-109 (1980).
23. B. L. Linder, A. Chernoff, K. L. Kaplan and D. S. Goodman,
    Release of platelet-derived growth factor from human platelets
    by arachidonic acid, Proc. Nat. Acad. Sci. USA, 76:4107-4111
    (1979).
24. H. N. Antoniades, Ch. D. Scher and Ch. D. Stiles, Purification
    of human platelet-derived growth factor, Proc. Nat. Acad. Sci.
    USA, 76:1809-1813 (1979).
25. C. H. Heldin, B. Westermark and A. Wasteson, Platelet-derived
    growth factor. Isolation by a large-scale procedure and analysis
    of subunit composition, Biochem. J., 193:907-913 (1981).
26. W. J. Pledger, Ch. D. Stiles, H. N. Antoniades and Ch. D. Scher,
    Induction of DNA synthesis in Balb/c-3T3 cells by serum compo-
    nents:reevaluation of the commitment process, Proc. Nat. Acad.
    Sci. USA, 74:4481-4485 (1977).
27. D. R. Clemmons, J. J. van Wyk and W. J. Pledger, Sequential ad-
    dition of platelet factor and plasma to BALB/c 3T3 fibroblast
    cultures stimulates somatomedin-C binding early in cell cycle,
    Proc. Nat. Acad. Sci. USA, 77:6644-6648 (1980).
28. C. H. Heldin, B. Westermark and A. Wasteson, Specific receptors
    for platelet-derived growth factor on cells derived from con-
    nective tissue and glia, Proc. Nat. Acad. Sci. USA, 78:3664-3668,
    (1981).
29. J. L. Goldstein and M. S. Brown, The low-density lipoprotein
    pathway and its relation to atherosclerosis, Ann. Rev. Biochem.,
    46:897-930 (1977).
30. L. D. Witte and J. A. Cornicelli, Platelet-derived growth factor
    stimulates low density lipoprotein receptor activity in cultured
    human fibroblasts, Proc. Nat. Acad. Sci. USA, 77:5962-5966 (1980).

31. G. R. Grotendorst, H. E. J. Seppa, H. K. Kleinman and G. R. Martin, Attachment of smooth muscle cells to collagen and their migration toward platelet-derived growth factor, Proc. Nat. Acad. Sci. USA, 78:3669-3672 (1981).

32. R. R. Botti and O. D. Ratnoff, The clot-promoting effect of soaps of long-chain saturated fatty acids, J. Clin. Invest., 42: 1569-1577 (1963).

33. J. C. Hoak, A. A. Spector, G. L. Fry and E. D. Warner, Effect of free fatty acids on ADP-induced platelet aggregation, Nature, 228:1330-1332 (1970).

34. R. Farbiszewski and K. Worowski, Enhancement of platelet aggregation and adhesiveness by betalipoprotein, J. Atheroscler. Res., 8:988-990 (1968).

35. A. Nordøy, Lipids as triggering factors in thrombosis, Thrombos. Haemostas., 35:32-48 (1976).

36. H. C. Kwaan, J. A. Colwell, S. Cruz, N. Suwanwela and J. C. Dobbie, Increased platelet aggregation in diabetes mellitus, J. Lab. Clin. Med., 80:236-246 (1972).

37. B. C. O'Malley, W. R. Timperley, J. D. Ward, N. R. Porter and F. E. Preston, Platelet abnormalities in diabetic peripheral neuropathy, Lancet, 2:1274-1276 (1975).

38. A. S. Ward, N. Porter, F. E. Preston and V. Morris-Jones, Platelet aggregation in patients with peripheral vascular disease, Atherosclerosis, 29:63-68 (1978).

39. P. P. Steele, H. S. Weily, H. Davies and E. Genton, Platelet function studies in coronary artery disease, Circulation, 48:1194-1200 (1975).

40. F. Dreyfuss and J. Zahavi, Adenosine diphosphate-induced platelet aggregation in myocardial infarction and ischaemic heart disease, Atherosclerosis, 17:107-120 (1973).

41. G. Danta, Second phase platelet aggregation induced by adenosine diphosphate in patients with cerebral vascular disease and in control subjects, Thromb. Diath. Haemorrh., 23:159-169 (1970).

42. Z. Kalendovsky, J. Austin and P. P. Steele, Increased platelet aggregability in young patients with stroke, Arch. Neurol., 32:13-20 (1975).

43. K. K. Wu and J. C. Hoak, Increased platelet aggregation in patients with transient ischemic attacks, Stroke, 6:521-524 (1975).

44. L. A. Anderson and J. Gormsen, Platelet aggregation and fibrinolytic activity in transient cerebral ischemia, Acta neurol. scand., 55:76-82 (1976).

45. J. W. Ten Cate, J. Vos, H. Oosterhuis, D. Prenger and C. S. P. Jenkins, Spontaneous platelet aggregation in cerebrovascular disease, Thrombos. Haemostas., 39:223-229 (1978).

46. A. C. A. Carvalho, R. W. Colman and R. S. Lees, Platelet function in hyperlipoproteinemia, New Engl. J. Med., 290:434-438 (1974).

47. J. H. Daugherty, D. E. Levy and B. B. Weksler. Platelet activa-
    tion in acute cerebral ischemia - serial measurements of plate-
    let function in cerebrovascular disease, Lancet, 1:821-824
    (1974).
48. K. L. Mettinger, D. Nyman, K. G. Kjellin, A. Sidén and C. E.
    Söderström, Factor VIII related antigen, antithrombin III,
    spontaneous platelet aggregation and plasminogen activator in
    ischemic cerebrovascular disease. A study of stroke before 55,
    J. Neurol. Sci., 41:31-38 (1979).
49. D. R. Rosing, D. R. Redwood, P. Brakman, T. Astrup and S. E.
    Epstein, Impairment of the diurnal fibrinolytic response in
    man. Effects of aging, type IV hyperlipoproteinemia, and coro-
    nary artery disease, Circ. Res., 32:752-758 (1973).
50. J. R. O'Brien, M. D. Etherington and S. Jamieson, Acute plate-
    let changes after large meals of saturated and unsaturated fats,
    Lancet, 1:878-880 (1976).
51. J. R. O'Brien, M. D. Etherington and S. Jamieson, Effect of a
    diet of polyunsaturated fats on some platelet-function tests,
    Lancet, 2:995-997 (1976).
52. S. Renaud, R. Morazain, L. McGregor and F. Baudier, Dietary
    fats and platelet functions in relation to atherosclerosis and
    coronary heart disease, Haemostasis, 8:234-251 (1979).
53. T. W. Meade, W. R. S. North, R. Chakrabarti, Y. Stirling, A. P.
    Haines, S. G. Thompson and M. Brozovic, Haemostatic function
    and cardiovascular death : early results of a prospective study,
    Lancet, 1:1050-1054 (1980).
54. P. Brakman, T. Astrup, R. I. Levy and D. S. Fredrickson, Rest-
    ing levels of blood fibrinolysis in hyperlipoproteinemia,
    J. Appl. Physiol., 36:430-433 (1974).
55. I. Lipinska, B. Lipinski and V. Gurewich, Lipoproteins, fibrino-
    lytic activity and fibrinogen in patients with occlusive vascu-
    lar disease and in healthy subjects with a family history of
    heart attacks, Artery, 6:254-264 (1979).
56. P. Andersen, Hyperlipidaemia and reduced fibrinolytic activity
    associated with thromboembolic complications in a family, Acta
    Med. Scand., 200:289-291 (1976).
57. I. D. Walker, J. F. Davidson, I. Hutton and T. D. V. Lawrie,
    Disordered "fibrinolytic potential" in coronary heart disease,
    Thrombos. Res., 10:509-520 (1977).
58. R. K. Dube, P. K. Saha, B. Dube, B. C. Katiyar and P. V. B. Rao,
    Alterations in blood fibrinolysis in occlusive stroke, Indian
    J. Med. Res., 68:492-494 (1978).
59. L. O. Pilgeram, A. N. Chee and G. von dem Bussche, Evidence for
    abnormalities in clotting and thrombolysis as a risk factor for
    stroke, Stroke, 4:643-657 (1973).
60. S. Isacson and I. M. Nilsson, Defective fibrinolysis in blood
    and vein walls in recurrent "idiopathic" venous thrombosis,
    Acta Chir. Scand., 138:313-319 (1972).

EPIDEMIOLOGY OF ATHEROSCLEROTIC HEART DISEASES

Guy G. De Backer

Senior Research Associate
National Fund for Scientific Research
Belgium

1. INTRODUCTION

Epidemiological studies of atherosclerotic heart diseases are concerned with the patterns of the occurrence of these diseases in human populations.
These patterns may indeed vary with time, with place and with individual characteristics. Therefore epidemiology is also concerned with the factors that are related with these patterns. For instance, within a population one can try to determine whether there has been a change of the frequency of the disease over the years or whether individuals with coronary heart disease (CHD) are or were different from those without it. Between populations the frequency of certain conditions can be compared and related to personal and community characteristics of the populations concerned.

2. GENERAL PURPOSES

Epidemiological studies are of great importance in evaluating the scope and the impact of atherosclerotic heart diseases on the community, in elucidating the cause, especially by comparing results observed by different research methods and in developing and evaluating preventive approaches and public health practices.

3. METHODOLOGY

The occurrence of atherosclerosis in the population can be studied using mortality and morbidity data. The case fatality rate of certain disease entities as myocardial infarc-

tion is indeed so high that the national ischaemic heart
disease (IHD) mortality rates reflect quite well the differences in incidence of myocardial infarction between communities
as was documented in the myocardial infarction register study
(1). Regarding morbidity studies and surveys of factors that
could be associated with the occurence of CHD, various methodo-
logical problems should be considered. Only methods that were
thoroughly validated should be used. General guidelines have
been presented (2). Since epidemiological studies are often
prolonged over time great attention should be given during the
course of the study to continuous monitoring of the accuracy
and precision of the methods that are used.

4. MORTALITY STATISTICS

The great advantage of mortality statistics is that they
are cheaply available in most Western countries. They therefore provide a readily available basis for the study of changes
in IHD mortality over time and between countries. In Belgium
for instance a decrease in cardiovascular mortality has been
observed in both sexes when the period 1969-1976 is considered.
In order to prove that a decrease in cardiovascular mortality
is not producing a similar increase in other types of mortality
the total mortality rates should be looked for. In Belgium
total mortality also decreased significantly in both sexes
during the period 1969-1976.

A more pronounced decline in IHD mortality has been
observed in the U.S. and in other countries.
In the meantime other countries are reporting an increase of
IHD mortality while others remain stable over the last decade.
These wide variations in the evolution of IHD mortality rates
between countries is unexplained and requires detailed information on the incidence of various disease entities. Changes in
mortality rates over time or differences in mortality rates
between countries can indeed be related to various conditions.
Changes may be related to the revision of the ICD code. Errors
can occur in the establishment of the denominator. Changes and
differences can be artifactual due to changes or differences in
diagnostic procedures which may be reflected in the accuracy of
completing the death certificates. Assuming that the changes
over time or the differences between countries are real and
after having ruled out differences in the age distribution of
the populations either by age standardisation or by looking
into age specific groups, several explanations are still
available : a decline may indicate a decrease of the case
fatality rate related to better medical care or may be due to a
lower disease incidence which by itself may again be the
result of genetic or environmental factors. If the decrease in
mortality is due to a change in incidence then one should

determine whether this is related to changes in risk factors, behavior or socioeconomic characteristics of the population. A multinational monitoring of trends and determinants in cardio-vascular diseases is actually in preparation in different European, American and Australian communities.

The marked international differences in mortality rates from coronary heart disease have been confirmed by internatio-nal morbidity studies as the Seven Countries study (3). In addition these studies have shown that a high proportion of the differences in IHD frequency between countries could be attri-buted to differences in coronary risk factors.

Whether these differences in mortality rates are related to the environment or to genetic factors has also been studied by the obervation of the migration of people from one country to another with different IHD mortality experience. If indeed environmental factors are of prime importance then one should expect that the mortality rates among migrants would approxima-te the mortality experience of the country of adoption and would become different from the mortality rate of the country of origin. On the contrary, if genetic factors are of the greatest importance one would expect that the mortality among the migrants should not differ from that in their country of origin and should remain different from the mortality rate in the country of adoption.
Various kinds of such migrant studies have been carried out (4, 5, 6). From these studies it can be concluded that environmen-tal factors exceed the genetic ones in explaining the differen-ces in mortality experience. However one should consider that the premigration environment, the age at the time of migration and selective forces may have influenced the later outcome.

Not only between countries interesting differences in IHD mortality have been observed but also and even to a greater extent within countries. Regional differences in IHD mortality may again be artifactual due to errors in numerator or denomi-nator. However frequently the data are derived from an identi-cal source (national statistics) and based on a population with comparable health care facilities and similar diagnostic practices of physicians. As an example observations made in Belgium are presented. Belgium is what is called an industria-lized country of 11.781 square miles; the greatest distance from one frontier to another is only 180 miles. A particulari-ty of the country is the existence of two different cultural communities, a dutch speaking one in the north and a french speaking one in the south. Both communities are not different in health care system or in health facilities. However each community has his own network of information i.e. radio, T.V., newspaper etc.

Table 1. Ratio's (%) of observed mortality rates from ischae-
         mic heart disease (A83) in Northern (N) and Southern
         (S) regions over the observed national IHD mortality
         rates. Males aged 40-59 yrs. 1972-1975.

| | 40 - 44 | | 45 - 49 | | 50 - 54 | | 55 - 59 | |
	N	S	N	S	N	S	N	S
1972	98	120	93	112	87	123	90	115
1973	103	119	91	129	92	127	93	115
1974	82	131	95	124	83	123	98	112
1975	93	131	90	130	94	115	97	112

In table 1 the ratio's of the observed IHD mortality rates in
the northern and southern regio's over the observed national
IHD death rates are presented for the years 1972-1975 for males
aged 40-59 years.
Consistent and important differences between north and south
are observed in all age groups in all different years.

The likelihood that these differences between north and
south are real can greatly be enforced when results obtained by
different ways of enquiries are consistent with these findings.
In table 2 results observed in a population study among male
subjects aged 40-59 years, are presented. In the table the
prevalence rates of ECG abnormalities as determined on a
resting electrocardiogram are presented. Minnesota code
I_{1-2-3} and IV_{1-2-3}, V_{1-2-3} reflect either myocardial necrosis
or ischaemia. The prevalence rates are lowest in the north and
highest in the south. The ratios of the observed prevalence
rates in the regions over the national rates are significantly
different between north and south.

Prevalence rates derived from cross sectional studies have
some limitations and should therefore be confirmed by observa-

Table 2. The Belgian Heart Disease Prevention Project.
         Prevalence rates of ECG abnormalities and ratios of
         regional over national prevalence rates in different
         regions.

ECG abnormalities	North-East	North-West	Brussels	South
Prevalence (%)	5.7	7.4	7.2	8.1
Ratio (%) of reg. prev. rate / nat. prev. rate	80	103	102	115

tions made in prospective surveys. From 1973 to 1979 a cohort
of more than 11.000 men aged 40-59 years at the start was
followed for cardiovascular mortality as a control group of a
multifactorial controlled intervention trial (7). The follow-
up was ensured by a standardized protocol. All fatal and
non-fatal cardiac events were scrutinized by one team of
investigators using the available information from hospital
records, general practitioners etc. The six year cumulative
death rates from fatal myocardial infarction and sudden death
were 12.8°/.. and 16.3 °/.. for respectively the northern
and southern regions, i.e. a significant difference of 24%.
It is of interest to relate these differences to results on
coronary risk factors in both regions. In that respect other
investigations (8, 9) have demonstrated significant differences
in cholesterol distribution between both regions. At the
baseline examination of the Belgian heart disease prevention
project this difference was confirmed by analysing the coronary
risk factors in samples of males aged 40 to 59 years employed
by various factories in both communities. Results of the
baseline survey were presented (10) and are summarized in table
3. A significant difference between regions was observed in
mean cholesterol levels. This difference was unexplained by
differences in other risk factors or by socioprofessional
class. In table 3 the expected annual CHD incidence is also
given, derived from a multiple logistic function (MLF) including age, systolic blood pressure, cholesterol, smoking
and physical activity. For each region the ratio is presented
of the number of expected cases based on a MLF of the regional
population over the number of expected cases based on a MLF of
the total population. These ratios are strikingly similar to
the ratios calculated for the regional differences in ECG
abnormalities (table 2).

Table 3. The Belgian Heart Disease Prevention Project.
         Prevalence of coronary risk factors and multiple
         logistic function in different regions.

	North-East	North-West	Brussels	South
Cholesterol (m $\pm$ sd)	226 $\pm$ 39	233 $\pm$ 35	239 $\pm$ 37	247 $\pm$ 40
Systolic BP (m $\pm$ sd)	140 $\pm$ 17	142 $\pm$ 20	140 $\pm$ 18	141 $\pm$ 19
Smoking (%)	69	65	59	61
Expected annual incidence (MLF) (%)	4.31	5.34	4.96	6.37
$\frac{\text{Exp. cases region}}{\text{Exp. cases total}}$ x100	87	108	100	128

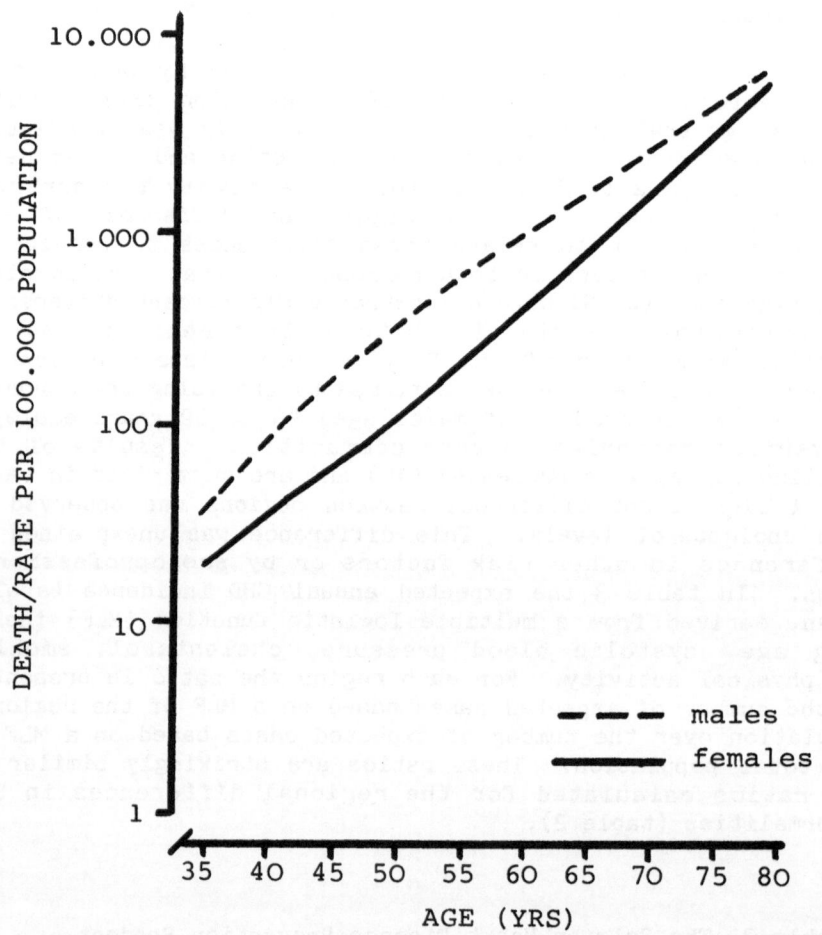

Fig. 1. Age specific mortality rates per 100.000 from cardiovascular diseases (code 390-458) for males and females in
Belgium, 1978.

So, the differences in mortality rates between both
commmunities are in accordance with differences in morbidity
rates observed in a cross-sectional survey, are consistent with
findings from a prospective survey and with the prediction of
risk according to the classical coronary risk factors.

Besides time and geographical differences, mortality rates can also be looked for by individual characteristics. In most national statistics however, the information on personal factors is limited to age, sex and color. In some countries occupational class and marital status are available. Interesting relations between these personal characteristics and the frequency of IHD have been observed. As an example data on age and sex are presented in figue 1. In this figure the age specific mortality rates from cardiovascular diseases (codes 390-458) for males and females in Belgium are given for the year 1978.

The death rates for both males and females increase with age but the difference between the high rates for males and the lower one for females decreases with age beginning at age 55 and continuing to decline until the male and female rates approximate each other.

Comparable trends in death rates from ischaemic heart disease by age and sex have been observed in the U.S. and England. Although these observations could be influenced by a 'cohort effect' they are in accordance with results from recent studies indicating that at the age of 55 men loose a factor that had previously put them at extra risk for developing CHD. The data do not support the idea that women loose protection from CHD after the menopause. During recent years there have been some studies indicating indeed that male sex hormones may play a role in the pathogenesis of CHD.

5. MORBIDITY DATA

Almost no national data exist on CHD morbidity statistics. The divergences in changes of mortality rates between countries clearly underline the need for such data. The information available today is based on epidemiological studies of certain population groups. These studies were mainly undertaken to determine whether coronary heart disease differed in different populations or in relation to suspected etiological factors.

A. OBSERVATIONAL STUDIES

1. Cross sectional surveys

When one has a good reason to study a particular characteristic in relation to IHD in the population one starts with identifying subjects who have or do not have IHD. Among these individuals the factor of interest is studied. Such a design is often called a case-control study although that term can also be applied to prospective studies. In atherosclerosis case-control studies are frequently used in post-infarct patients who are compared with normal controls. In such studies the

independent discriminant value of a new factor can be
analysed.   As an example results from a case-control
study, reported elsewhere (11), are summarized in tables
4 and 5.   In table 4 seventy male post-infarct patients
are compared with 70 controls matched for age and for
body mass index.

The purpose of the comparison was to study the discriminant value of the apoproteins A_1, A_2 and B.   In the
table cases are compared with controls in various lipid
and apoprotein measurements as well as in ratios derived
from these measurements.   Significant differences are
observed.   In table 5 the independence of the discriminant value of each variable is studied using a stepwise

Table 4. Comparison of cases and controls in lipids,
         apoproteins and derived ratios.

	Infarct patients n = 70	Controls n = 70	t
Total chol mg%	254	242	1.7°
HDL chol mg%	46	57	6.2[xxx]
Apo A_1 mg%	111	125	3.5[xxx]
Apo A_2 mg%	46	43	1.9°
Apo B mg%	143	113	6.3[xxx]
$\frac{HDL-C}{Tot\ C}$%	18	24	6.3[xxx]
$\frac{Apo\ B}{Apo\ A_1}$%	134	93	7.4[xxx]
$\frac{Apo\ A_2}{Apo\ A_1}$%	42	35	6.2[xxx]

° : p not significant; [xxx] p < 0.001

Table 5. Results from a stepwise discriminant function
analysis between cases and controls.

Variables	% correctly classified	F
Apo B/Apo A_1	72	18.8^{xxx}
HDL-C	77	6.3^{x}
Apo A_2/Apo A_1	80	4.9^{x}
Tot chol	80	0.3
HDL-C/TC	82	2.1

^{xxx} $p < 0.001$; ^{x} $p < 0.05$

discriminant function analysis. From that analysis it
can be seen that 3 variables discriminate significantly
and independently between cases and controls. The
overall exact classification of cases and controls was
82%. Data derived from such cross-sectional case-control
studies can generate further working hypotheses for
elucidating the etiology an pathogenesis of CHD. One of
the disadvantages of a cross-sectional approach is that
one does not know whether the factor that discriminate
between cases and controls preceeded the onset of the
disease of followed it. Another disadvantage of case-
control studies is selection bias when hospital patients
are used. Furthermore when fatal cases are excluded as
in the example on post-infarct survivors a selection bias
may again influence the outcome of the study. Therefore
the limitations of interferences derived from retrospective studies make it desirable to confirm associations
observed in case-control studies by means of prospective
surveys.

2. Prospective studies

Numerous prospective studies of IHD incidence have
been conducted in selected groups of the population
in the Western world. In these studies different
individual and group characteristics have been found
statistically associated with the incidence of IHD.
One should be cautious in the interpretation of such
associations; one should specifically consider some
particular characteristics of such associations before
drawing conclusions about the nature of the relationship.
Among the characteristics to be considered are the
consistency of the association, the strength of the
relationship, the specificity of the association with the
disease that is concerned, the temporal relationship of

the observed association and the coherence of that
association with known facts from experimental and
clinical pathological studies. Furthermore, from the
point of view of prevention some factors as for instance
age and sex are less interesting. The most interesting
factors for further application in preventive studies
should be related to a life style or environment and be
susceptible to change. So, from a long list of factors
that were found significantly associated with IHD incidence a small number can be derived that are both interesting from a preventive point of view likely to be
considered as causal.

A first set of risk factors concerns the relationship food habits-serum lipids and IHD. Besides a few
exceptions, numerous studies in different populations
have shown that the risk of CHD increases throughout the
range of plasma cholesterol levels. The link between
dietary fat and serumcholesterol in epidemiology is also
clearly present when one looks in large heterogeneous
populations with a broad range of dietary habits. In
such studies (3, 12, 13) much of the difference in CHD
incidence between countries could be attributed to
habitual diet difference in saturated fat. Similarly
most of the differences in average serumcholesterol level
could be explained by differences in habitual diet.
However when it comes to studies of individuals within a
single population some paradoxal results have been
observed. Several studies have failed to detect a
relationship between an individuals intake of saturated
fat and his level of serumcholesterol or his risk of CHD.
This apparent paradox can be explained by the fact that
individuals vary markedly from day to day in their fat
intake. Therefore it is difficult to characterize
precisely a persons diet. It has been calculated that
one needs to collect data over more than a full week
period to characterize a single individuals diet with
some precision (14). So, the intra-individual variability in dietary habits is certainly one of the reasons why
an association between diet and cholesterol is less
apparent within a single population. A second factor is
the much narrower range of fat intake within one population than between populations. Therefore one expects to
see a lower order correlation between dietary fat and
serumcholesterol within a single population, than between
populations where the range of fat intake is broader.
However not all studies have failed to detect a significant relationship within a single population.

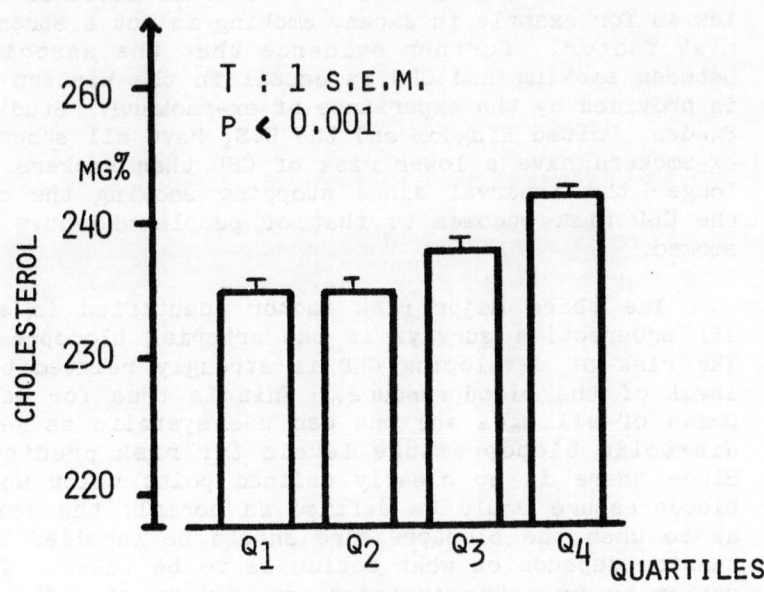

BELGIAN HEART DISEASE PREVENTION PROJECT
DIETARY BEHAVIOR - SERUMCHOLESTEROL

FINAL EXAMINATION - CONTROL GROUP N=6749

Fig. 2.   In figure 2 results are presented observed in a
survey in Belgium where a simple qualitative dietary
questionnaire was used in a large population survey
in men aged 46-65 years. From that questionnaire a
fat consumption score was calculated based on the
consumption of saturated and polyunsaturated fats.
In the figure the population is divided in quartiles of
fat consumption score. A higly significant gradient was
observed between fat consumption score and serumcholesterol. Recently others (15) have published a clear
association between results from dietary surveys and the
cholesterol level in a population from Chicago; they
also found prospectively a clear association between
dietary habits and the incidence of CHD over an 18 year
period.

A second major factor that has been identified as a possible causal factor in CHD is smoking of cigarettes. Several prospective studies in many different countries have shown that smokers have a greater IHD risk than non-smokers and that there is a dose-response relationship. However it should be noted that in countries where other risk factors and mainly the diet-lipid factor are lacking and where the overall level of CHD is low as for example in Japan, smoking is not a strong CHD risk factor. Further evidence that the association between smoking and CHD is causal in the Western world is provided by the experience of ex-smokers. Studies in Sweden, United Kingdom and the U.S. have all shown that ex-smokers have a lower risk of CHD than smokers. The longer the interval since stopping smoking the closer the CHD risk becomes to that of people who have never smoked.

The third major risk factor identified in almost all prospective surveys is the arterial bloodpressure. The risk of developing CHD is strongly related to the level of the bloodpressure. This is true for men and women of all ages and one can use systolic as well as diastolic bloodpressure levels for risk prediction. Since there is no clearly defined point below which a bloodpressure could be defined as normal, the decision as to when the bloodpressure should be labelled hypertension depends on what action is to be taken. If the action to be taken is treatment with hypotensive drugs one must worry about the side effects of the drugs and the cost of treatment. In other words one must balance the possible benefits of therapy against the social, medical and personal costs. On the benefit side results from different studies are accumulating suggesting that even treatment of 'mild' hypertension is beneficial in CHD risk reduction (16, 17). On the cost side one must consider the number of people that would need to be treated; the favorable results of the latest studies stimulate further preventive action with the emphasis on the primary prevention of the development of hypertension and on the question of lowering bloodpressure by hygienic means.

One of the most important characteristic of the three major coronary risk factors - cholesterol, smoking and arterial bloodpressure - is their independence in risk prediction. The more risk factors an individual has the greater is his level of risk. This cumulative effect has been clearly demonstrated in different prospective surveys. In the Framingham study

(18) it was further clearly demonstrated that the additive effect of a slight elevation of the three major risk factors is as worse as a single extreme cholesterol or bloodpressure elevation.

Serumcholesterol, cigarette smoking and arterial bloodpressure have been designated major risk factors because of their strong and consistent relationship with CHD frequency. However they only account for a part of the known variation the occurrence of CHD between and within populations. Other factors may be of great interest in explaining a part of the unexplained variation in CHD risk. Excellent reviews on the importance of these other factors have been published (12, 13, 18, 19-22).

Physical activity and psychosocial factors have been the subject of different studies. An inverse association between the degree of physical activity at work and the incidence of CHD has been shown in some studies. Men in the most active jobs had the lowest CHD risk. However there is some question as to the selective forces that determine the type of job a person chooses. For instance a man who is less fit and who is at greater risk for CHD for other reasons may choose to enter a less active occupation. Furthermore in Western societies where CHD is most common fewer jobs require more physical activity. It is therefore the amount of physical activity in leisure time that discriminates more active individuals from those less active. Recent studies indicate that CHD risk is inversely related to vigorous leisure time activities (23). This association was shown to be independent from smoking habits, body mass and arterial bloodpressure. However there have been studies that failed to show an association between physical activity and CHD risk. These negative results may have been partly due to difficulties in the accurate classification of the degree of physical activity. Recent studies suggest a threshold effect, that means that only vigorous activities appear to be protective. Failure to appreciate this threshold phenomenon may have accounted for negative results in some studies. More research with validated methods also involving the actual physical capacity levels are needed and actually underway (24).

It has long been believed by clinicians and lay people that psychosocial factors including stress are important in the pathogenesis of CHD. However there has been great difficulty in defining precisely

the nature of the psychosocial factors and whether they
arise from the personality of the individual or from the
social and cultural environment. One of the strongest
pieces of evidence linking psychosocial factors to the
risk of CHD comes from the studies of the so called type
A or coronary-prone behavior pattern. Type A behavior
is characterized by striving, aggressiveness, feeling of
time urgency and struggle to get ahead. The Western
collaborative groupe study (25) in the U.S. showed that
in men who's behavior was described as type A the
incidence of CHD over an 8 1/2 year period was twice
that in men who's behavior was not type A. This increasing risk was independent of the major coronary risk
factors. However, although this association is important it is not clear to what extend the behavior pattern
is an integral part of the individuals personality and
to what extent it is promoted by the social environment.
In our own experience in the Belgian Heart Disease
Prevention Project there was a clear association between
type A behavior pattern and socioprofessional class
(26). However, independent of socioprofessional class
type A behavior pattern was clearly associated with the
prevalence of CHD (27). A preliminary analysis of the
prospective data also indicates an independent association between type A behavior pattern and the incidence
of CHD (28).

B. EXPERIMENTAL STUDIES

In experimental epidemiology the investigator can
specify the conditions in which the study is to be conducted. He controls the method of assigning subjects to either
an exposed or non-exposed group. Such an experimental
design is called a clinical trial or a community trial
depending on various characteristics of the study design.
Community trials are frequently used in preventive cardiology research. An overview of such preventive trials in the
primary and secondary prevention of CHD is given elsewhere
in this monograph.

6. INTERFERENCES FROM EPIDEMIOLOGICAL STUDIES

Epidemiological studies can be used to elucidate the
etiology of coronary heart disease; they can provide a basis
for developing and evaluating preventive procedures and public
health practices; statistical relationships should be analysed
with great caution. Assuming that selection bias and methodo-
logical bias is ruled out, an observed association between a
factor and CHD can always be indirect. One should always
remember that in elucidating the etiology of CHD, inferences

from epidemiological studies should not be made in isolation. They must take into account all relevant biological information. The epidemiological and other evidences can accumulate to a point where a causal hypophesis becomes highly probable. Such a causal hypothesis can be sufficiently probable to provide a reasonable basis for preventive trials or public health action.

REFERENCES

1. World Health Organization, Myocardial Infarction Community Registers, Public Health in Europe, WHO Copenhagen (1976).
2. G. Rose, and H. Blackburn, Cardiovascular survey methods, WHO Geneva, monograph series n° 56 (1968).
3. A. Keys,, ed., Coronary heart disease in Seven Countries, Circulation, 41:suppl. 1 (1970).
4. H. Kato, J. Tillotson, M.Z. Nichaman, G.G. Rhoads, H.B. Hamilton, Epidemiologic studies of coronary heart disease and stroke in Japanese men living in Japan, Hawai and California, Am. J. Epid. 97:372 (1973).
5. M. Toor, A. Katchalsky, J. Agmon, D. Allalouf, Atherosclerosis and related factors in immigrants in Israel, Circulation, 22:265 (1960).
6. D.E. Krueger, I.M. Morijama, Mortality of the foreign born, Am. J. Publ. Hlth 57:496 (1967).
7. G. De Backer, M. Kornitzer, C. Thilly, A.M. Depoorter, The Belgian multifactor preventive trial in CHD : design and methodology, Hart Bulletin 8:143 (1977).
8. J.V. Joossens, K. Vuylsteek, E. Brems-Heyns, J. Carlier, J.H. Claes, G. De Backer, M. Graffar, H. Kesteloot, M. Kornitzer, J. Lequime, R. Pannier, A. Raes, O. Van Houte, M. Vastesaeger, G. Verdonk, The patterns of food and mortality in Belgium, Lancet I:1069 (1977).
9. O. Van Houte, H. Kesteloot, An epidemiological survey of risk factors for ischaemic heart disease in 42.804 men. I. Serumcholesterol value, Acta Cardiol. 27:527 (1972).
10. M. Kornitzer, G. De Backer, M. Dramaix, C. Thilly, Regional differences in risk factor distributions, food habits and coronary heart disease mortality and morbidity in Belgium, Int. J. Epid. 8:23 (1979).
11. G. De Backer, M. Rosseneu, J.P. Deslypere, Discriminative value of lipids and apoproteins in coronary heart disease, Atherosclerosis (in press).
12. J. Stamler, Lifestyles, major risk factors, proof and public policy, Circulation 58:3 (1978).
13. A. Keys, Coronary heart disease - the global picture, Atherosclerosis 22:149 (1975).
14. K. Liu, J. Stamler, A. Dyer, J. McKeever, P. McKeever, Statistical methods to assess and minimize the role of intraindividual variability in obscuring the relationship

between dietary lipids and serumcholesterol, J. Chron. Dis. 31:399 (1978).

15. R.B. Shekelle, A. McMillan Shryock, O. Paul, M. Lepper, J. Stamler, S. Liu, W.J. Raynor, Diet serumcholesterol and death from coronary heart disease : the Western Electric Study, New Engl. J. Med. 304:65 (1981).

16. Hypertension Detection and Follow-up Program Cooperative Group. Five-Year findings of the hypertension detection and follow-up program, JAMA 242:2562 (1979).

17. The Australian Therapeutic trial in mild hypertension, Lancet I:1261 (1980).

18. W.B. Kannel, Some lessons in cardiovascular epidemiology from Framingham, Am. J. Cardiol. 37: 269 (1976).

19. J.H. Fuller, M.J. Shipley, G. Rose, R.J. Jarrett, H. Keen, Coronary-heart-disease risk and impaired glucose tolerance, Lancet I:1373 (1980).

20. B.V. Stadel, Oral contraceptives and cardiovascular disease, New. Engl. J. Med. 304:672 (1981).

21. V. Froehlicher, A. Battler, M. Dan McKirnan, Physical activity and coronary heart disease, Cardiology 65:153 (1980).

22. Review panel on coronary-prone behavior and coronary heart disease : a critical review, Circulation 63:1199 (1981).

23. J.N. Morris, M.G. Everitt, R. Pollard, S.P.W. Chave, A.M. Semmence, Vigorous exercise in leisure time : protection against coronary heart disease, Lancet II:1207 (1980).

24. J. Sobolski, G. De Backer, S. Degré, M. Kornitzer, H. Denolin, Physical activity, physical fitness and cardiovascular diseases : design of a prospective epidemiologic study, Cardiology 67:38 (1981).

25. R.H. Rosenman, R.J. Brand, R.I. Sholtz, M. Friedman, Multivariate prediction of coronary heart disease during 8.5 year follow-up in the Western Collaborative Group Sudy, Am. J. Cardiol. 37:903 (1976).

26. F. Kittel, M. Kornitzer, G. De Backer, M. Dramaix, Metrological study of psychological questionnaires with reference to social variables, J. Beh. Med. (in press).

27. M. Kornitzer, F. Kittel, G. De Backer, M. Dramaix, The Belgian Heart Disease Prevention Project : type A behavior and prevalence of coronary heart disease, Psychosom. Med. 43:133 (1981).

28. G. De Backer, F. Kittel, M. Kornitzer, M. Dramaix, Behaviour, stress and psychosocial traits as risk factors, Prev. Med. (in press).

HYPERLIPIDEMIA AS A RISK FACTOR

M. Mancini and P. Rubba

Center for Arteriosclerosis and Metabolic Disease
Semiotica Mecica, 2nd Faculty of Medicine
University of Naples, Naples
Italy

Hyperlipidemia plays a key role in the pathogenesis of atherosclerosis and its clinical manifestation (coronary heart disease, stroke, lower limb gangrene etc.). Evidence will be presented from several sources (epidemiological research, pathology, clinical investigation) on the relationship between plasma lipid or lipoprotein abnormalities and atherosclerotic cardiovascular disease.

THE ATHEROSCLEROTIC LESION

Atherosclerosis is a pathologic process affecting the intima of the aorta and the larger distributing arteris (1, 2). It takes the form of focal thickenings or plaques of fibrous and fatty material, which often enough encroach on the lumen of the vessel and, particularly when complicated by thrombosis may lead to impairment of the arterial circulation and ischaemia of the supplied tissues. Circulatory impairment has important clinical effects mainly at three sites in the body : the heart, the brain and the lower limbs. The lesions of atherosclerosis are most common in the aorta, where they range from flat or slightly elevated yellow spots or streaks to large raised greyish nodules or plaques.

In the fatty streak the lipid is more superficial and is found mostly in the cytoplasma of smooth muscle cells; the tunica media underlying the fatty streak shows very little change. The fatty streak may be seen frequently in the posterior wall of the aorta from childhood while always by the age of 20 some evidence of atherosclerosis can be found on careful inspection of the aorta.

The microscopical appearence of a typical raised plaque is characterized by intimal accumulation of lipids. Lipids are found deeply in the intima, often as a central pultaceous mass of necrotic material and free fat, which contains visible cholesterol crystals. The fatty material is mostly cholesterol and its esters, but it also contains phospholipid and a variable amount of glyceride. Proliferation of fibroelastic tissue is usually most prominent in the more superficial layers of the intima. The fatty streak and the raised plaque are thought to represent successive stages in a single pathologic process having as a distinctive feature the accumulation of lipids in the intima.

The relationship between hyperlipoproteinemic states and lipid accumulation in the arterial intima has been studied by a variety of techniques. By using a sensitive rocket immunoelectrophoresis method the concentration of some lipoprotein constituents (apolipoprotein B and C) has been determined in plasma and in aortic biopsies, obtained during vascular surgery. A strong direct correlation could be demonstrated between the concentration of apo B or apo C in plasma and that in the arterial intima (3). Because there is no evidence that apolipoproteins may be synthesized in situ, it seems reasonable that plasma lipoproteins or their metabolic products can enter the arterial intima and achieve concentrations directly proportional to their blood levels.

The great importance of lipid accumulation in relation to atherogenesis is further supported by studies in experimental animals (4). Although susceptibility to experimental atherosclerosis varies very much among different species it has been found possible in many instances to reproduce typical atherosclerotic lesions by feeding diets very rich in cholesterol. Herbivorous animals (in particular rabbit) are very sensitive to this dietary change. Other animals require some additonal procedure. For example sodium cholate should be combined with cholesterol feeding in order to produce arterial lesions in the rat. In rhesus monkey experimental atherosclerosis has been produced by feeding a diet enriched in cholesterol and saturated fat (butterfat).

In summary animal study have given strong support to the lipid theory of atherogenesis.

IMPORTANT LESSONS FROM EPIDEMIOLOGY

In general retrospective observations in groups of patients who have suffered one or more episodes of myocardial infarction have shown only slightly higher levels of blood lipids as compared to normal controls (5-9). It is probable that most patients with very high lipid levels have not survived the acute episode, not being examined therefore in a survey of this type.

Several well known cross-sectional studies have demonstrated that populations who differ in their habitual dietary intake of saturated fat and cholesterol also differ markedly in serum cholesterol levels and in the incidence and prevalence of coronary heart disease (10)   This is one of the most serious manifestations of the atherosclerotic process, being responsible of a sizeable fraction of total deaths in most populations.   One of these studies was initiated more than 20 years ago in southern Italy with a pilot survey in Nicotera, a small village in Calabria region. This study was under the leadership of Dr. Ancel Keys who has recently published results on the follow-up of 10.000 men in seven different countries (11). A much lower plasma cholesterol concentration and coronary mortality was demonstrated in the Mediterranean countries, where olive oil is habitually consumed and dietary intake of saturated fatty acids is lower than in northern Europe and the United States. This study therefore supported the theory relating plasma cholesterol to atherosclerotic cardiovascular disease.

Further evidence in this direction came from another epidemiological study, which pooled results from eight different prospective studies (12) and involved over twelve thousand men (mostly of middle age). Mean length of follow up was eight years. During this time over eight hundred first major coronary events occurred. In this study once again plasma cholesterol was found to be consistently and strongly related to coronary heart disease. Over the range of values that many clinical laboratories stil designate as within normal limits (220-280 mg/dl), risk is proportional to the cholesterol level. Although an optimal value cannot be precisely identified it should be somewhere under 200 mg/dl (12).

In conclusion epidemiological data, especially those coming from prospective studies have unequivocally demonstrated that hyperlipidemia or hyperlipoproteinemia are important risk factors for the complications of atherosclerosis in human beings.

CLINICAL OBSERVATION

Every day's clinical experience with hyperlipidemic patients reinforces the concept that increased lipid concentration in plasma is an important etiological factor for atherosclerosis. The physician therefore needs to be familiar with nomenclature and properties of the main plasma lipoprotein fractions.

The plasma lipoproteins are macromolecular complexes composed of a heterogenous mixture of proteins and lipids, whose function is to transport lipids in the circulation. The major human plasma lipoproteins are defined, on the basis of their flotation rate in salt solutions, into following density classes : high density

lipoproteins or HDL (d=1.063-1.210), low density lipoproteins or
LDL (d=1.006-1.063, very low density lipoproteins or VLDL (d=0.95-
1.006) and chylomicrons (d $<$ 0.95).

LDL have been further subdivided into intermediate density
lipoproteins or IDL (d=1.006-1.019), with LDL redefined as
the 1.019-1.063 density fraction.

VLDL and chylomicrons are mainly involved in triglyceride
transport, LDL and HDL in cholesterol transport and metabolism
(13). The apoprotein or apolipoproteins together with polar
lipids (phospholipid) facilitate the solubilization of the apolar
lipids (cholesterol, cholesteryl esters, triglyceride).

The plasma concentration of the main lipoprotein classes may
vary among different populations. It was found that LDL and
VLDL were lower in southern Italy as compared to Northern Europe,
whereas HDL concentration did not differ (14). It should be
pointed out that available data suggest a lower fat consumption
and a lower coronary mortality in Italy (15). Here the 90th
percentile for the lipid distribution in the normal population is
equal to 6.32 mmol/l for total serum cholesterol and to 1.88
mmol/l for total serum triglyceride.

The knowledge of the distribution of lipid concentration in
the health population is a prerequisite for defining hyperlipoproteinemia. The increase of plasma lipoproteins (and therefore of
plasma lipids) above normal limits is called hyperlipoproteinemia
(or hyperlipidemia). More than ten years ago the W.H.O. has
proposed a typing system for the different forms of primary
hyperlipoproteinemia in man. Types do not reflect well defined
disease entities but rather represent a short-hand nomenclature,
useful for description of plasma abnormalities (16); in particular
types are not indicative of the genetic abnormality underlying
hyperlipoproteinemia. For a genetic typing more detailed family
studies and more sophisticated biochemical procedures are needed.

The close observation of cases with marked elevation of blood
lipids is certainly convincing that the circulating lipids are
very important for atherogenesis (16). This is particularly true
for the genetic disease called familial hypercholesterolemia (FH)
characterized by type II hyperlipoproteinemia and marked increase
of plasma concentration of LDL (17). This plasma abnormality is
found not only if FH but, although of a lesser degree, in combined
hyperlipidemia and poligenic hypercholesterolemia also (18).

The first of these conditions is the best characterized both
from a metabolic and genetic standpoint (19). It is trasmitted as
an autosomal dominant trait. Homozygous cases have almost double
increase in LDL concentrations as compared to heterozygous (table

1) they always show xantelasma, precocious arcus cornealis, tendon and tuberous xanthomata. These pathologic findings together with extensive and premature atherosclerosis results from tissue accumulation of cholesterol. Familial hypercholesterolemia, although very interesting for elucidation of the pathogenesis of premature atherosclerosis however accounts for only a minority of cases of hypercholesterolemia in the population.

A form by far so common is combined hyperlipoproteinemia (18). Its phenotypic expression is highly variable, in most instances being represented by a type II B pattern. This is due to the simultaneous increase of LDL and VLDL which both carry a sizeable proportion of the so called 'atherogenic cholesterol' (LDL-VLDL cholesterol). In this form of hyperlipoproteinemia a reduction in the plasma concentration of the non atherogenic HDL has been observed.

Another form of hyperlipidemia which is associated with high risk of premature atherosclerotic complications is type III hyperlipoproteinemia (20). This type of hyperlipoproteinemia is identified through demonstration of a broad beta band in the electrophoretic pattern of whole serum and/or of a floating beta in VLDL fraction. This type of hyperlipoproteinemia has been found to be strongly associated, if untreated, to premature development of arterial stenosis or occlusion in the coronary, aortoiliac or femoral district (fig. 1).

Type IV hyperlipoproteinemia (charcterized by VLDL increase) is less associated to premature atherosclerosis; however this plasma abnormality is so common in the population that it nevertheless rank the first place among lipoprotein disorders, which are associated with clinical signs of coronary or peripheral atherosclerosis (7, 8). Type V hyperlipoproteinemia (chylomicron plus VLDL increase) is a relatively rare abnormality, for which association with premature atherosclerosis has not been so far extensively documented.

The clinical evaluation of patients with different forms of hyperlipoproteinemia, especially type II, III and IV demonstrate the strong relationship between plasma lipid and lipoprotein abnormalities and clinical disturbances arising from arterial stenosis or obstruction.

REGRESSION OF ATHEROMA

Extensive work in non human primates has suggested that after induction of atherosclerosis by dietary means, it is possible to obtain marked regression, even of advanced lesions, through effective correction of hyperlipidemia (21, 22). Increasing evidence in this direction is also being collected in man.

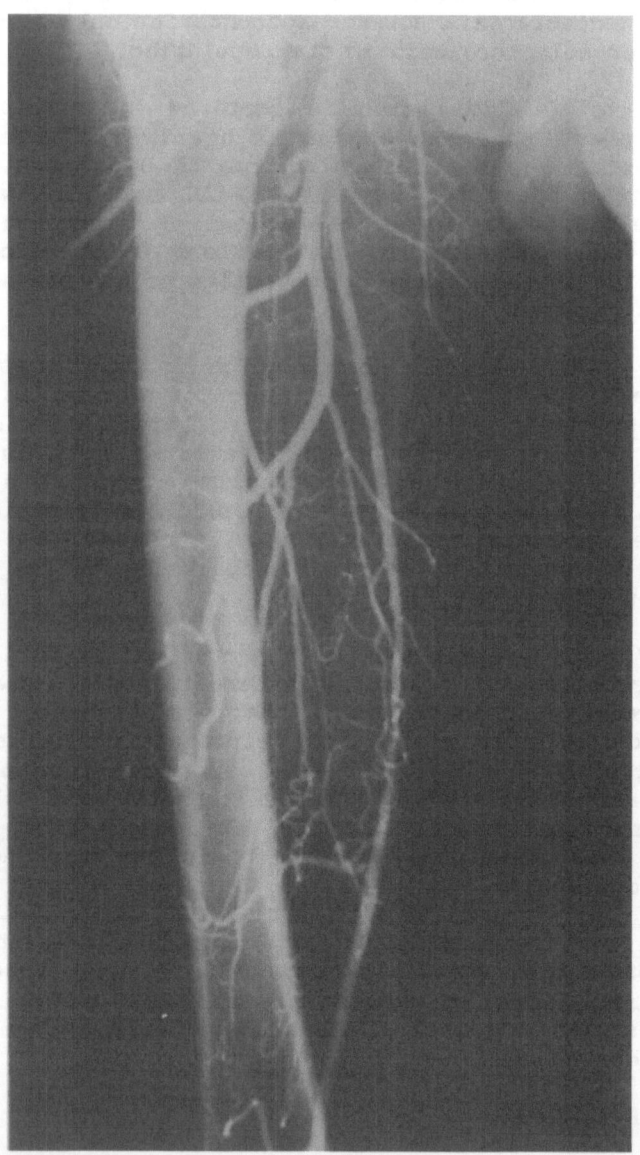

Fig. 1. Patient M.T., age 40, blood pressure 140/80 mmHg, 20
        cigarettes/day, plasma cholesterol = 9.85 mmol/l, trigly-
        ceride = 4.89 mmol/l. Angiography : stenosis of right
        superficial femoral artery (see arrows).

Table 1 : Mean lipoprotein concentration (mmol/l) in familial
         hypercholesterolemia.

		LIPOPROTEINS		
	VLDL		LDL	HDL
	Chol	TG	Chol	Chol
Homozygous (1M, 4F)	.40	.17	16.90	.96
Heterozygous (4M, 8F)	.53	.60	9.61	1.34
NLP (74 M)	.47	.66	2.72	1.22

Barndt and colleagues in fact have demonstrated (23) by angiography regression of early atherosclerotic plaques in the femoral
arteries, after two years of effective lipid lowering treatment in
middle age hyperlipidemic patients.

We have assessed peripheral atherosclerosis of the lower
limbs by digital pulse plethysmography with pulse wave analysis, a
non invasive method, which is extremely sensitive for diffuse non
obstructive atherosclerosis. Inclination time (IT) of the pulse
wave is almost always abnormal in type II B hyperlipoproteinemia
and often in type II A, III and IV (24). After a basal examination all the patients were given dietary and/or pharmacological
advice. In the following year the adherence to the prescribed
regimen was very good in some of them, less good in others.
Fortytwo patients (table 2) were then reexamined three years after
the first observation. Some of them showed a worse (more prolonged) IT of the pulse wave while others has a shorter IT, suggesting some degree of atherosclerosis regression. Hyperlipidemic
men showing circulatory improvement or deterioration did not
differ (table 3) in their baseline characteristics (serum cholesterol and triglyceride body weight and blood pressure). Those
later showing progression probably smoke a few cigarettes more,
although the difference did not reach statistical significance.

When evaluating change in plasma lipids (table IV) three
years later as compared to baseline, it was found that those
showing worsening of IT (suggesting atherosclerosis progression)
had not modified significantly their plasma cholesterol concentration. On the other hand IT improvement (suggesting atherosclerosis regression) was associated with a significant cholesterol

Table 2 : Hyperlipidemic men who have been reexamined after 3
          years on lipid lowering treatment.

IT	Type of hyperlipidemia				
	IIA	IIB	III	IV	V
Improved	5	5	1	8	2
Worsened	8	4	0	9	0
All	13	9	1	17	2

Table 3 : Plasma lipids, BWI, blood pressure and smoking : base-
          line values in hyperlipidemic men showing improvement or
          disease progression.

	Improvement n = 21	Progression n = 21
Chol (mmol/l)	7.69 ± .64	7.28 ± .52
TG (mmol/l)	6.51 ± 3.86	4.16 ± .82
BMI (Kg/cm-100)	1.09 ± .03	1.11 ± .02
DP (mmHG)	84 ± 2	86 ± 2
Smoking (cig./day)	13 ± 2	18 ± 3

reduction, of about 20%. These data give further support to the
idea that atherosclerosis regression may be possible, provided the
control of hypercholesterolemia be adequate and precocius. They
do encourage the effort of early detection and treatment of
hyperlipoproteinemia.

    Many dietary and pharmacological means are nowadays available
for effective management of the different forms of hyperlipidemia. Even in the condition of extreme elevation of plasma cholesterol concentration as in FH, promising results are being obtained
through the procedure of periodic plasmapheresis. After plasma
exchange marked cholesterol reduction is achieved, lasting about
two weeks (25). Interestingly enough immediately after plasmapheresis there is a pronounced hemodinamic improvement. The rapidity
of circulatory changes suggests the possibility of improvement in
some way of hemoreological properties of blood through prevalent
removal of the high molecular weight LDL or of some plasma constituent, so far unidentified.

Table IV : Effect of lipid lowering treatment in hyperlipidemic
          men improving or showing peripheral vascular disease
          progressesion.

	Chol (%)	TG (%)	BWI (Kg/cm-100)
Improvement n = 23	-18 ± 5[a]	-19 ± 10	-.023 ± .014
Progression n = 21	- 1 ± 4	-16 ± 11	-.043 ± .018

a : p < .0.1 $\overline{X}$±SEM

However parietal changes, although unlikely, cannot by
excluded. Plasmapheresis therefore offer some hope for the
management of the most malignant form of human hyperlipoproteinemia, which, if untreated, leads to coronary death within the third
decade.

    In conclusion epidemiological studies, experimental pathology
and clinical experience all indicate that hyperlipidemia plays a
very important role in the pathogenesis of atherosclerosis.
Several forms of treatment are nowadays available for the management of hyperlipidemic patients and there is convincing evidence
that effective correction of lipid and lipoprotein abnormalities
is useful for the prevention of the ischaemic complications of
atherosclerotic disease.

REFERENCES

1. R. Ross, J.A. Glomset, The pathogenesis of Atherosclerosis
   (First of two parts), The New England J. Medicine, 295:369
   (1976).
2. R. Ross, J.A. Glomset, The pathogenesis of Atherosclerosis
   (Second of two parts), The New England J. Medicine, 295:420
   (1976).
3. A.C. Onitiri, B. Lewis, H. Bentall, C. Jamieson, J. Wisheart,
   I. Faris, Lipoprotein concentrations in serum and in biopsy
   samples of arterial intima - A quantitative comparison,
   Atherosclerosis, 23:513 (1976).
4. P. Costandinides, Experimental Atherosclerosis, Elsevier,
   Amsterdam (1965).
5. R.M. Greehalgh, B. Lewis, D.S. Rosengarten, J.S. Calman, I.

Mervant, P. Martin, Serum lipids and lipoproteins in peripheral vascular disease, Lancet, 2:957 (1971).

6. J.L. Goldstein, W.R. Hazzard, H.G. Schrott, E.L. Bierman, A.G. Motulski, Hyperlipidemia in coronary heart disease. I. Lipid levels in 500 survivors of myocardial infarction, J. Clin. Invest., 52:1533 (1973).

7. L.A. Carlson, M. Ericsson, Quantitative and qualitative serum lipoprotein analysis. II. Studies in male survivors of myocardial infarction, Atherosclerosis, 21:417 (1975).

8. A. Lewis, A. Chait, C.M. Oakley, I.D.P. Wootton et al., Serum lipoprotein abnormalities in patients with ischemic heart disease : comparison with a control population, Brit. Med. J., 3:489 (1974).

9. S. Panico, E. Farinaro, G. Riccardi, P. Rubba, Lipid and lipoprotein levels in survivors of myocardial infarction, in :'International Conference on Atherosclerosis', L.A. Carlson et al. (eds.), 709, Raven Press, New York (1978).

10. A. Keys, Coronary heart disease in seven countries, Circulation, 41 supplement 1, (1970).

11. A. Keys et al. (eds.), Seven countries. A multivariate analysis of coronary heart disease and death, Harvard University Press, Cambridge Massachusetts (1980).

12. The Pooling Project Research Group, Relationship of blood pressure, serum cholesterol, smoking habit, relative weight to incidence of major coronary events : final report of the Pooling Project, J. Chron. Dis., 31:201 (1978).

13. J.D. Brunzell, A. Chait, E.L. Bierman, Pathophysiology of lipoprotein transport, Metabolism, 27:1109 (1978).

14. B. Lewis, M. Mancini, L.A. Carlson, H. Micheli et al., Serum lipoproteins in four European communities : a quantitative comparison, Eur. J. Clin. Invest., 8:165 (1978).

15. World Health Organization, World Health Statistics Annual 1973-76, vol 1, WHO Geneva (1976).

16. P. Rubba, E. Farinaro, A. Postiglione, P. Strazzullo, P. Oriente, M. Mancini, Multiple lipoprotein abnormalities in primary hyperlipidemia in Naples, in : 'International conference on Atherosclerosis', L.A. Carlson et al., (eds.), 117, Raven Press, New York (1978).

17. J. Slack, Risk of ischemic heart disease in familial hyperlipoproteinemias, Lancet, 2:1380 (1969).

18. J.L. Goldstein, H.G. Schrott, W.R. Hazzard, E.L. Bierman, A.G. Motulsky, Hyperlipidemia in coronary heart disease. II. Genetic analysis of lipid levels in 176 families and delineation of a new inherited disorder, combined hyperlipidemia, J. Clin. Invest., 52:1544 (1973).

19. J.L. Goldstein, M.S. Brown, Lipoprotein receptors, cholesterol metabolism and atherosclerosis, Arch. Pathol., 99:181 (1975).

20. J. Morganroth, R.I. Levy, D.S. Fredrickson, The biomedical, clinical and genetic features of type III hyperlipoprotein-

emia, Ann. Int. Med., 82:158 (1975).

21. G. Weber, Regression of arterial lesions : Facts and problems, in : 'International Conference of Atherosclerosis', L.A. Carlson et al., (eds.), 1, Raven Press, New York (1978).

22. R.W. Wissler, D. Vesselinovitch, Animal models of regression, in : 'Atherosclerosis IV', G. Schettler, Y. Goto, Y. Hata, G. Kloss, (eds.), 377, Springer Verlag, New York (1977).

23. R. Barndt, P.W. Blankenhorn, S.H. Brooks, Regression and progression of early femoral atherosclerosis in treated hyperlipoproteinemic patients, Ann. Int. Med., 86:139 (1977).

24. P. Rubba, S. Panico, F.R. Piantadosi, A. Postiglione, M. Mancini, Early signs of peripheral atherosclerosis of the lower limbs in asymptomatic primary hyperlipoproteinemia, Artery, 6:59 (1979).

25. A. Postiglione, P. Rubba, N. Scarpato, A. Iannuzzi, M. Mancini, Increased blood flow to lower limbs in two patients with familial hypercholesterolemia, Atherosclerosis, in press.

DIABETES : IS IT A RISK FACTOR FOR ATHEROSCLEROSIS?

M. Mancini, G. Riccardi and A. Rivellese

Center for Arteriosclerosis and Metabolic Disease
Semiotica Medica, 2nd Faculty of Medicine
University of Naples, Naples
Italy

Diabetic patients are more prone to develop atherosclerosis and its complications than non diabetics. This is demonstrated by several clinico-pathological and epidemiological observations (1-3). One of the most accurate of these is the Framingham study which clearly demonstrates that the average annual incidence of vascular disease is higher in diabetics at all age groups, in both sexes and in all main arterial districts (4).

Although diabetes is often associated with atherosclerosis, the mechanism of this association is still unclear. The question is whether any other factor beside hyperglycemia can be responsible for the increased risk of atherosclerosis in diabetes. A recent survey in diabetic patients from various countries on the prevalence of ecg abnormalities related to coronary atherosclerosis (Q waves and ST/T changes) can answer the question (5). The variation in the frequency of these abnormalities between different population groups is very large (fig. 1) : about 3 times higher for USA versus Japanese men and USSR women versus Polish ones. As the degree of hyperglycemia was comparable in all the groups under study, the possible association of other factors such as hypercholesterolemia, hypertension, thrombophilia, etc. might explain the variable frequency of atherosclerotic complications in diabetic patients in various parts of the world (5). In this regard many authors have tried to define the role of the classical risk factors in the development of atherosclerotic complications in diatbetic patients (4, 6, 7).

In the Framingham study (4) the possible influence of hypercholesterolemia, arterial hypertension, cigarette smoking on CHD incidence was evaluated in both sexes in diabetics with both uni-

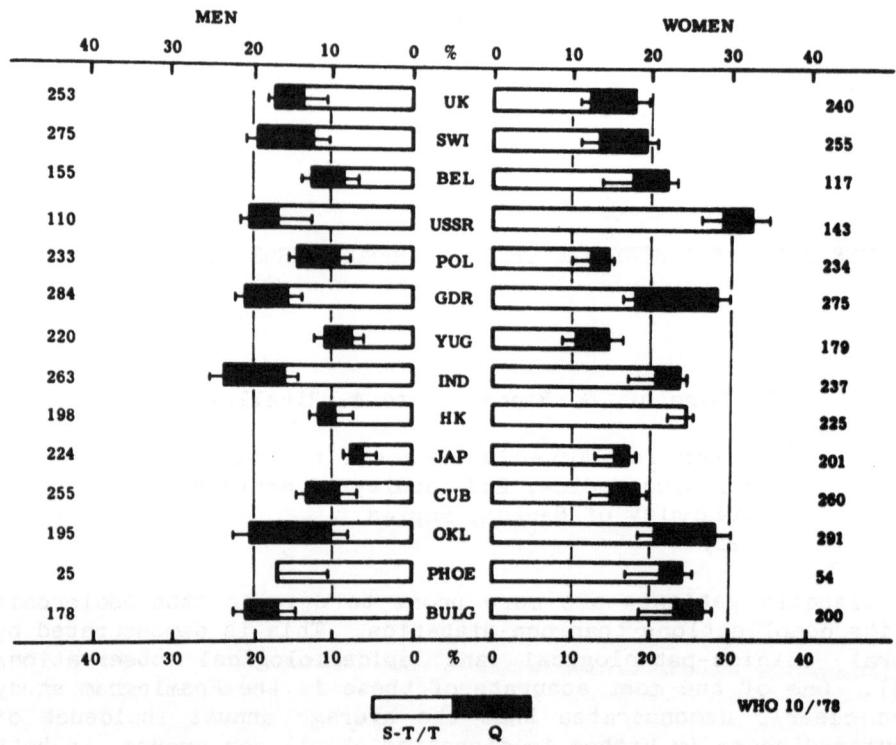

Fig. 1 : Frequency distribution of ECG abnormality rates adjusted
        for age (ref. 5).

variate and multivariate analysis. A significant association was
found in men between CHD incidence and a low serum level of HDL
cholesterol, a high serum level of LDL cholesterol and a high
systolic blood pressure. The presence of diabetes in men, independently from other risk factors, did not influence the incidence
of coronary events. In women, on the contrary, diabetes resulted
an important additional risk factor for CHD.

     That the level of blood glucose has little or no influence on
atherogenesis is not unanimously believed. From the Whitehall
study (7), in fact, a threshold level of blood glucose (200 mg/dl)
has been identified above which the incidence rate of CHD is
almost doubled without any further increase of morbility and
mortality by increasing the values of blood glucose.

     Atherosclerosis of the lower limbs is also very frequent in
diabetic patients (4) but in general the level of blood glucose
and the duration of diabetes is not correlated with its incidence
rate as is instead the value of systolic blood pressure and of
total serum cholesterol. Only for distal localization of arterial

occlusions, below the knee, serum cholesterol has not any more predictive importance while the duration of diabetes and the level of blood glucose are strongly correlated with the severity of vascular disease (8). In other words, while proximal localization of arterial occlusion in the lower limbs of diabetic patients is mainly associated to the same risk factors as in non diabetic persons, distal localization was mainly maximally affected by hyperglycemia.

Another possible explanation of the frequent association between diabetes and atherosclerosis can be found in the type of antidiabetic treatment. In a recent study diabetic patients treated with insulin presented a mortality rate 8 times higher compared to non diabetic controls while those under oral drugs had a risk of death only 1.5 times higher. The relative risk of death for vascular causes, i.e. the vascular death rate for diabetics as compared with non-diabetics, was six times higher for diabetic patients treated with insulin (10).

The importance of high blood level of insulin as a risk for atherosclerosis has been assessed also in non diabetics subjects. In the Helsinky policemen study (11) the whole population has been divided in five quintiles on the basis of increasing values of serum insulin (fasting, 1 hour after an oral standard glucose load, 2 hours after and sum) and for each quintile the 5 years incidence rate of CHD has been evaluated. It appeared that in the higher quintile of serum insulin there was an increased incidence of cardiovascular events (fig. 2). In the same study the relationship between various possible risk factors and the incidence of CHD has been evaluated by multivariate analysis. If plasma insulin was not included in the analysis, then blood glucose appeared as a significant predictor of CHD events. This was not the case if, instead, plasma insulin was included, due to the strong correlation between blood glucose and serum insulin in anormal population. This does suggest that the correlation found in some studies between blood glucose and atherosclerotic complications may, in fact, be due to the strong relationship between blood glucose and insulin, the latter being very likely responsible for the accelerated atherogenesis.

How insulin excess may stimulate atherogenesis has been postulated by Stout (12). He thinks that insulin may act as a growth factor for smooth muscle cells of arterial wall that, when stimulated, may well induce a rapid progression of atherosclerotic lesions.

Two more questions need to be considered : 1) are patients with diabetes but without hyperlipidemia, hypertension or smoking habit at higher risk of developing atherosclerosis than non diabetic individuals? 2) Is there an additive effect when two or

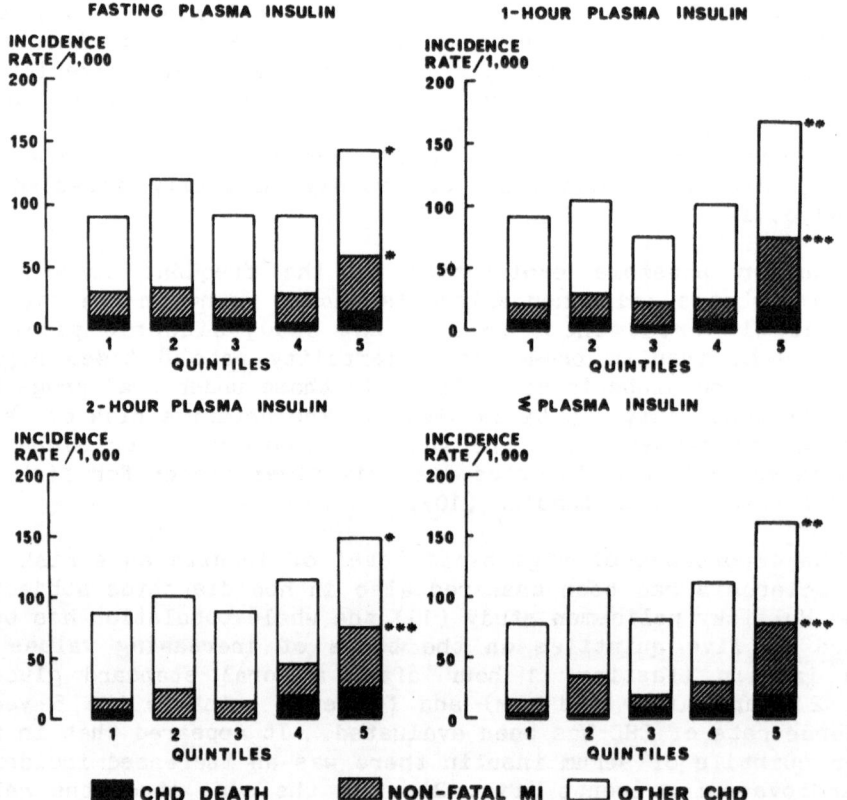

Fig. 2 : 5-yr incidence of CHD death, nonfatal MI, and other CHD
by quintiles of plasma insulin levels.
* p < .05, ** p <.01, *** p < .001, χ^2 test, top
quintile compared with combined lower quintiles
(Pyörälä, Helsinki, Policemen Study, ref. 11).

more of these factors are concomitant in the same subjects?

To answer these questions we have studied 54 non insulin
dependent diabetic male patients, age 40 to 59 years, with a body
weight index (Kg/cm-100) of 1.13 ± .17. None of them had clinical
signs of PVD or history of intermittent claudication. All the
patients were investigated by digital pulse plethismography
measuring the inclination time (IT) of the pulse wave in both the
second toes and using the more abnormal value for statistical
analysis. This simple measurement has proved to be a reliable
index of atherosclerosis in non obliterated arteries (13). Normal
values of IT are > 130 msec (13).

Table 1 : Influence of different types of hyperlipidemia on IT
values.   (M±SD)

GROUPS	N	CHOL (mg/dl)	TG (mg/dl)	IT (msec)
1)	8	260±30	317±110	148±54
2)	6	249±30	154± 36	163±54 °
3)	8	191±26	372±134	120±42
4)	27	171±31	114±131	126±29

°p < 0.05; °°p < 0.01; °°°p < 0.01 vs normolipidemic (group 4)

The influence of hyperlipidemia on peripheral atherosclerosis, judged by the value of IT, is reported in tab. 1. Patients are divided into four groups according to their serum cholesterol and triglyceride values : 1) high total serum cholesterol and triglyceride; 2) high serum cholesterol; 3) high serum triglyceride; 4) normal serum lipid values. Only diabetic patients with hypercholesterolemia (group 2) had IT values significantly higher than normolipidemic diabetic patients (group 4). The difference between group 1 (high cholesterol and triglyceride) and group 4 (normal lipid values) was of borderline significance. The group with hypertriglyceridemia alone had a similar IT as the group with normal lipid values. Age, duration of diabetes, systolic blood pressure and smoking habits were similar in all groups. It appears therefore that in diabetic patients hypercholesterolemia but not hypertriglyceridemia is an important risk factor for peripheral atherosclerosis.

The influence of different types of antidiabetic treatment on IT values is evaluated in tab. 2 : IT is signficantly higher in patients on insulin treatment compared with those either on oral drugs or on diet. Once again other parameters known to influence IT (blood lipid values, blood pressure and smoking habits) are similar in the three groups of patients. Although different treatment may reflect different degree of severity of diabetes, it is interesting that again insulin appears associated with more advanced atherosclerosis.

A subgroup of our diabetic patients free of other known cardiovascular risk factors was compared with a similar group (once again without risk factors) of non diabetic individuals. The two groups showed a very similar IT level suggesting that diabetic patients without hypercholesterolemia, hypertension or smoking habit have a risk to develop atherosclerosis similar to that of a group of non diabetic persons (tab. 3).

Table 2 : IT values and possible risk factors for PVD in diabetics
on different types of hypoglicemic treatment. (M+SD)

TYPE OF TREATMENT	AGE (years)	SBP (mmHG)	CHOL (mg/dl)	DURATION (years)	CIG. (n/day)	IT (msec)
DIET (n = 9)	51 + 3	138+17	181+53	3 + 4	12+12	129+40
ORAL DRUGS (n = 14)	50 + 5	138+18	200+50	10 + 7	18+8	122+25
INSULIN (n = 15)	53 + 5	147+20	147+20	11 + 7	11+6	155+41°

°p < .05 (One way analysis of variance)

Table 3 : Comparison between diabetics and controls in absence of
risk factors. (M+SD)

	AGE (years)	CHOL (mg/dl)	SBP (mmHg)	CIG. (n/day)	IT (msec)
Controls n = 19	50.7 + 6.9	173.6 + 29.2	128 + 11	17.5 + 16.2	116.2 + 15
Diabetics n = 19	50.8 + 4.2	170.7 + 34	133.7 + 15	13.3 + 10	119.2 + 27

The combined influence of more than one factor on PVD was
also evaluated in this study. When one or more of the principal
risk factors are present together in the same patient, IT is
worsened in a progressive fashion suggesting that these factors
have an additive effect (fig. 3).

Ongoing research work indicates the possible atherogenic role
of new factors in diabetes. It has recently been found, for
instance, that excessive glycosilation can take place for several
proteins (14) beside serum hemoglobin : albumin, tissue elastin
and serum LDL have been found partially glycosilated in diabetic
patients. It is therefore tempting to speculate that increased
levels of blood glucose in diabetics induce glycosilation of
various proteins in plasma and in arterial wall, thus accelerating
the progression of atherosclerosis (15).

In the last years much importance has been given to some

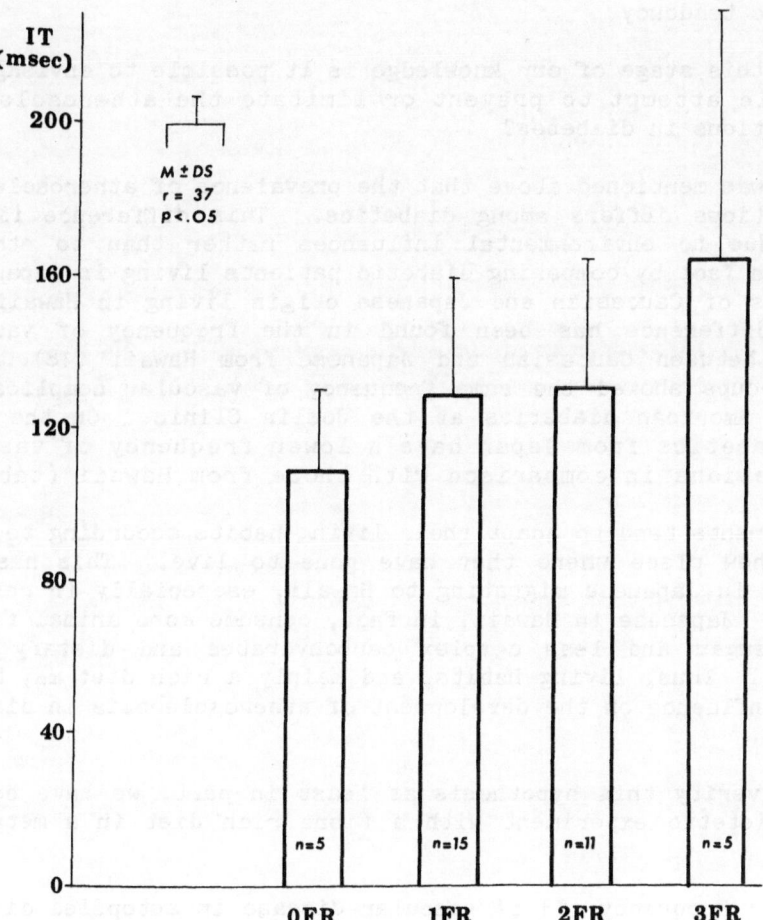

Fig. 3 : Relationship between the number of risk factors and early signs of peripherale atherosclerosis.

hemostatic variables, which might have pathogenic influence in the atherosclerotic process. It is known that blood clotting is favoured in diabetic patients either of type I or type II as factor VII, VIII and fibrinogen are increased (16). Moreover platelet adhesiveness is higher in these patients compared with non diabetics. All this abnormal hemostatic functions favour trombotic tendency.

At this stage of our knowledge is it possible to envisage any realistic attempt to prevent or limitate the atherosclerotic complications in diabetes?

It was mentioned above that the prevalence of atherosclerotic complications differs among diabetics. This difference is very likely due to environmental influences rather than to ethnical ones. In fact by comparing diabetic patients living in Japan with diabetics of Caucasian and Japanese origin living in Hawaii very little difference has been found in the frequency of vascular disease between Caucasian and Japanese from Hawaii (18). Both these groups showed the same frequency of vascular complications seen in American diabetics at the Joslin Clinic. On the other hand diabetics from Japan have a lower frequency of vascular complications in comparison with those from Hawaii (tab. 4).

Migrants tend to adapt their living habits according to those of the new place where they have gone to live. This has been observed in Japanese migrating to Hawaii, escpecially in relation to diet. Japanese in Hawaii, in fact, consume more animal fat and simple sugar and less complex carbohydrates and dietary fiber (tab. 5). Thus, living habits, and mainly a rich diet may have a strong influence on the development of atherosclerosis in diabetic patients.

To verify this hypothesis at least in part, we have carried out a dietetic experiment with a fibre rich diet in a metabolic ward.

Table 4 : Frequency (%) of vascular disease in autopsied diabetic patients.

| | JOSLIN CLINIC | HAWAII | | JAPAN |
| | | Caucasians | Japanese | |
	4097 cases	128 cases	251 cases	1885 cases
Total	77.1	75.8	74.5	51.0
Brain	12.4	18.0	21.9	18.3
IHD	39.8	32.8	32.7	9.7
Other cardiac	13.8	15.6	8.8	6.9
Renal	9.1	8.6	10.6	16.1

(Kawate et al. 1979, ref. 18)

Table 5 : Mean nutrient intake (g) in Japanese people from Hawaii
        and Japan.

NUTRIENT	HAWAII	HIROSHIMA
N. of subjects	210	188
Total Intake (cal)	2.175	2.258
Proteins	91	74
animals	62	37
vegetable	29	37
Fats	72	43
animal	42	19
vegetable	30	24
Carbohydrates	265	349
simple	94	36
complex	171	313

(Kawate et al. 1979, ref 18)

Six insulin dependent and eight non insulin dependent diabetic patients of both sexes have participated to the study.
Patients were hospitalized and they accepted to follow, in a
random order, three weight maintaining diets (diet A, B, C) for
ten days each. Diet A and B were very similar except for the
content of fiber : 16 g for the first and 54 g for the second
one. Diet C was low in fibre (20 g) and low in CH (40% of total
calories). More details on the three diets have been published
elsewhere (19).

Blood glucose levels during the three diets are reported in
tab. 6. During the high fibre diet post prandial blood glucose
and average daily blood glucose profile were significantly reduced

Table 6 : Blood glucose (BG) levels after each dietary period.
                                                        (M±SD)

| | DIETS | | |
	A	B	C
2h post prandial BG (mmol/l)	9.05 ±2.94	6.83 ±2.72	8.71 ±3.89
average daily BG (mmol/l)	7.77 ±2.0	6.38 ±2.16	7.49 ±1.55

Significance compared with B : °p < .025; °°p < .01; °°°p < .005

in comparison both with diet A (low in fibre) and with diet C (low in fibre and CH).

The effect of the fibre rich diet on lipoprotein composition was also interesting : during the high fibre diet (B) both total and LDL cholesterol were reduced by 30 to 40% and they increased again during the low CH diet (C).

There was only a significant increase of HDL during the fibre rich diet but then keep constant during the low CH diet (tab.7). This study clearly shows that a high fibre diet can well controll both blood glucose and blood lipid concentration thus indicating that it could be considered the diet of choice to prevent athero-sclerosis in diabetic patients.

Table 7 : Lipoprotein composition at the end of the three dietary periods.   (M+SD)

Diets	CHOLESTEROL (mmol/1)				TRIGLYCERIDE (mmol/1)	
	TOT.	VLDL	LDL	HDL	TOT.	VLDL
A	5.88 °°	.67 °	3.81 °	1.40	1.61	1.05
	±1.30	± .36	±1.27	± .4	± .71	± .64
B	4.66	.52	2.85	1.36	1.51	.88
	± .67	± .26	± .67	± .34	± .59	± .50
C	5.57 °°°	.49	3.57	1.53 °°°	1.38	.84
	± .96	± .28	± .80	± .44	± .54	± .39

°p <.05, °°p < 0.1, °°°p < .001 (significance vs B)

REFERENCES

1. L.D. Ostrander, J. jr. Francis, N.S. Hagner, M.D. Mjelsberg, and F.V. Epstein, The relationship of cardiovascular disease to hyperglycemia, Ann. Intern. Med., 62:1188 (1965).
2. M.J. Garcia, P.M. Mc Namara, and R. Gordon, Morbidity and mortality in diabetics in the Framingham population, sixteen years follow up study, Diabetes, 23:105 (1974).
3. J.M.B. Bloodworth, Vascular disease and Diabetes Mellitus in : 'Diabetes Mellitus', Diagnosis and treatment, vol II,

Hamwi, G.J., Danowski, T.S. (eds.), American Diabetes Association, New York (1967).

4. W.B. Kannel, and D.L. McGee, Diabetes and glucose tolerance as risk factors for cardiovascular disease : The Framingham study, Diabetes Care, 2:120 (1979).

5. H. Keen, and R.J. Jarrett, The WHO multinational study of vascular disease in Diabetes : 2. Macrovascular Disease prevalence, Diabetes Care, 2:187 (1979).

6. L.D. Ostrander, D.E. Lamhpiear, W.J. Carmen, and G.W. Williams, Blood glucose and risk of coronary heart disease, Arteriosclerosis, 33 (1981).

7. K.W. Beach, J.D. Brunzell, L.L. Conquest, and D.E. Strandness, The correlation of arteriosclerosis obliterans with lipoprotein in insulin-dependant and non insulin-dependent diabetes, Diabetes , 28:836 (1979).

8. V. Janka, E. Standl, and H. Mehnert, Peripheral vascular disease in Diabetes Mellitus and its relation to cardiovascular risk factors : screening with the Doppler ultrasonic Technique, Diabetes Care, 3:207 (1980).

9. J.H. Fuller, M.J. Shipley, G. Rose, R.J. Jarrett, and H. Keen, Coronary Heart Disease risk and impaired glucose tolerance, Lancet, I:1373 (1980).

10. E.A. Dupree, and M.B. Marter, Role of risk factors in complications of diabetes mellitus, Am. J. Epid., 112:100 (1980).

11. K. Pyorala, Relationship of glucose tolerance and plasma insulin to the incidence of coronary heart disease : results from two population studies in Finland, Diabetes Care, 2:131 (1979).

12. R.W. Stout, Diabetes and Atherosclerosis. The role of Insulin., Diabetologia, 16:141 (1979).

13. S. Zattersquist, V. Bergvell, B. Linde, and B. Pernow, The validity of some conventional methods for the diagnosis of obliterative arterial disease in the lower limbs as evaluated by arteriography, Scand. J. Clin. Lab. Invest., 33:633 (1971).

14. R. Fluckiger, and K.H. Winterhalter, In vitro synthesis of hemoglobin A_{1c}, FEBS Lett., 71:356 (1976).

15. A. Cerami, V.J. Stevens, and V.M. Monnier, Role of non enzymatic glycosilation in the development of sequelae of diabetes mellitus, Metabolism, 28 (Suppl. 1):431 (1979).

16. J.H. Fuller, H. Keen, R.J. Jarrett, T. Omer, T.W. Meade, R. Chakrabarti, W.R.S. North, and Y. Stirling, Haemostatic variables associated with diabetes and its complications, Br. M. J., 2:964 (1979).

17. C.T. Dollery, L.A. Friedman, C.N. Hansby, E.M. Kohner, P.J. Lewis, M. Porta, and J. Aebster, Circulating prostacyclin may be reduced in diabetes, Lancet, 2:1365 (1979).

18. R. Kawate, M. Yamakido, Y. Nishimoto, P.H. Bennett, R.F. Hammon, and W.C. Knowler, Diabetes Mellitus and its vascular complications in Japanes Migrants on the Island of

Hawaii, _Diabetes Care_, 2:161 (1979).

19. A. Rivellese, G. Riccardi, A. Giacco, D. Pacioni, S. Genovese, P.L. Mattioli, and M. Mancini, Effect of dietary fibre on glucose control and serum lipoproteins in diabetic patients, _Lancet_, II:447 (1980).

ATHEROSCLEROSIS

G. A. Gresham

Professor of Morbid Anatomy
University of Cambridge

CLINICAL FEATURES PREVENTION AND REGRESSION

Clinical Features

Myocardial infarction is nowadays a common and well recognised sequela of coronary atherosclerosis and yet it was only first described clearly in the second decade of this century. Over the period 1950-1973 the total mortality rate for England and Wales had declined in both sexes and in all age groups. However the cause specific pattern of mortality also changed alarmingly. The four major groups of chronic disease (heart disease, stroke, respiratory disease and cancer) in 1977 represented a greater proportion of total mortality than in 1951. In middle aged men heart disease accounted for 20% of deaths in 1951 and 40% in 1971 (Figure 1). This could not be explained by the three revisions of the International Classification of Disease from 1950 - 1973 since the revisions did not include any major change in the method of coding heart diseases. It is true that the diagnostic class of "myocardial degeneration" has largely disappeared from the official nomenclature. However this cannot explain the spectacular rise in the incidence of ischaemic heart disease. Many cases classified as myocardial degeneration now fall into the category of the various cardiomyopathies.[1]

From the clinicopathological point of view the clinical features of ischaemic heart disease can be classified as due to:-

    a)   Pump failure (muscle and valves)

    b)   Electrical failure (cardiac conduction)

    c)   Events in the diseased coronary arteries

1950 - 1973

(ENGLAND AND WALES)

TOTAL MORTALITY RATE FELL:-
(FOR BOTH SEXES AND ALL AGE GROUPS)

HEART DISEASE IN MIDDLE AGED MEN:-

1951 - 20% OF ALL DEATHS

1971 - 40% OF ALL DEATHS

MYOCARDIAL DEGENERATION AS A DIAGNOSIS
HAS LARGELY DISAPPEARED

Figure 1

Patients dying from ischaemic heart disease are found to have thrombosed coronary arteries in one third of the cases. Two thirds have coronary arteries which have the lumen reduced by as much as 85% and multiple stenoses affecting all the main arteries are frequent.

A common manifestation of ischaemia of the myocardium is sudden death. Of all deaths between 15 to 30% are sudden. They are most frequent in males and the most frequent cause is atherosclerotic disease of the coronary arteries. A large proportion of such deaths occur outside the hospital environment so that it is not always easy to determine the precise pathophysiology (Figure 2). For example when 50,000 people or so are gathered in a stadium there is a strong possibility that one of them will drop dead suddenly. This phenomenon of "stadium death" is well recognised. In the few cases where terminal electrocardiograms have been obtained about half had ventricular arrest and half had ventricular fibrillation. Death is therefore due to electrical failure (Figure 3). Post mortem examination usually reveals severe coronary arterial narrowing. However myocardial changes are not always visible to the naked eye. Occasionally old

infarcts with more recent infarction are found. In
others a few small subendothelial scars are found and in
others the myocardium appears macroscopically normal.
However histochemical methods may show microscopic
evidence of myocardial damage (Figure 4).

SUDDEN DEATH

15 to 30% OF ALL DEATHS ARE SUDDEN

MOST OCCUR OUTSIDE HOSPITAL:-

4% OCCUR WHILST DRIVING

5% OCCUR DURING EXERCISE

THE MAJORITY OCCUR DURING SLEEPING HOURS

50% HAVE CONSULTED THEIR DOCTORS RECENTLY

SUDDEN DEATH IS ASSOCIATED WITH:-

STRESS

ALCOHOL CONSUMPTION

SMOKING

SUDDEN ELECTRICAL CARDIAC FAILURE

TERMINAL E.C.G. SHOWS:-

ASYSTOLE IN 50%

VENTRICULAR FIBRILLATION IN 50%

TERMINAL E.C.G. EVENTS ARE PRECEDED BY:-

ECTOPIC BEATS

REENTRANT PHENOMENA

INVOLVEMENT OF THE CONDUCTING SYSTEM

Figures 2 and 3

The reports of the incidence of coronary thrombosis
in such cases of sudden death are very variable.
Roberts[2] found thrombi infrequently in cases of
infarction. Other workers have found thrombi more often.
Serial sections of the coronary arteries of hearts

showing infarction revealed proximal thrombi in 80% of
the cases and 90% of these were associated with rupture
of an atheromatous plaque.[3]

PATHOLOGY OF SUDDEN DEATH

CORONARY ARTERIES MAY SHOW:-

NARROWING

THROMBI IN 80%

PLAQUE RUPTURE IN 90% WITH THROMBI

NOTHING AT ALL

MYOCARDIUM MAY SHOW:-

SUBENDOTHELIAL SCARS

AN OLD INFARCT

OLD AND RECENT INFARCTS

NOTHING AT ALL

Figure 4

Sudden death is often defined as unexpected death
occurring in persons without previous symptoms. Others
include patients with a previous history of angina
pectoris or of myocardial infarction. For all of these
three groups the so called risk factors appear to be
the same. The frequency is greatest in the male and
increases with age. About 50% of those that die suddenly
have consulted their doctors recently. Retrospective
consideration of their symptoms which are often
interpreted by the patient as indigestion suggest that
they may have had angina. About 4% occur whilst driving
vehicles, 5% during exercise but the vast majority occur
during the sleeping hours. Psychological stress,
alcohol ingesting and smoking have all been associated
with sudden death.[4]

The ultimate cause of sudden death is dysrhythmia.
This is often generated by a focus of ischaemic muscle
generating ectopic beats or reentrant phenomena. A
small proportion may be associated with abnormality of
the conduction system. This is particularly associated
with thrombosis of the right coronary artery which is

followed by a transient atrioventricular block which
may persist for a few days. During this period a fatal
block may develop. This phenomenon was thought to be
due to blockage of the atrioventricular nodal artery.
Others have suggested that diffusion of potassium ions
from ischaemic muscle adjacent to the node disturb its
function. For this reason the right coronary artery
has been named the artery of sudden death. However the
epithet could be equally applied to the left coronary
artery because thrombosis of this vessel causes infarction
of 60% of the left ventricular myocardium leading to
massive pump failure.

There is a curious group of cases of sudden death
associated with some coronary artery narrowing but not
with thrombosis nor with lesions in the conduction
system. The postulate has been that small platelet
thrombi form in the coronary microcirculation leading
to widespread ischaemia. Such thrombi have been found
in some cases of sudden death and raise the possibility
that they may be distal emboli from proximal coronary
artery disease or may have formed 'in situ'. However
they arise, such aggregates initiate a self perpetuating
ischaemia by the release of endoperoxides forming
thromboxane A2. This, in turn, produces vascular spasm
and further aggregation of platelets.[5]

The situation has been mimicked in experimental
animals either by the injection of platelets into the
coronary tree or ADP which is a powerful platelet
aggregating agent. The literature on this subject has
been extensively reviewed by Haerem.[6]

Other causes of sudden death from ischaemic heart
disease are less common than electrical failure. They
are rupture of the infarcted myocardium and papillary
muscle rupture. The latter is rare and occurs in about
1% of all people dying with myocardial infarcts. The
effect depends upon the extent of rupture. If both heads
of the papillary muscle give way then the mitral
incompetence that develops is acutely fatal. If one
head ruptures the effects may not prove fatal. The
muscle most often affected is the posterior papillary
muscle of the mitral valve.

Rupture of the ventricular wall may involve the
lateral wall or the ventricular septum. Rupture of the
lateral wall tends to occur within four days of
infarction at the time when proteolysis has softened
the necrotic muscle. It usually affects the entire

wall of the ventricle and is rapidly fatal from cardiac
tamponade due to the haemopericardium in 25% of cases.
Previous old pericardial adhesions may localise the
rupture and prevent a fatal outcome. Septal rupture
may prove rapidly fatal or the patient may survive long
enough to enable surgical repair of the hole. In
general the survival depends on the size of the hole in
the septum: the smaller it is the longer the survival
post-rupture (Figure 5).

Turning now from the syndrome of sudden death to the
more chronic conditions that may follow myocardial
ischaemia. The first point to recognise is that even
after complete recovery the possibility of a subsequent
infarct is always present. Angina pectoris is another
chronic clinical manifestation of coronary
atherosclerosis and its description by William Heberden
in 1772 long antecedes the account of myocardial
infarction. The main clinical feature is chest pain on
exertion though the pain can occur in sites other than
the chest such as the jaw and the arm. It is an
expression of inadequate oxygenation of the heart
muscle and is associated with major narrowing of at
least one coronary artery in 90% of the subjects.
Despite the relatively static nature of the coronary
disease the symptoms are variable. Variant angina, as
it is called, is probably an expression of atherosclerotic
narrowing coupled with spasm or platelet emboli in small
coronary arterial branches. If the symptoms increase
steadily in severity to a crescendo they often indicate
the development of infarction. Infarcts may not be
present in the myocardium in about two thirds of patients
with angina but statistics show that 25% of males with
angina will develop infarction in five years and 30%
of males with angina over the age of 55 years will die
within eight years.

Not all patients with severe coronary artery
stenosis develop angina. This is to some extent
determined by the length of the narrowed segment of the
artery and also by the vascular resistance beyond it.
This, in turn, is determined by the extent of development of the collateral circulation which develops
pari passu with main coronary artery sclerosis
(Figure 6).

Chronic myocardial conditions that may follow
cardiac ischaemia are aneurysm and cardiomyopathy and
both may lead to congestive cardiac failure.
Ventricular aneurysms are largely fibrous sacs

developing at the site of old infarcts. Very little
muscle remains in them and they consequently stretch
under the influence of the intraventricular pressure.
The adjacent unaffected muscle is usually hypertrophied.
The degree of hypertrophy may be considerable so that
the left ventricular function is reasonably normal. If
however the aneurysm is large congestive cardiac
failure may develop. In addition thrombosis usually
develops within the aneurysmal sac and may provide a
source of emboli into the systemic circulation in
subsequent years. Old sclerotic ventricular aneurysms
rarely rupture.

PUMP FAILURE AS A CAUSE OF SUDDEN DEATH

MYOCARDIAL RUPTURE MAY INVOLVE:-

LATERAL WALL OF THE LEFT VENTRICLE
1 - 4 DAYS POST INFARCTION: 25% HAVE A
HAEMOPERICARDIUM

VENTRICULAR SEPTUM: SPEED OF DEATH
DEPENDS ON THE SIZE OF THE HOLE

PAPILLARY MUSCLES IN 1%.USUALLY THE
POSTERIOR MUSCLE. RUPTURE OF BOTH IS
RAPIDLY FATAL

Figure 5

Ischaemic cardiomyopathy is a condition of diffuse
ischaemic fibrosis leading to heart failure. During
life the condition is often regarded as a congestive
cardiomyopathy because there are no symptoms of chest
pain and the electrocardiographic appearances are normal.
It is only at autopsy that the diffuse fibrosis and
extensive narrowing of the coronary arteries is revealed.[8]
About 18% of the mortality from ischaemic heart disease
is due to chronic congestive cardiac failure.

Finally a word about the Dressler syndrome which
is an unusual sequel of myocardial infarction. It is
the development of pleurisy, pulmonary consolidations
and pericarditis after a few weeks. It can readily be
confused with myocardial reinfarction or with
pulmonary infarction. It does however readily respond
to steroid therapy and is thought to be an autoimmune

response to the initial cardiac infarction [9] (Figure 7).

ANGINA PECTORIS PATHOLOGY

SEVERE NARROWING OF AT LEAST ONE
MAIN CORONARY ARTERY IN 90% OF CASES

66% DO NOT HAVE INFARCTS

28% OF MIDDLE AGED MEN WITH ANGINA
WILL DIE WITHIN 8 YEARS

NOT ALL PATIENTS WITH SEVERE
CORONARY NARROWING HAVE ANGINA

THIS IS DETERMINED BY:-

THE LENGTH OF THE NARROWED ARTERIAL
SEGMENT

THE RESISTANCE BEYOND IT

THE EXTENT OF THE COLLATERAL
CIRCULATION

Figure 6

Consequences of atherosclerotic disease of the
coronary arteries themselves as opposed to effects on
the myocardium are relatively uncommon. One example
is aneurysm of the atherosclerotic artery. The lesion
was found in about 1% of angiograms made of patients
selected for prospective coronary by-pass surgery for the
relief of angina. The aneurysms were both saccular and
fusiform and were located on one vessel in seven and
on multiple vessels in four patients. The right
coronary artery followed by the left circumflex were the
most frequently involved. The left main coronary was not
affected in this series. When there is not severe
occlusion of the diseased arteries the clinical features
may be bizarre. Small thrombi or platelet clumps
derived from turbulent blood in the sac may shower into
the coronary tree and produce atypical clinical effects.
Sometimes the aneurysm may rupture into the pericardial
sac though this is very rare. Occasionally a flap of
diseased intima may be dissected off the inside of the
aneurysm and acting like a hinged door shut off the
lumen of the main artery. [10,11]

CHRONIC CONSEQUENCES OF
CARDIAC ISCHAEMIA

VENTRICULAR ANEURYSM MAY LEAD TO:-

VENTRICULAR HYPERTROPHY

CONGESTIVE CARDIAC FAILURE

THROMBOSIS WITH SUBSEQUENT EMBOLISM

CARDIAC RUPTURE WHICH IS VERY
UNUSUAL

ISCHAEMIC CARDIOMYOPATHY

THIS IS CONGESTIVE CARDIAC FAILURE
WITHOUT CLINICAL OR ELECTROCARDIO-
GRAPHIC EVIDENCE OF ISCHAEMIA

DRESSLER SYNDROME

PLEURISY,PERICARDITIS, PULMONARY
CONSOLIDATIONS ARISING ABOUT 4
WEEKS AFTER MYOCARDIAL INFARCTION.
IT IS PROBABLY AN AUTOALLERGIC
PHENOMENON

Figure 7

Prevention of Coronary Atherosclerosis

We have already indicated that prevention of
coronary atherosclerosis must be begun in childhood. To
do this it is essential to examine all the risk factors
that are known to be associated and to eliminate them
wherever possible. This is not always easy because
social customs die hard and genetic influences are
difficult to reverse. Compliance in youth, in any form
of prophylaxis or treatment is difficult as death and
illness seem to be many years away. Many attempts to
initiate programmes of prevention have failed because the
approach has not been subtle enough. The theme must be
to promote healthier living and not to initiate
procedures which are crudely said to postpone the age of
dying.

Another problem has been the fact which we have
already stated that only 50% of the incidence of
ischaemic heart disease is explicable in terms of the
known risk factors.

Extensive clinicopathological, experimental and epidemiological evidence has accumulated over the years to show that multiple factors act in concert to promote atherogenesis. A number of these factors have been clearly identified by one method or another that have been used and we shall consider them.

That a strong hereditary effect exists is indicated by racial differences and familial susceptibility within races of people. It is difficult sometimes to separate genetic influences from social habits in family groups. A study was made of workers in the Finnish paper industry half of whom came from the East which has the highest incidence of ischaemic heart disease in the world and half came from the South. The expected clustering of coronary heart disease was confirmed, the increase in risk being fourfold amongst the brothers of men with ischaemic heart disease but only twofold amongst fathers and no relation was established with the mothers. In these families the difference in incidence in heart disease between the East and South disappeared. This appeared to be a ceiling effect. The Finnish workers concluded that the familial effect was due to a clustering of polygenic factors such as hypertension and hyperlipidaemia.[12]

In such cases as the Finnish group the early recognition of hypertension and hyperlipidaemia and its subsequent treatment might be expected to prove useful against the later development of coronary artery disease.

The next point to consider is the incidence of the disease in the various social classes. In the past the coronary prone individual was often portrayed as the obese, stocky, anxious, overworked professional. In recent times as shown by the Whitehall study of 17,530 London civil servants the incidence of ischaemic heart disease has shifted. It is now more prevalent in the lowest social group V. This was associated with smoking, short stature, high blood pressure, obesity and lower levels of glucose tolerance.[13] Some of these factors are correctable but not all.

Another approach has consisted of attempts to define specific personality traits that might be associated with the development of ischaemic heart disease. The problem here is that many of the studies have been done on patients who already have manifest cardiovascular disease and their personalities may well have been modified by their disease. A detailed study was made of white males between the ages of 40

to 74 in Evans County Georgia. They were classified
into three groups according to serum cholesterol and
blood pressure levels. The low risk had low levels of
pressure and cholesterol. The medium group had one or
other parameter elevated and the high risk group had
both factors raised. A separate group consisted of
people with diagnosed coronary artery disease. A
psychological test composed of the anxiety scale,
repression scale and lie scale was applied to samples
from each group. It was found that the coronary group
was less hostile, more anxious and repressed than the
other groups. There was no gradient between the low and
high risk non-coronary groups which led to the inference
that the psychological changes followed rather than[14]
preceded the coronary attack.

      Obesity is often quoted as a risk factor for
ischaemic heart disease though it must be remembered
that obesity and overweight are not necessarily the
same. Increased weight can also be due to water
retention which is a feature of some hypertensive
subjects. Clearly such overweight bears a close
relation to the development of ischaemic heart
disease as does hypertension itself. The most
disappointing aspect of our ignorance about obesity is
that the nature of the association between obesity
and ischaemic heart disease is still far from clear.
In Western society most overweight people are obese
and indices of relative weight such as weight/height
squared gives a good measure of body fat. However
laboratory methods for measuring body fat such as
densitometry, total body water and potassium are all
subject to considerable error.

      Another problem about assessing the role of
obesity in ischaemic heart disease is that many
factors are interrelated. Body weight increases with
age and with the cessation of smoking. A study of
patients with probable or overt ischaemic heart
disease showed no relation to total body fat as
estimated by measurements of total body water using
tritium dilution. In this sense the smoking habits
were not considered so that the result may have been
an artefact in that some patients with the disease were
cigarette smokers which itself is related to low body
weight. A simple artefact arises in attempting to
relate obesity to hypertension. The 22 cm
sphygmomanometer band in use in Britain fails
completely to encircle the arms of many people and
this leads to falsely high blood pressure readings.

However intraarterial pressure measurements do reveal
an association between increasing obesity and rising
blood pressure. But, as we have already indicated,
this may in part be due to water rather than fat
accummulation.

Studies of the relative importance of different
risk factors for ischaemic heart disease done
prospectively indicate that overweight is only of
importance by virtue of its association with blood
pressure, serum cholesterol and glucose intolerance.
However in considering a preventative programme it is
important to realise that factors which are useful in
predicting future disease are not necessarily the most
appropriate to tackle in prevention.

Blood pressure, blood glucose and serum cholesterol
all tend to fall in people who lose weight. For each
10% reduction of weight we might expect a 20% reduction
in the incidence of ischaemic heart disease. However
we do not know the answer to this prediction nor do
we know the risk to smokers and non smokers if they
are 20%, 40% or 60% overweight. However sufficient is
known to indicate that if good patterns of nutrition
and physical exercise are established in childhood,
at least in whom there are associated risk factors,[15]
benefit might accrue.

The role of exercise in relation to heart disease
is a topic of considerable debate. Studies of
marathon runners have proved interesting in this
regard. In 1961 an article in the New England Journal
of Medicine suggested that the coronary arteries of a
man who used to run the conventional marathon distance
of 42 kilometres were two to three times wider than
normal and showed minimal atherosclerosis. Two
subsequent reports supported this view. However
one of the cases died of myocardial infarction and the
other of a hypertrophic cardiomyopathy though in both
examples the coronary arteries were normal. However
four subsequent reports showed severe coronary artery
disease in marathon runners.[16] Clearly no conclusions
about the effects of marathon running can be culled
from these isolated reports.

Epidemiological surveys have not yet provided
evidence that physical inactivity is a risk factor
for ischaemic heart disease. This may be due to the
difficulty of measuring it as compared to blood
pressure, serum cholesterol or the number of

cigarettes smoked. It does seem that physical activity
taken in leisure time diminishes the incidence of first
heart attacks. But several factors interact in persons
who do that. Marathon runners for example tend to be
well educated, lean non-smokers without hypertension
and the levels of high density lipoproteins, which are
thought to be anti-atherosclerotic are raised by
exercise.

The effect of exercise on the coronary arteries
may be to prevent the development of atherosclerosis
or to inhibit its progression once it is established.
Serial coronary angiograms in patients with ischaemic
heart disease who exercised confirmed the latter view.[17]
This may be brought about by improvement in the
collateral circulation and this has been confirmed in
physically conditioned experimental animals. In
addition the bradycardia induced by regular exercise
might improve diastolic filling of coronary arteries
and reduce myocardial oxygen needs.

However dysrhythmias may occur during or after
physical exercise, and levels of norepinephrine, lactic
acid and potassium are all elevated. A case could
therefore be made that the marathon runner is at a
greater risk of cardiovascular death when running and
has a greatly reduced risk when he is not.[18]

Diet has been related to atherogenesis for many
years. Cholesterol feeding produces the disease in
animals and elevated blood cholesterol levels in man
are a well recognised risk factor. On the basis of this
a vast literature has grown up on the subject and
several preventative trials have been launched in
various countries aiming to reduce the intake of
cholesterol and animal fats. This vast problem of
diet and arterial disease will be dealt with elsewhere in this course so it is not proposed to deal
with it in detail here. Suffice to say that a wide
variety of dietary factors other than cholesterol have
received attention in this regard. Examples are hard
and soft water, dietary fibre, sucrose, milk, total
caloric intake, wine, garlic and contraceptive pills.

A number of trials have been concerned with
changing the type of fat in the diet from saturated to
polyunsaturated. This sort of diet can lead to a fall
of serum cholesterol by as much as 30 mgm/100 ml within
a year and the effect is maintained on the diet for the

trial period of six years. This was associated with a
significantly lower incidence of coronary heart disease
in the experimental group. Other workers propose the
value of periods of fasting on the principle that this
utilises the body stores of lipid for energy purposes
and hence reduces the level of serum cholesterol.[19]

A diametrically opposed view is that hyperlipidaemia
is a secondary event in ischaemic heart disease and is
not a major cause of coronary artery disease in man.
Such workers lay the blame on dietary sucrose which is
a principle source of calories and leads to a
functional hyperinsulinism.[20] Evidence in support of the
role of dietary sucrose comes from a variety of sources
Many patients with ischaemic heart disease give a history
of excessive intake of sucrose and cyclic attacks of
angina pectoris can be induced by sugar-induced
hypoglycaemia. Abnormally high plasma insulin responses
have been shown following a dose of glucose to patients
who have had myocardial infarcts. The peculiar resistance
of the Masai to heart disease despite a high intake
of fat is explained by the absence of sucrose from their
diet. Whereas a high intake of sucrose increased the
blood concentration of cholesterol. When the dietary
carbohydrate is replaced by bread as in Dutch Trappist
monks the cholesterol levels are low. This and a good
deal more evidence incriminating dietary sucrose in
atherogenesis is contained in the paper by Roberts.[20]

Various sorts of polyunsaturated fats have been
fed in order to modify the incidence of ischaemic heart
disease. The work was based on the notion that
essential fatty acid deficiency existed in atheromatous
subjects and this predisposed to a reduced glucose
tolerance. Another mode of action of the unsaturated
fatty acids might be related to the mechanisms of blood
coagulation. Deaths from ischaemic heart disease are
rare in Eskimos who consume a good deal of fish
containing eicosapentaenoic acid. This substance is the
precursor of the prostaglandin (PGI_3). This is an agent
which prevents platelet aggregation. If platelets are
important in atherogenesis then this approach might
be fruitful. It certainly is a sensible way of tackling
the thrombotic complications of coronary atherosclerosic
disease.[21]

The relationship between obesity diet and abnormal
response to carbohydrates are linked in the disease
diabetes mellitus. There is a well known association
between disease of large and small arteries and

diabetes. Here again however several atherogenic factors interact. One study of diabetics revealed hypertension in 75% with a greater proportion of females affected. This is the reverse in non-diabetics. So there is an increased tendency to hypertension in diabetics particularly in those over the age of 50 years.[22]

Other changes present in diabetics that may work together to enhance the atherosclerotic process are endothelial and platelet malfunction and lipoprotein disturbances. Endothelial injury is suggested by high plasma levels of van Willebrand factor, a glycoprotein found only in endothelial cells, platelets and megakaryocytes. This leads to increased permeability of vessels in the diabetic as is confirmed for example by fluorescein leakage from vessels in the eye of diabetics. This increased permeability coupled with a smooth muscle stimulating factor in diabetics provides a foundation for atherogenesis.[23]

The role of soft water in the production of arterial disease is debated. Mortality from heart disease is higher in areas with soft water, and furthermore it rises if the water supply of the area is artificially softened. It may not be a direct effect of the water itself. For example vegetables boiled in soft water lose their mineral content which can be restored in part by the addition of salt. This is suggested by the fact that residents in soft water areas excreted more sodium in their urine than those from hard water areas. A number of surveys have supported the "soft water" effect though precisely how it is mediated is unknown. By promoting salt intake and encouraging hypertension ischaemic heart disease mortality will rise but this is probably only part of the soft water story.[24,25]

Contraceptive pills are in such common use nowadays that they might be regarded almost as part of the diet of women. The evidence linking myocardial infarction with the contraceptive pill is convincing. Non-fatal myocardial infarction in women in the third decade is of the order of about 2 per 100,000. Those taking the pill had an incidence of 5.4. Myocardial infarction in these women often occurs with little coronary artery disease. It may be that the hormone is producing effects by its action on platelets. Women on the pill who develop thrombotic episodes have been shown to have antibodies to ethinyloestradiol in their plasma.

This may be a useful indication of women at risk. Use
of contraceptive pills increases the risk of myocardial
infarction threefold in women in the fourth decade.[26]

Other atherogenic factors are altered by ingestion
of contraceptives. Thus cholesterol, low density
lipoproteins, very low density lipoproteins and
triglycerides were all elevated and related to the
oestrogen content of the pill.[27]

Smoking is epidemiologically a well established
risk factor in atherosclerosis. Intimal fibrosis
with or without lipid deposition has been shown in the
coronary arteries of heavy cigarette smokers. Measurement of the levels of carboxyhaemoglobin in the blood
of smokers was not as good to prognosticate for the
occurrence of atherosclerotic disease as the smoking
history. However the blood levels did show a strange
association with myocardial infarction. In addition
the inhalation of tobacco smoke either by the person
smoking or by people in the vicinity of smokers can
precipitate angina pectoris.[28]

Another interesting observation was the increased
incidence of aortic aneurysms in smokers.[29] It has been
postulated that such aneurysms are due to medial hypoxia
in arteries with atherosclerotic disease and may indicate
one of the ways in which smoking produces arterial
damage. Other possibilities are vasospasm from
nicotine, allergy to the tobacco glycoprotein, by the
activation of Factor XII or even by a mutagenic effect
if the monoclonal view of atherogenesis is accepted.

A refreshing view about prevention of atherosclerosis
was the suggestion that alcohol consumption showed a
strong negative correlation with the tendency to develop
arterial disease and the entire alcohol effect was due
to wine.[30] Even this view was damped by the suggestion
that countries having a high intake of wine also
consumed garlic and the effect might be due to this.

If risk factors can be eliminated some effect on
atherogenesis can be expected in young people. Will
the disease also regress in older subjects? There is
good evidence from populations that fasted or were
starved that this might be so. War time studies, studies
of victims in concentration camps and studies of persons
with wasting disease all point to the possibility that
lipid may come out of the lesion.[31]

REFERENCES

1. D. G. Clayton and A. G. Shaper, Trends in heart
    disease in England and Wales 1950-1973,
    Health Trends 9:1 (1977).
2. W. C. Roberts, Relationship between coronary
    thrombosis and myocardial infarction, Mod.
    Concepts Cardiovasc. Dis. 41:2 (1972).
3. T. Horie, M. Sekiguchi and K. Hirosawa, Coronary
    thrombosis in pathogenesis of acute myocardial
    infarction, Brit. Heart J. XL:153 (1978).
4. M. J. Davies and A. Popple, Sudden unexpected
    cardiac death - a practical approach to the
    forensic problem, Histopathology 3:255 (1979).
5. N. El-Maraghi and E. Gentom, The relevance of
    platelet and fibrin thromboembolism of the
    coronary microcirculation, with special
    reference to sudden cardiac death, Circulation
    62:936 (1980).
6. J. W. Haerem, Sudden unexpected coronary death.
    The occurrence of platelet aggregates in the
    epicardial and myocardial vessels of man,
    Acta. Path. et. Microbiol. Scand. Sect. A
    Supp. 265 (1978).
7. W. T. Hayes, H. Bernhardt and J. M. Young, Rupture
    of interventricular septum following myocardial
    infarction, Southern. Med. J. 60:25 (1967).
8. G. E. Burch, C. Y. Tsui and J. M. Harb, Ischaemic
    cardiomyopathy, Amer. Heart J. 83:840 (1972).
9. E. J. Levin and D. Bryk, Dressler syndrome
    (postmyocardial infarction syndrome),
    Radiology 87:731 (1966).
10. M. J. Lipton, J. F. Feifer, M. G. Lopes and
    H. N. Hultgren, Aneurysms of the coronary
    arteries in the adult. Clinical and
    angiographic features, Radiology 117:11 (1975).
11. H. A. Berkoff and G. G. Rowe, Atherosclerotic
    ulcerative disease and associated aneurysms
    of the coronary arteries, Amer. Heart J.
    90:153 (1975).
12. Why does coronary heart disease run in families ?
    Leader, Brit. Med. J. 11/11 :415 (1977).
13. G. Rose and M. G. Marmot, Social class and
    coronary heart disease, Brit. Heart J.
    45:13 (1981).
14. M. A. Ibrahim, C. D. Jenkins, J. C. Cassel,
    J. R. McDonough and C. G. Hames, Personality
    traits and coronary heart disease, J. Chron.
    Dis. 19:255 (1966).

15. How dangerous is obesity? Leader, <u>Brit. Med. J.</u>
     1/1:1115 (1977).
16. T. D. Noakes, L. H. Opie, A. G. Rose and P. H. T.
     Kleynhans, Autopsy proved atherosclerosis in
     marathon runners, <u>New Eng. J. Med.</u> 301:86 (1979).
17. R. Selvester, J. Camp and M. Sanonarco, Effect of
     exercise training on progression of
     documented coronary arteriosclerosis in men,
     <u>Amer. N. Y. Acad. Sci.</u>301:495 (1977).
18. T. G. Pickering, Jogging, marathon running and the
     heart, <u>Amer. J. Med.</u> 66:717 (1979).
19. A. M. Immerman, Fasting and diet restriction in the
     treatment of cardiovascular disease,
     <u>A.C.A. J. of Chiropractice</u> 14:42 (1980).
20. H. J. Roberts, Are the massive diet fat - heart
     coronary drug studies justified? <u>Angiology</u>
     19:652 (1968).
21. D. V. Hamilton, E. J. A. Lea and S. P. Jones,
     Dietary fatty acids and ischaemic heart
     diseases, <u>Acta Med. Scand.</u> 208:337 (1980).
22. H. T. Blumenthal, M. Alex and S. Goldenberg,
     A study of lesions of the intramural coronary
     artery branches in, diabetes mellitus,
     <u>Arch. Pathol.</u> 70:13 (1960).
23. J. A. Colwell, Atherosclerosis in diabetes mellitus,
     <u>J. Chron. Dis.</u> 34:1 (1981).
24. A. G. Shaper, R. G. Packham and S. J. Pocock,
     The British regional heart study:cardiovascular
     mortality and water quality, <u>J. Environmental
     Path. and Toxicol.</u> 3:89 (1980).
25. G. W. Comstock, The epidemiological perspective:
     water hardness and cardiovascular disease,
     <u>J. Environmental Path. and Toxical</u> 3:9 (1980).
26. J. I. Mann, W. H. W. Inman and M. Thorogood,
     Oral contraceptive use in older women and
     fatal myocardial infarction, <u>Brit. Med. J.</u>
     II:445 (1976).
27. R. B. Wallace, J. Hoover, E. Barrett-Conner,
     B. M. Rifkind, D. B. Hunninghake, A. Mackenthun
     and G. Heiss, Altered plasma lipid and
     lipoprotein levels associated with oral
     contraceptives and oestrogen use, <u>Lancet</u>
     II;111 (1979).
28. W. S. Aronow, Smoking, carbon monoxide and coronary
     heart disease, <u>Circulation</u> XLVIII:1169 (1973).
29. O. Auerbach and L. Garfinkel, Atherosclerosis
     and aneurysm of aorta in relation to smoking
     habits, <u>Chest</u> 78:805 (1980).

30. A. S. StLeger, A. L. Cochrane and F. Moore,
     Factors associated with cardiac mortality in
     developed countries with particular reference
     to the consumption of wine, <u>Lancet</u> I :1017
     (1979).
31. A. L. Immerman, Fasting and diet restriction in
     the treatment of cardiovascular disease.
     <u>A.C.A. J. of Chiropractice</u> 14:42 (1980).

PREVENTION OF CORONARY HEART DISEASE

PART I. PRIMARY PREVENTION OF CORONARY HEART DISEASE

Marcel Kornitzer

Laboratory of Epidemiology and Social Medicine
Free University of Brussels, Campus Erasme, CP.590
808 Route de Lennik, 1070 Brussels – Belgium

INTRODUCTION

Atherosclerosis or better said athero-thrombosis is the pathological basis for coronary heart disease (CHD). Several epidemiologic autopsy studies have shown the correlation between prevalence of atherosclerotic complicated lesions and incidence of CHD at the population level.

As for the evolution of atherosclerosis, fatty streaks start early in life, even during the first decade and develope during the second and third decade whilst fibrotic and complicated lesions appear at a subclinical level. Starting during the third and increasing during the following decades clinical CHD appear it is the classical tip of the iceberg.
Ideal, and for the moment (utopic), prevention would rest on the total disappearance of atherosclerosis, at least fibrotic and complicated lesions, at the population level. A less ambitious goal would be the persistance of atherosclerosis at a subclinical level during at least 6 or 7 decades of mens'life delaying the appearance of clinical manifestations like angina, myocardial infarction or sudden death.

A brief recall of the most important coronary risk factors which have already been presented to you (Table 1).

The first two risk factors have a special status as they are not subject to modification : age and sex. Three risk factors have been found in most of the epidemiological prospective studies : high serum cholesterol, high blood pressure and smoking (cigarettes). Suffice to enumerate the other ones,

315

Table 1.   Coronary Risk Factors

Age	Blood viscosity
Sex	Heart Rate
Serum cholesterol	Sedentarity
Blood pressure	Water hardness (/-/)
Cigarette smoking	Oral contraceptives
HDL-cholesterol (/-/)	Urbanisation
Triglycerides	Type "A" behavior pattern
Glucose intolerance	Neuroticism
Diabetes	Stress
Obesity	Genetic factors
Nutrition (Fibers /-/; Linoleic Acid /-/)	

knowing that for some of them the assumption of a causal relationship with CHD is still weak or controversial. HDL-cholesterol presents a negative correlation with risk of CHD so that this factor is called a protective one; triglycerides, glucose intolerance, diabetes, obesity. Specific nutritional items like fiber and linoleic acid bear also a negative correlation with CHD. Blood viscosity, heart rate, sedentarity, water hardness (also a negative correlation). Oral contraceptives, urbanisation, Type "A" behavior pattern, neuroticism, stress and genetic factors. For most of those risk factors, the assumption of causal relationship rests on the so-called 8 criteria for inference of causality :

1. The power of association : relative risk should be elevated
2. A dose effect relationship
3. A temporal relationship : the factor should preceed the event
4. Same observations should have been in several epidemiological studies
5. The factors should be independently associated with the event : multivariate analysis will solve this question
6. The factor should bear a predictive power : it should predict the incidence of CHD in other population studies
7. Same observations in animal studies : experimental studies should have come to the same results
8. There should be a logical pathogenic mechanism

The inference of causal relationship should rest if possible on randomized controlled preventive trials.

Those trials rest on a working hypothesis : X is a causal factor for CHD (Table 2).

If X is reduced (or eliminated) in the experimental group→ incidence of CHD should be reduced as a consequence (compared to

Table 2. Primary Prevention of Coronary Heart Disease

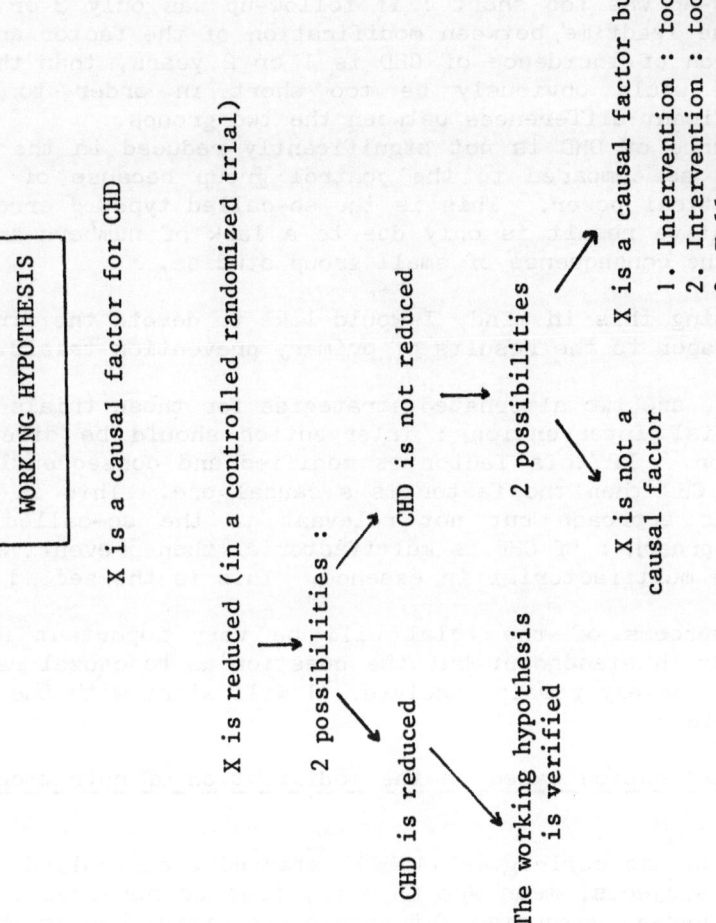

incidence in the control group). In that case, the working
hypothesis is verified. The other possibility is that incidence
of CHD is not significantly reduced in the experimental as
compared to the control group. The most straightforward explanation is that X in not a causal factor for CHD. Nevertheless,
alternative explanations should be taken into consideration : X
is a causal factor but
1) Intervention started too late in life (40 yr and over) when
   atherosclerotic lesions have a high prevalence
2) Intervention was too weak, thus the level of the risk factor
   was insufficiently reduced.
3) Follow-up was too short : if follow-up was only 3 or 4 years
   and the leadtime between modification of the factor and modification of incidence of CHD is 1 or 2 years, than the trial
   period would obviously be too short in order to observe
   significant differences between the two groups.
4) Incidence of CHD is not significantly reduced in the experimental as compared to the control group because of lack of
   statistical power. This is the so-called type β error where
   a negative result is only due to a lack of numbers and is in
   fact the consequence of small group studies.

   Keeping this in mind, I would like to devote the first part
of this paper to the results of primary prevention trials.

   There are two alternated strategies for those trials :
Unifactorial intervention : intervention should be directed at
one factor. If this factor is modified and consequently incidence of CHD than the factor is a causal one. This is a sound
scientific approach but not relevant to the so-called public
health approach : if CHD is multifactorial than preventive trials
should be multifactorial in essence. This is the second strategy.
Here a success of the trial will be very important from the
public health standpoint but the question as to causal relationship will largely remain unsolved. I will start with the unifactorial trials.

Primary prevention based on the modification of nutrition (Table
3)

   Dayton and colleagues (1959), started a controlled trial on
846 male subjects, mean age 65.5 yr, free or non-free of CHD at
start. Whereas saturated fat intake was diminished in the experimental group, the polyunsaturated fats were increased so that
the P/S ratio was far above 1 (around 3) which in fact is not a
physiological ratio. Compared tot the control group, serum
cholesterol level was reduced by 12.7% in the experimental one.
Fatal atherosclerotic events were significantly reduced in males
aged 54-65 whereas morbidity was not.

Table 3.   Primary Prevention of CHD: Nutrition

TRIAL	METHODOLOGY	ACTING ON	MORTALITY	MORBIDITY
Dayton et al.(V.A. 1959 →) (N: 422 + 424; M̄ Age 65.5)	↓↓ Saturated fats ↑↑ Polyunsaturated fats → P/S ≥ 1	Serum cholesterol (↓ 12.7%)	Fatal atherosclerotic events 54-65 ↓ P < 0.01 66-88 → NS	NS Mortality + Morbidity → P < 0.01
Turpeinen et al. (Helsinki Mental Hospitals 1958 →) (Cross-over technique)(2x 6yrs) Males and Females Hospital N : 234 Ss Age Range 34-64 Hospital K : 172 Ss (M̄ : 51)	↓↓ Saturated fats ↑ Polyunsaturated fats	Serum cholesterol (↓ 9 %)	Total : NS CHD Males : S Females :NS	Minnesota Code ↑ significant differences
Christakis et al. (Anti-Coronary Club N.Y. 1957 →) Males 40-59 N = 814 Free of CHD at entry Control group : Cancer deterction	"Prudent diet" ↓↓ Saturated fats ↑ Polyunsaturated fats P/S ≈ 1.35	Serum cholesterol (↓ 11.5%)		Experimental: 3.39 °/°° Control: 9.80 °/°° P < 0.02
Frantz et al. (The Minnesota Coronary Survey)	"Cholesterol lowering diet"	↓ Serum cholesterol	SD - MI Strokes (Males < 50yr) Experim.: 2.5°/°° Control : 8.9°/°° Total mort.: NS.	

Total atherosclerotic events were also significantly reduced.
All causes mortality was not signficantly different in the two
groups and this was due to an excess of carcinoma in the experimental group.

    Turpeinen and colleagues (1968), started a cross-over rando-
mized trial in two mental hospitals in the vicinity of Helsinki.
 Each phase lasted 6 years and at start Hospital N and K counted
respectively 234 and 172 subjects, aged 34-64, mean age 51. In
the experimental hospital, saturated fats were reduced with
partial replacement by polyunsaturated fats. Serum cholesterol
was reduced by 9% in the experimental group.

Table 4 gives some of the results (Miettinen et al., 1972) :
During the first period, male all-causes mortality (per 1000 per-
son-year) in diet and control hospitals were respectively 34.6
and 40.2 (-13.9%) and CHD mortality 5.7 and 15.2 (-62%). During
the second period, the figures were, for total mortality, respectively 35.1 and 38.8 (-9.5%) and for CHD mortality 7.5 and 13
(-42.5%).

In females total mortality, during the first period, was increased in the experimental group by 20%, compared to the control
group, but CHD mortality was reduced by 33%. During the second

Table 4. Age-Adjusted Death-Rates from Certain
Causes per 1000 Person-Years

MALES	CHD	All Causes
Hospital N, period 1 (diet)	5.72	34.56
Hospital N, period 2 (control)	12.97	38.78
Hospital K, period 1 (control)	15.18	40.20
Hospital K, period 2 (diet)	7.50	35.12
Pooled diet periods*	6.61	34.84
Pooled control periods**	14.08	39.50
FEMALES		
Hospital N, period 1 (diet)	3.96	31.08
Hospital N, period 2 (control)	7.74	32.13
Hospital K, period 1 (control)	8.06	25.89
Hospital K, period 2 (diet)	6.46	30.66
Pooled diet periods*	5.21	30.87
Pooled control periods**	7.90	29.01

* Hospital N, period 1, and Hospital K, period 2
** Hospital N, period 2, and Hospital K, period 1
From: Miettinen et al., 1972, Lancet, ii.

Table 6. Primary Prevention of CHD:
          Smoking (G. Rose and J.S. Hamilton 1968 →)

- Randomized controlled trial

- 1445 male smokers → 51% of experimental group reporting
                          being ex-smokers at one year

Mortality Follow-up on Average 7.9 years.

Results TOTAL MORTALITY   Control   1.63/100 men-years
                           Intervention   1.74/100 men-years

Controlled Trials on Smoking (Table 6)

One published trial can be referred here, that of Rose and
Hamilton (1978) which was initiated in 1968 in 1445 male smokers. At one year, 51% of the experimental group reported being
ex-smoker. Average mortality follow-up was 7.9 years. No
significant differences in total mortality have yet been observed in that trial. CHD mortality have not yet been published.

Controlled Trials on Hypertension (Table 7)

Five important trials have been published.
- The V.A. Cooperative Trial started in 1963. The first publication concerned 143 males (Veterans Administration Cooperative
Study Group on Antihypertensive Agents, 1967). Mean ages were
respectively 51.4 (control) and 50 (experimental). Administered
drugs were : hydrochlorothiazide, reserpine and hydralasine. In
the 143 subjects with entry diastolic blood pressure between 115
and 129 mmHg, the trial had to be stopped early because of a
significant excess of cardiovascular events (mortality and morbidity) in the control group, directly related to hypertension.
In 380 males with entry diastolic blood pressure between 90 and
114 mmHg, total mortality was reduced by 50% in the experimental
group, cardiovascular- and CHD mortality were reduced whereas
non significant differences were observed for total CHD incidence (Veterans Administration Cooperative Study Group on Antihypertensive Agents, 1970). This trial was in fact not meant to show
differences in CHD incidences as it was stopped when differences
in other target end points were reached.

- The U.S. Public Health Cooperative Study Group, initiated a
randomized trial in 389 subjects, with mild hypertension, mean
age 44, in 1964 (McFate Smith, 1977). Administered drugs :

Table 7.   Primary Prevention of CHD: Hypertension

T R I A L	S I Z E	DEFINITION OF HT	D R U G S	TOTAL MORTALITY	CV MORTALITY	CHD MORTALITY	MORBIDITY
V.A.Coop Study 1963 → (1)	N=143 Males (70+73) Age M̄ : Cont. 51.4 Int . 50	115-129 (diastolic)	Hydrochlorothiazide Reserpine Hydralasine	Cont. 4 Int . 0	4		Placebo : 27 Interv : 2 P < 0.01
V.A.Coop Study 1963 → (2)	N=380 Males	90-114 (diastolic)	Same drugs	Cont. 21 Int . 10	Cont. 19 Int . 8	Cont. 11 Int . 6	(Tot.CHD) Cont . 13 Int . 11 NS
U.S.Public Health Coop Study Group 1964 →	N=389 Males+Females Age M : 44	> 90 (diastolic)	Chlorothiazide Reserpine		Cont. 4 Int . 2	Cont. 2 Int . 2	(Tot.CHD) Cont . 7 Int . 8 NS
Australian Therapeutic Trial in Mild Hypertension 1973 →	N=3427 Cont . 1706 Int . 1726 Males+Females Age M̄ : 50.4	95-109 (diastolic) with systolic < 200	Chlorothiazide + Methyldopa Propranolol Pindolol + Clonidine Hydralasine	Cont. 35 Int . 25	Cont. 18 Int . 8	Cont. 11 Int . 5	(CHD Total hard end points) Cont. 33 Int . 33 NS
H.D.F.P. 1970 →	N=10940 Males+Females Age : 30-69 yr SC versus RC	> 90-104 (diastolic) 105-114 115+ (diastolic)	Diuretics Antiadrenergic Vasodilator	C C : 6.4% R C : 7.7% – 17%	Reduction -18.8%	Reduction -15%	
Oslo Study 1973 →	N=785 Age : 40-49		Hydrochlorothiazide Methyldopa or Propranolol		Mortality + Morbidity Sign.Red.		(Total CHD) NS

chlorothiazide and reserpine.   No differences in cardiovascular
and CHD mortality were observed, nor was there any difference between the two groups in total CHD incidence.

- The Australian Therapeutic Trial in Mild Hypertension (1980),
was initiated in 1973 in 3427 subjects mean age 50.4 years.
Definition of hypertension : diastolic blood pressure between 95
and 105 with systolic blood pressure under 200 mmHg. Administered drugs : first chlorothiazide, than methyldopa or propranolol
or pindolol was added than (eventually) clonidine or hydralasine. A reduction of 29% in total mortality was observed in the
experimental group.   Important reductions in cardiovascular and
CHD mortality were also oberved whereas total CHD hard end
points were not significantly different in both groups.

- The Hypertension Detection and Follow-up Programme was initiated in the U.S. in 1979; 10940 subjects (males + females) aged
30-59 yr were randomized by strata of diastolic blood pressure
(90-104; 105-114; 115 +) into a Stepped Care and Referred Care
Group. Administered drugs : diuretics, antiadrenergic, vasodila-
tators. After 5 yr follow-up, a significant reduction in total
mortality of 17% was observed.   In the subgroup, with entry
pressures between 90 and 104 mmHg, reduction of total mortality
of 20% (P < 0.01) was achieved.
Preliminary results concerning specific mortalities are favorable total cardiovascular -18.8%; total CHD mortality -15%; cerebrovascular mortality - 45%.

- The Oslo Study initiated in 1973 a trial in 785 males aged 40-
49 at entry (Helgeland et al., 1980).   Administered drugs :
hydrochlorothiazide, methyldopa or propranolol.   A significant
reduction in cardiovascular mortality + morbidity has been observed whereas the reduction in total CHD hard event was non
significant.

Multifactorial Approach
The North Karelia Project (Table 8)
     Was established after a population petition to reduce the
extremely high CVD rates in North Karelai (Tuomilehto, 1980).
It was initiated in 1972 (Salonen et al., 1979).
Principles : 1. Controlled but not randomized
             2. Multifactorial aiming at life-style modification.
Risk factors were reduced in North Karelia as compared to the
reference area.   Reduction in serum cholesterol was 4.1% in
males and 1.2% in females. For systolic blood pressure, figures
were respectively -3.6% and -4.8%.   For prevalence of smokers
-1.3.% and -0.7%.
The coronary risk profile (computed by means of the multiple
logistic function) was reduced by 17.4% in males and 11.5% in
females.

M. KORNITZER

Table 8. Primary Prevention of CHD:
Multifactorial Prevention - The North Karelia Project

"The North Karelia Project was established after a population petition to reduce the extremely high CVD rates in
North Karelia" - J. Tuomilehto. Period : 1972 → 1977.
Principles : 1. Controlled but not randomized
               2. Multifactorial intervention aiming at life-style modification

RISK FACTOR MODIFICATION

	Serum cholesterol	Systolic blood pressure	Prevalence of smokers	MLF
25-59 yrs Males	-4.1% (11 mgr/dl)	-3.6% (5.3 mmHg)	- 1.3%	-17.4%
Females	-1.2% (3 mgr/dl)	-4.8% (7.2 mmHg)	- 0.7%	-11.5%

MODIFICATION OF MORTALITY

	All causes		Cardiovascular mortality		Coronary Disease		Stroke	
	M	F	M	F	M	F	M	F
30-64 yrs North Karelia	-5%	-13%	-13%	-31%	-16%	-5%	-38%	-50%

COMPARISON OF NORTH KARELIA AND REFERENCE AREA

MODIFICATION OF MORTALITY (Δ)
6 yrs incidence °/oo

	M	F			M	F
All causes - N.K.	2.2	0.9		Cardiovascular N.K.	1.4	0.8
Ref.	2.2	1.2		Ref.	1.9	0.9

Important reduction in cardiovascular coronary and stroke mortalities were observed. But as some reductions were also observed
in the reference area, the differences were not statistically
significant. This trial has shown that it is possible to modify
the coronary risk profile and consequently CHD incidence in an
area of over 200000 citizens by means of an integrated approach
using mass media and individual counselling.

The Oslo Study (Hjerman et al., 1980)
    Was initiated in 1973 and is aimed at the reduction of both
serum cholesterol and smoking in high-risk (HR) subjects; 1232
HR subjects were randomized and in the experimental group subjects were given face-to-face counselling. First published
results show a reduction of 50% in total 5 year cardiovascular
incidence in the experimental group as compared to the control
group.

Other ongoing studies.
    A serie of studies are about to publish their results in
1982. They are :
1. The Göteborg Study : 30000 subjects were randomized in one
   experimental and two control groups (Wilhelmsen et al., 1972).
2. The Multiple Risk Factor Intervention Trial or MRFIT : Individual randomization of high-risk subjects (highest decile of
   the MLF distribution curve), (The Multiple Risk Factor Intervention, 1976).
3. The WHO European Collaborative Trial in the Prevention of
   Cardiovascular Disease include groups from Belgium, Italy,
   Poland and United-Kingdom (World Health Organization European
   Collaborative Group, 1974).
   Principle : randomization of factories. Fourty-four pair of
              factories were randomized (63.732 male subjects,
              age 40-59 at entry). Both individual and mass-me-
              dia counselling are provided.

REFERENCES

Christakis, G., Rinzler, S.H., Archer, M., Kraus, A., 1966,
      Effect of the anti-coronary club program on coronary
      heart disease. Risk-factor status, JAMA, 198:129.
Dayton, S., 1971, Rationale for use of lipid-lowering drugs,
      Federation Proceedings, 30:849.
Frantz Jr., I.D., Dawson, E.A., Kuba, K., Brewer, E.R., Gate-
      wood, L.C., Bartsch, G.E., 1975, The Minnesota coronary
      survey : Effect of diet on cardiovascular events and
      deaths, Circulation, supp. II-4, 51/52:No6.
Hypertension Detection and Follow-up Program Cooperative Group,

1979,Five-year findings of the hypertension detection and follow-up program.
I. Reduction in mortality of persons with high blood pressure, including mild hypertension, JAMA, 242:2562.
II. Mortality by Race-sex and age, JAMA, 242:2572.
Helgeland, A., Hjermann, I., Holme, I., Lund-Larsen, P.G., Leren, P., 1980, Treatment of mild hypertension : A five-year intervention trial. The Oslo Study. Abstracts VIII Europ. Congress of Cardiol., p. 123.
Hjermann, I., Helgeland, A., Holme, I., Lund-Larsen, P.G., Leren, P., 1980, A randomized intervention trial in primary prevention of coronary heart disease. The Oslo Study. Abstracts VIII Europ. Congress of Cardiol., p. 164.
McFate Smith, W., 1977, Treatment of mild hypertension. Results of a ten-year intervention trial, Circ. Res., 40, Supp. I.:98.
Miettinen, M., Turpeinen, O., Karvonen, M.J., Elosua, R., Paavilainen, E., 1972, Effect of cholesterol-lowering diet on mortality from coronary heart disease and other causes, Lancet, ii:835.
Oliver, M.F., Heady, J.A., Morris, J.N., Cooper, J., 1978, A cooperative trial in the primary prevention of ischaemic heart disease using clofibrate, Brit. Heart J., 40:1069.
Oliver, M.F., Heady, J.A., Morris, J.N., Cooper, J., 1980, WHO cooperative trial on primary prevention of ischaemic heart disease using clofibrate to lower serum cholesterol : Mortality follow-up, Lancet ii:379.
Oliver, M.F., 1978, Cholesterol, coronaries, clofibrate and death, N. Engl. J. Med., 299:1360.
Rose, G., Hamilton, J.S., 1978, A randomized controlled trial of the effect on middle-aged men of advice to stop smoking, J. Epidem. Community Hlth., 32:275.
Salonen, J.T., Puska, P., Mustaniemi, H., 1979, Changes in morbidity and mortality during comprehensive community programme to control cardiovascular diseases during 1972-7 in North Karelia, Brit. Med. J., 2:1178.
Turpeinen, O., Miettinen, M., Karvonen, M.J., Roine, P., Pekkarinen, M., Lehtosuo, E.J., Alivirta, P., 1968, Dietary prevention of coronary heart disease : Long-term experiment. I. Observations on male subjects., Am. J. Clin. Nutr., 21:255.
The Australian Therapeutic Trial in Mild Hypertension, 1980, Report by the Management Committee, Lancet, i:1261.
The Multiple Risk Factor Intervention (MRFIT), 1976, A national study of primary prevention of coronary heart disease, JAMA, 235:825.
Tuomilehto, J., 1980, The most recent lesson from community control of cardiovascular diseases, Acta Cardiol., 35:251.
Veterans Administration Cooperative Study Group on Antihypertensive Agents, 1967, Effects of treatment on morbidity in

hypertension.

I., Results in patients with diastolic blood pressure averaging 115 through 129 mmHg, JAMA, 202:1028,1970.

II., Results in patients with diastolic blood pressure averaging 90 through 114 mmHg, JAMA, 213:1143.

Wilhelmsen, L., Tibblin, G., Werko, L., 1972, A primary preventive study in Gothenburg, Sweden, Prev. Med., 1:153.

World Health Organization European Collaborative Group, 1974, An international controlled trial in the multifactorial prevention of coronary heart disease, Inter. J. Epidemiol., 3:219.

PREVENTION OF CORONARY HEART DISEASE

PART II. SECONDARY PREVENTION OF CORONARY HEART DISEASE

Marcel Kornitzer

Laboratory of Epidemiology and Social Medicine
Free University of Brussels, Campus Erasme, CP.590
808 Route de Lennik, 1070 Brussels - Belgium

INTRODUCTION

I would like to focus this paper on the secondary prevention of coronary heart disease (CHD). Secondary prevention includes those activities that alter favorably the natural history of clinical CHD, that is angina pectoris and myocardial infarction. One should also include all therapeutic manoeuvres that decrease the case fatality rate during the acute phase of a myocardial infarction (MI).

In other words, secondary prevention of CHD needs a comprehensive approach.
On table 1, I have tried to summarize the different stages of CHD. In symptomfree subjects, we should speak of primary prevention. In stable angina, it should be worthwhile to act on the classical risk factors : serum cholesterol, blood pressure and cigarette smoking. Indeed, I would like to remind you that in the Whitehall Study, those risk factors were still powerful predictors of CHD in subjects either with angina on the standardized Rose Questionnaire or minor ECG modifications (Rose et al., 1977). In stable, as well as in unstable angina, the surgical approach will be reviewed. Prevention of MI in subjects with unstable angina should maybe include drug treatment. In the prehospital phase of a myocardial infarction, health education and well equiped ambulance should be able to shorten the delay between onset of symptoms and admission in the coronary care unit (CCU), although, 2 controlled studies have questionned the evidence for CCU treatment in all patients with an acute MI (Mather et al., 1971; Mather et al., 1976). We should review the available evidence in favor of systematic drug administration in

331

Table 1.

PRIMARY PREVENTION	SECONDARY PREVENTION			
- Symptom-free populations - High-risk subjects	Stable angina → Unstable angina → Myocardial Infarction → Hospital Phase → Post-Hospital Phase			
		Pre-Hospital Phase		

Risk-factor modification
 	
Smoking   Cholesterol
Nutrition   Obesity
Physical activity
(Salt reduction)
Hypertension
 	
Non Drug
 	
Drug
	- Risk-factor modification ?
	- Drug treatment
	  . β blockade ?
	  . Anti-coagulation?
	  ."Anti platelet aggregation "?
		- Health education
		- Ambulance
		- Anti-arrhythmic drugs
			- Anticoagutation
			- Anti-arrhythmic drugs
			- Infarct size Limiting drugs
			- Physical revalidation
			- Smoking modification
			- Diet
				D R U G S
				- Anticoagulation
				- Anti platelet aggregation.
				- Anti-arrhythmic
				
				NON DRUG
				- Physical revalidation
				- Diet

order to reduce the case fatality rate for a MI. Last but not least, we should deal with secondary prevention in patients in the chronic stage of MI.

I would like to summarize some epidemiological wellknown facts concerning the natural history of CHD.
1. Incidence of a major coronary event (MI or sudden death) is 3 to 5 times higher in angina patients as compared to that in the "normal" population.
2. Ten procent of MI patients who are discharged from the hospital will die within one year. Thereafter, the death rate remains about 3-4%/year.
3. More than 50% of patients with a recurrent MI will die sudden-

Table 2.   CORONARY DRUG PROJECT
            Factors influencing long-term prognosis after recovery
            from myocardial infarction

            Placebo group (N = 2789 ♂) - 3 year Mortality

ENTRY - VARIABLES (N = 20)	t- Values (adjusted)
1. ST Depression	5.17
2. Cardiomegaly (X-Ray)	5.07
3. Functional class (N Y H A)	2.81
4. Ventricular cond.def.	3.88
5. Diuretics	2.87
6. Intermittent claudication	3.11
7. Cholesterol	3.88
8. Frequent ventr.ect.beats	2.81
9. Inactivity (leisure time)	2.73
10. Q / QS (ECG)	2.61
11. Heart rate	2.24
12. Number of myocardial infarction	2.32
13. Systolic blood pressure	2.96
14. Diastolic blood pressure	-2.15
15. Use of oral med. for hyperglycemia	2.17
16. Cigarettes	2.06

From: Coronary Drug Project Research Group, 1974, J.Chron.Dis.,27:267

ly, whereas 20-25% of subjects with a first MI will never reach the hospital.

Factors influencing long-term prognosis after recovery from MI were reported for the placebo group of the Coronary Drug Project (1974). As can be seen on table 2, 16 entry variables were predictors of 3 year mortality. Of those, at least six (1, 2, 3, 4, 10, 12) are not or poorly modifiable within a secondary prevention program, hence this should reenforce the idea of a more efficient primary prevention. Serum cholesterol and hypertension are still powerful predictors but cigarette smoking is the last significant entry variable.

Treatment of stable angina

For stable angina, there are 3 randomized trials. The V.A. Cooperative Coronary Surgery Study randomized 1015 subjects (Detre, 1977). Four year survival rate is significantly higher in surgical subjects with 3 vessel disease and abnormal left ventricular function, when the left main artery is stenoted. Surgical survival is also higher in left main artery disease. No significant differences between medically and surgically treated patients is observed in the absence of left main disease (Table 3).

Table 3.   STABLE ANGINA

V A COOPERATIVE CORONARY SURGERY STUDY (1970 → 1974)(N = 101

Four-year cumulative survival-rates (%) ±S.E. by extent of disease.

	LEFT MAIN INCLUDED		LEFT MAIN EXCLUDED	
	Med.	Surg.	Med.	Surg.
All patients	83 ± 2	86 ± 2	86 ± 2	85 ± 2
3 Vessels, abnormal L.V.F.	74 ± 4	87 ± 3*	79 ± 5	84 ± 4
2 & 3 Vessels, abnormal L.V.F.	78 ± 3	84 ± 3	81 ± 3	82 ± 3
1 Vessel, abnormal L.V.F. & 1, 2, 3 Vessels, normal L.V.F.	95 ± 2	92 ± 3	96 ± 2	93 ± 3
Left main artery	64 ± 8	93 ± 4**		

* P < 0.025 ;   ** P < 0.005.
From : Detre et al., 1977, The Lancet, ii.

Table 4.   STABLE ANGINA

THE EUROPEAN CORONARY SURGERY STUDY GROUP (1973 → 1976)(N = 768)

Five-year cumulative survival-rates (%) by extent of disease

	MEDICAL	SURGICAL
All patients	84.1	93.5[*]
Left-main artery disease	61.7	92.9[**]
3-Vessel disease	84.8	94.9[***]
2-Vessel disease	87.5	91.6 [N.S.]

[*]$P < 0.001$; [**]$P = 0.037$; [***]$P < 0.001$; N.S. = Not Significant
From : The Lancet ii, 1979.

Kloster et al., (1979), randomized 100 patients to surgical or medical treatment. No statistical difference in major cardiac events after 3 yrs were observed although surgical subjects with 3 vessel disease had statistically fewer major events as compared to medical subjects.

In the European Coronary Surgery Study Group (1979), five-year survival was higher in subjects with left main artery disease and 3 vessels disease (Table 4). Those results in favor of surgical treatment cannot be discarded, although all those trials are not without flaws.

Treatment of unstable angina

The natural history in patients with unstable angina is rather depressive (Table 5).

In Gazes'Study (1973), more than half of the patients died within ten years, the 8 months incidence of MI being 21% with a case fatality rate of 41%. In high-risk subjects with untractable pain and ST changes the 5 year survival rate was 27%, the 3 month incidence of MI 35% with a case-fatality rate of 63%.

Very recently, Telford and Wilson (1981), published the first controlled trial of unstable angina in 214 patients using only medical treatment. During the trial period, transmural myocardial infarction developed in 9 (17%) out of 54 patients on placebo, 8 (13%) out of 60 on atenolol, 1 (2%) out of 51 on

Table 5.   UNSTABLE ANGINA

N A T U R A L H I S T O R Y	
A. <u>140 PATIENTS</u>	– Five-year survival : 61% – Ten-year survival : 48% – Incidence of M.I. : 21% (8 months) → Mortality : 41%
B. <u>HIGH-RISK GROUP</u> (Pain ◆◆ ; ST changes)	– One-year survival : 57% – Five-year survival : 27% – Incidence of M.I. : 35% (3 months) → Mortality : 63%

From : Gazes et al., 1973, <u>Circulation</u>, 48: 331.

heparin, and 2 (4%) out of 49 on heparin and atenolol combined
(P = 0.024).   The improved prognosis in the heparin treated
patients was maintained at follow-up.   The authors stated that
intravenous heparin was beneficial in preventing myocardial infarction in patients with the "intermediate coronary syndrome".

In a non-randomized control study, Scanlon et al., (1973),
observed a higher mortality in medically treated subjects (Table
6).

Table 6.   UNSTABLE ANGINA

	Surgical Treatment	Medical Treatment
– Scanlon et al. (1973) (N = 85) Mortality	10.0%	27.0%
– Conti (Review) (1977) (N=1268) Mortality	7.0%	7.3%
– Conti (1978) (N= 269) Mortality	8.6%	6.2%

In a review of several studies with a total of 1268 subjects, no difference between surgery and drug treatment was observed (Conti, 1977). The same was true for a cooperative randomized trial (Conti, 1978).

In summary, unstable angina although poorly defined is a lethal entity where surgery is not indicated. Other controlled trials using heparin should be advocated.

Acute phase of myocardial infarction (Table 7)

Prognosis of a myocardial infarction is determined very early in the acute phase as 61% of all deaths occur within one hour in both males and females under ager 65. Thus, several authors focused their attention on the promotion of early and rapid prehospital coronary care : in Seatlle, Cobb et al. (1976) developed mobile CCU's manned exclusively by paramedical personnel. In Belfast, Pantridge (1974) developed a mobile ambulance system in the early seventies. The primordial aim of this rescue team is the timely defibrillation of primary ventricular fibrillation (Adgey et al., 1969; Eisenberg et al., 1979; Liberthson et al., 1974; Pantridge and Geddes, 1974). As for the hospital care, the first coronary care units (CCU) made their appearance in the U.S. 20 years ago and still there is a controversy concerning their utility. Indeed, whereas Chapman (1979), is strongly advocating the use of CCU on the basis of favorable results from non-randomized control studies, Mather and his group published two randomized trials, both of them essentially negative (Mather

Table 7. Acute Phase of a Myocardial Infarction

PREHOSPITAL CORONARY CARE

- SEATTLE (Cobb et al.)   : Mobile CCU (Paramedical personnel)
- BELFAST (Pantridge et al.) : Mobile Ambulances

  Aim : Timely defibrillation of primary ventricular fibrillation

HOSPITAL CARE

- Coronary Care Units (CCU)

  Two controlled randomized trials showed no significant difference between home care and CCU.

et al., 1971, 1976); 30% and 70% of all patients were randomized
in respectively the first and second study. Survival of patients
allocated to CCU was not better than that of patients remaining
at home. In summary, it can be said that the question is not
solved and that in 1981 a randomized trial is unthinkable given
the unwarranted position that all MI patients should be treated
in coronary care units. In any case, historical controls are of
no use given the modification over time of the natural history
of acute MI (Rose, 1975; Hunt et al., 1977; Craig et al., 1978).

Hospital phase of acute myocardial infarction

Coming to the hospital phase of acute MI, we summarized 6
controlled trials using anticoagulation (Carleton et al., 1960;
Wasserman et al., 1966; Assessment of short-term anticoagulant
administration after cardiac infarction, 1969; Drapkin and
Merskey, 1972, Handley et al., 1972; Anticoagulants in acute
myocardial infarction, 1973) (Table 8).

Most of those were performed 10 to 20 years ago. No one
showed a significant reduction in case fatality rate mostly
because lack of numbers. Taken as a whole they showed a 21%
significant reduction in case fatality rate and a 48% reduction
in clinically diagnosted thromboembolism. Those studies were
done before the introduction of coronary care units, preventive
treatment of arrhythmias and last but not least, before the
quasi systematic physical rehabilitation programmes including
early ambulation (West and Henderson, 1979; Harpur et al.,
1971). Selzer (1978) has rightly pointed to the fact that those
studies are not relevant to the acute MI in the seventies where
clinical thromboembolic complication is less than 1%!
A more timely approach could be early administration of
beta-blockers as MI size-limiting drugs or even, as shown in 2
controlled trials, in order to prevent the instalment of a MI
(Norris et al., 1978; Yusuf et al., 1980) (Table 9).
Maroko et al. (1977) published results of a controlled trial
using hyaluronidase and showing its size-limiting effect.

In the early seventies, the first randomized trials concerning the use of antiarrhythmic drugs were published (Pitt et
al., 1971; Valentine et al., 1974; Lie et al., 1974; Jennings et
al. 1976; Zainal et al., 1977) (Table 10).

Here the aim is to prevent the major arrhythmias like
ventricular tachycardia or fibrillation. While in all those
trials a significant reduction in arrhythmias was indeed observed, most of them lacked the power to detect statistical difference in early mortality.
Nevertheless, in two of those trials, a significant reduction in
early mortality has been observed, one using lidocaine (Valenti-

Table 8. Secondary Prevention:
Anticoagulation – Hospital Phase

R E S U L T S

A U T H O R S		NUMBER	CASE FATALITY (%)		THROMBOEMBOLISM (%)	
			Treatments	Controls	Treatments	Controls
Carleton et al.	(1960)	92	28.9	38.3	24.4	30.0
Wasserman et al.	(1966)	147	15.6	21.4	1.3	3.3
M R C Coop.	(1969)	1427	16.2	18.0	14.5	24.1
Drapkin et al.	(1972)	1136	14.9	21.2	18.8	24.6
Handley et al.	(1972)	53	7.4	7.7	0.0	26.9
Anticoagulants study	(1973)	999	9.6	11.2	7.8	18.8
TOTAL		3854	15.4	19.6	11.1	21.3
				– 21.4%		– 48%
				(P < 0.001)		(P < 0.001)

Table 9. Use of Beta-Blockers in the Acute Phase of a MI

A U T H O R S		NUMBER	D R U G	RESULTS
Norris et al.	(1978)	43	Propranolol (I.V + orally)	Pre-infarction → less frequent MI
Yusuf et al.	(1980)	214	Atenolol (I.V + orally)	Established MI → Size-limiting (Signif.) (Enzymes, ECG) Pre-infarction → Less frequent MI (signif.)

Table 10. Anti-Arrhythmic Drugs in the Acute Phase of a MI

A U T H O R S		NUMBER	D R U G	ARRHYTHMIAS	MORTALITY
Pitt et al.	(1971)	222	Lignocaine (IV infusion)	Signif.red.	N.S.
Valentine et al.	(1974)	269	Lidocaine (IM prehosp)		Signif.red.
Lie et al.	(1974)	212	Lidocaine (IV injection + infusion)	Signif.red.	N.S.
Jennings et al.	(1976)	95	Disopyramide (Per os)	Signif.red.	N.S.
Zainal et al.	(1977)	58	Disopyramide (Per os)	Signif.red.	Signif.red. (11 versus 1)

ne et al., 1974), the other disopyramide (Zainal et al., 1977).

I would like to stress that even oxygen administration during the acute phase of a MI has been tested in a randomized trial with a disappointing outcome (Rawles and Kenmure, 1976).

Secondary prevention of myocardial infarction : Chronic stage

Secondary prevention through diet was started more than 20 years ago as can be seen from the study of Morrison (1960) (Table 11).
In a low fat non randomized but controlled study, all patients in the control group were dead after 12 years. A collaborative group did not observe a significant reduction in recurrent MI (Research Committee, 1965). The same was true for the study of Rose et al. (1965), as well as the soyabeen study (Report of a Research Committee to the Medical Research Council, 1968).
The only important study with significant positive results was published by Leren (1966) : he observed a significant reduction in fatal + non-fatal MI in the treated group.

The most important controlled trial on lipid lowering drugs was the Coronary Drug Project (CDP) (Table 12) (Coronary Drug Project, 1970, 1972, 1973, 1975). Not one single drug used in that study was able to reduce CHD mortality : estrogens and dextrothyoxine had even an iatrogenic effect! In fact, the estrogen story started 20 years ago, when the groups of Marmorston et al. (1962) and Stamler et al. (1963) published the results of controlled trials in secondary prevention. The Stamler groups randomized 275 MI patients, the treatment group receiving 5mgr estrogens; five-year mortality rates were reduced by about 50% or more by hormone treatment. Mamorston et al. randomized patients recovering from an acute MI : 147 of them received a placebo, 120 received ethinyl estradiol, 85 received premarin (conjugated equine estrogens). Whereas ethinyl estra-diol did not improve survival this was the case for subjects receiving conjugated equine estrogens (Premarin) (Marmorston et al., 1962).
Interesting enough the V.A. Cooperative Urological Research Group (1967) published results concerning a randomized trial for the treatment of patients with cancer of the prostate. More than 2000 patients were enrolled. The Group concluded : although estrogen therapy (5mg) does cause a modest decrease in the morta-lity level from prostatic cancer, this decrease is outweighted by a substantial elevation in the mortality from other causes, primarily heart disease and cerebrovascular accidents.
Coming back to the CDP study, it should be noted that clofibrate (1.8gr/day) did not significantly reduce neither coronary morta-lity (fatal MI) nor morbidity (non-fatal MI). On the other hand, niacine (3gr/day) had a favorable effect on non-fatal MI, whereas it had not on coronary mortality.

Table 11. D I E T

	NUMBER	D I E T	RESULTS
Morrison (1960)	100	Low-fat	Significant reduction in mortality (12 yr).
Collaborative Group (1965)	264	Low-fat	Non significant reduction in fatal + nonfatal MI.
Rose et al. (1965)	80	Low-fat + corn-oil	Non significant increase in fatal + nonfatal MI (2 yr).
Leren (1966)	412	Low-fat + soya bean oil	Significant reduction in fatal + nonfatal MI.
Soya bean study (1968)	393	Low-fat + soya bean oil	Non significant difference

Table 12. Secondary Prevention:
Lipid Lowering Drugs

		DRUG	RESULTS
Coronary Drug Project	(1970)	Estrogen 5 mgr. (1119)	Iatrogenic : (Nonfatal MI)
Coronary Drug Project	(1972)	Dextrothyoxine 6 mgr. (1110)	Iatrogenic : (Sub-group : V.P.C.'s at entry) (Fatal MI; Nonfatal MI)
Coronary Drug Project	(1973)	Estrogen 2.5 mgr. (1101)	Iatrogenic : Thromboembolism, Cancer-Mortality.
Coronary Drug Project	(1975)	Clofibrate 1.8 mgr. (1103)	Fatal MI: N.S.; Nonfatal MI : N.S.
Coronary Drug Project	(1975)	Niacin 3 gr. (1119)	Fatal MI: N.S.; Nonfatal MI : Signif.reduction.
Physicians Newcastle	(1971)	Clofibrate (497)	Fatal MI: N.S.; SD : Signif.; Nonfatal MI : (P=0.055) Total morality : Signif.reduction.
Scottish Society Physiciants	(1971)	Clofibrate (717)	Base-line : Angina ↗ Signif.red. in Mortality ↗ N.S. red. in Nonfatal MI. Base-line : MI : N.S. red. in ↗ Fatal MI ↘ Nonfatal MI.
Carlson et al.	(1977)	Clofibrate + Nicotinic acid (558)	Total and CHD morality : N.S. Nonfatal MI : Signif.reduction.

The Newcastle study showed a significant reduction in total mortality and sudden deaths in subjects treated with clofibrate (Physicians of the Newcastle Study, 1971).

The Scottish study showed positive results for patients with angina at entry, that is a significant reduction in total mortality in subjects treated with clofibrate (Report by a Research Committee of the Scottish Society of Physicians, 1971).
In a randomized controlled study using clofibrate + niacine, Carlson et al. (1977) observed a significant reduction in non-fatal MI but not in total CHD mortality.

In may 1980, the International Society and Federation of Cardiology convened the councils of Rehabilitation, Atherosclerosis and Epidemiology in Kronberg, Federal Republic of Germany, in order to make a public policy report on secondary prevention (Secondary Prevention in Myocardial infarction survivors, 1980).
On lipids the pannel stated :
The controlled trial evidence justifying plasma lipid reduction in secondary prevention is very limited.
Advice may be given on the following theoretical reasons :

1. Hypercholesterolemia probably continues to aggravate CHD after MI.
2. To decrease progression of atherosclerosis and to support regression of existing arterial disease.
3. Changes in dietary fat intake may diminish liability to thrombosis.
4. To provide an education example to relatives of the patients.

Personally, I would stress the importance of point 4.

What about cigarette smoking in the secondary prevention?
The Coronary Drug Project study (1979), has shown, in the placebo group, an increase of about 25% to 30% for total mortality, cardiovascular mortality, sudden deaths, coronary mortality, non-fatal MI and fatal + non-fatal MI in smokers as compared to nonsmokers (Table 13).
Several nonrandomized, but controlled, studies have shown a significant decrease of between 30 to 50% in recurrent MI in subjects who quit at the acute stage of their MI (Jenkins et al., 1976; Mulcahy et al., 1975; Pohjola et al., 1979; Sparrow et al, 1978; Wilhelmsson et al., 1975).

The Kronberg Group made the following statement :
Non randomized trials report a favorable effect of cessation of smoking (subsequent fatal MI or SD reduced by 20-30%).
In fact, prevention is cheap, harmless and much easier to achieve than in symptomfree subjects.

Table 13.   Coronary Drug Project:
            Cigarette Smoking in Men with Myocardial Infarction

P L A C E B O G R O U P (N = 2789)			
	Smokers	Nonsmokers	Tation S/N.S.
Total mortality rate (5 yr. age adjusted)	24.3	18.8	1.29
Cardiovascular mortality	21.7	17.2	1.26
Sudden coronary death	10.2	8.0	1.27
Coronary mortality	18.5	14.8	1.25
Nonfatal MI	14.7	11.2	1.30
Fatal + nonfatal MI	29.7	24.1	1.23

From: The Coronary Drug Project Research Group, 1979, J.Chron.Dis., 32: 415.

As for physical rehabilitation after a sustained MI (Table 14), the Finnish Multifactorial Secondary Prevention Trial which was centered on physical rehabilitation has shown a significant reduction in coronary mortality and sudden deaths in the intervention group as compared to the control group (Kallio et al., 1979).   The National Exercice and Heart Disease Project (1980) which randomized 651 MI patients, observed no significant differences in total mortality and recurrent MI between intervention and control groups.   As for the WHO Study, results are still not available.

The Kronberg Group stated :
Physical rehabilitation and physical activity are advised in order to improve subjects' physical work capacity, to improve psychological status ("La joie de Vivre"), to enhance return to work and maybe to alter favorably the natural history of CHD.

Concerning long-term anticoagulation, we report here nine controlled trials as they were published by an ad-hoc collaborative group (An International Anticoagulant review Group, 1970) (Table 15).
Those trials randomized, between 1960 and 1966, 2205 males and 282 females.   Favorable results for the anticoagulated pooled groups were shown in males with a 20% reduction in death rate. Survivals at 2 years was significantly higher in subjects with antecedents of MI and/or angina.   A non significant reduction in

Table 14. Physical Rehabilitation

1. Kallio et al.(1979) - Multifactorial Intervention Programme - (N = 375)

	Coronary Mortality (3yr)(%)	Sudden deaths (%)	Reinfarctions
C. Gr.	29.4	14.4	
I. Gr.	17.5	5.5	
	(P.< 0.01)	(P.< 0.01)	N.S.

2. National Exercice and Heart Disease Project   (N = 651)

	Total Mortality (3yr)	Recurrent MI
C. Gr.	7.6%	7.2%
I. Gr.	5.0%	5.6%
	N.S.	N.S.

→ Favorable trend

3. WHO Randomized trial

No results available.

M. KORNITZER

Table 15. Long-Term Anticoagulation
Summary of Nine Controlled Trials[+] (2205 Males : 282 Females; 1950 → 1966)

	Anticoagulant series	Comparative series	Difference
MALES Death-rate/100/ months			
All	0.63	0.79	- 20% (P < 0.01)
With previous infarction < 55 yr.	0.64	0.95	
≥ 55 yr.	1.08	1.62	
Survival at 2 yrs (%)			
Neither angina nor MI	89	87	
With either or both angina/MI	83	76	P < 0.05
FEMALES Death-rate/100/ months	0.86	0.93	- 8% (N.S.)

[+]An International Anticoagulant review Group, 1970, Lancet i: 203.

death rate was observed in females. Again, we have to point
that these controlled trials were done 15 to 30 years ago.
Ancillary treatment of MI has undergone modifications since then,
although, it is right to state here that the new generation of
trials using platelet acting drugs are based on the same premi-
ses, namely to reduce a hypothetic hypercoagulable state in MI
patients.

In 1976, the so-called thrombosis services in the Nether-
lands started a controlled randomized trial concerning the long-
term anticoagulation in subjects aged 60 or over (Report of the
Sixty Plus Reinfarction Study Research Group, 1980). The outcome both in terms of total mortality and reinfarction was favorable to the anticoagulation group (table 16).

The Kronberg Group stated on long-term anticoagulation :
The evidence from controlled trials in not wholly consistent
although a reduction in the 2 year mortality is suggested
especially in high risk patients with recurrent infarction or
previous history of angina.
The question remains : Why is it that anticoagulation has fallen
in disuse in the United Kingdom, the United States and other
countries?

As for the use of beta-blockers, we have summarized 10
controlled trials with a total of more than 7000 patients
(Wilhelmsson et al., 1974; Multicenter International Study, 1975;
Ahlmark and Saertre, 1976; Barber et al., 1976; Evemy and
Pentecost, 1977; Burley et al., 1979; Andersen et al., 1979;
Lombardo et al., 1979; Baber et al., 1980; Norwegian Multicenter

Table 16. Long-Term Anticoagulation
Sixty Plus Reinfarction Study

Place	: The Netherlands	Size : 878 Patients
Time	: 1976 →	Age : 60 years or over
Follow-up	: 2 years	

Results :	Total Mortality		Reinfarction	
Anticoagulants	7.6%	P=0.017	5.7%	P=0.0001
Placebo	13.4%		15.9%	

Study Group, 1981), (Table 17). Four of them showed a significant reduction of total mortality in the treated group whereas
Barber and colleagues observe a significant reduction in subjects
with entry heart rate above 100/min.
All 3 studies using alprenolol were positive. The impact on
sudden death (SD) is not negligible. The Norwegian Multicenter
Study Group randomized 1884 patients in a timolol and placebo
group. Significant reductions in total mortality, SD and non-fatal MI were observed.

     The Kronberg Group stated :
Beta-blockers can reduce the risk of SD during the first 2 years
after MI. Not all trials have been positive. Many randomized
trials are under way.

     As for clinical trials with platelet-acting drugs, we summa-
rized 6 controlled studies using acetylsalicylic acid and one
using sulfinpyrazon (Elwood et al., 1974; Coronary Drug Project-
Aspirin, 1976; Elwood et al., 1979; Breddin, 1979; Aspirin
Myocardial Infarction Study Research Group, 1980; Persantine-
Aspirin Reinfarction Study (PARIS) Research Group, 1980; Anturance Reinfarction Trial Research Group, 1980), (Table 18).

     None of the aspirin trials showed a significant decrease of
total mortality although the drop in total mortality varied
between 17 and 42% in 5 trials whereas Elwood and colleagues
(1974) observed a significant decrease in total coronary incidence.
The Anturant Reinfarction Trial showed a significant decrease in
sudden death at 6 months.
The Kronberg Group concluded that the use of those drugs is
under active investigation and that no clear recommendations are
possible.
The Kronberg Pannel discussed 2 other factors : Hypertension and
Diabetes.
For hypertension they stated :
Treatment of hypertension should have a favorable influence on
angina pectoris and on heart function. The group observed
rightly that no controlled trials on longevity are available.
As for diabetes, the general principles of management are the
same as in patients without CHD :
1. Caloric restriction and exercice in overweight.
2. A low saturated fat, high complex carbohydrate diet.
3. Sodium restriction if hypertension or cardiac insufficiency
   are present.
As for stress as a secondary risk factor, there is an evident
lack of epidemiological data except that type A behavior subjects are prone to MI recurrence (Rosenman et al., 1967).

     We have tried to summarize here the "state of the art"

SECONDARY PREVENTION OF CORONARY HEART DISEASE

Table 17. Use of Beta-Blockers: Randomized Trials

AUTHORS	NUMBER	DRUG	TOTAL MORTALITY	FATAL MI	DUDDEN DEATH	NONFATAL	FATAL + NONFATAL
Wilhelmsson et al.(1974)	230	Alprenolol	Signif.red.		Signif.red.	N.S.	
Multicenter Intern.Study (1975)	3038	Practolol	Signif.red.	Sign.red.	Signif.red.	N.S.	Signif.red
Ahlmark & Saertre (1976)	162	Alprenolol	Signif.red.		Signif.red.	Sign.red.	
Barber et al.(1976)	298	Practolol	N.S.(H.R.> 100 Signif.red.)				
Evemy & Pentecost (1977)	94	Practolol	N.S.			N.S.	
Burley et al. (1979)	300	Oxprenolol			N.S.	N.S.	
Andersen et al. (1979)	480	Alprenolol	Signif.red.				
Lombardo et al. (1979)	260	Oxprenolol	N.S.				
Baber et al. (1980)	720	Propranolol	N.S.			N.S.	N.S.
Norwegian Multicenter Study Group (1981)	1884	Timolol	Signif.red.		Signif.ref.	Sign.red.	Signif.red

Table 18. Secondary Prevention:
Anti-Platelet Aggregation

AUTHORS	NUMBER	DRUG	RESULTS
Elwood et al., 1974	1239	A.S.A.	Total mortality : N.S. decrease (-25%)
Coronary Drug Project (Aspirin) (1976)	1529	A.S.A.	Total mortality : N.S. (-30%) Coronary mortality : N.S. (-27%) Fatal + Nonfatal MI : N.S. (-21%)
Elwood et al., 1979	1682	A.S.A.	Total mortality : N.S. (-17%) Coronary mortality : N.S. (-22%) Fatal + Nonfatal MI : (-28%) :Signif. Nonfatal MI : (-34%) :Signif.
Breddin (1979)	478	A.S.A.	Total mortality : N.S. (-42%)
Aspirin Myocardial Infarction Study (1980)	4534	A.S.A.	Total mortality : N.S. (+12.5%)
Persantine-Aspirin Reinfaction Study (1980)	1216	A.S.A.	Total mortality : N.S. (-17%)
Anturance Reinfarction Trial (1980)	1629	Sulfinpyrazon	Coronary mortality : N.S. (-17%) S.D. : Signifi.Decrease (P < 0.01)

concerning the secondary prevention of coronary heart disease conceptualising a comprehensive approach taking into account a continium with stable angina at one, and the chronic stage of myocardial infarction at the other end.

In some of those stages the surgical approach should not be dismissed, whereas drugs like beta-blockers will eventually find their place in the armamentum of the clinicians in search of ways to modify the natural history of coronary heart disease.

REFERENCES

Adgey, A.A.J., Nelson, P.G., Scott, M.E., Geddes, J.S., Allen, J.D., Zaidi, S.A., Pantridge, J.F., 1969, Management of ventricular fibrillation outside hospital, Lancet, i:1169.

Ahlmark, G., Saertre, H., 1976, Long-term treatment with beta-blockers after myocardial infarction, Europ. J. Clin. Pharmacol., 10:77.

Andersen, M.P., Bechsgaard, P., Frederiksen, J., 1979, Effect of alprenolol on mortality among patients with definite or suspected acute myocardial infarction : Preliminary results, Lancet, ii:865.

An International Anticoagulant revieuw group, 1970, Collaborative analysis of long-term anticoagulant administration after acute myocardial infarction, Lancet, i:203.

Anticoagulants in acute myocardial infarction : Results of a cooperative clinical trial, 1973, JAMA, 225:724.

Anturance Reinfarction Trial Research Group, 1980, Sulfinpyrazone in the prevention of cardiac death after myocardial infarction, N. Engl. J. Med., 302:250.

Aspirin Myocardial Infarction Study Research Group, 1980, A randomized controlled trial of aspirin in persons recovered from myocardial infarction, JAMA, 243:661.

Assessment of short-term anticoagulant administration after cardiac infarction, 1969, Report of the Working party on anticoagulant therapy in coronary thrombosis, Br. Med. J., 1: 335.

Baber, N.S., Wainwright, E.D., Howitt, G., 1980, Multicentre postinfarction trial of propranolol in 49 hospitals in the United Kingdom, Italy and Yugoslavia, Br. Heart J., 44:96.

Barber, J.M., Boyle, D., Chaturvedi, N.C., Singh, N., Walsh, M.J., 1976, Practolol in acute myocardial infarction, Acta Med. Scand., suppl. 587:213.

Breddin, M., 1979, Multicenter two-years prospective study on the prevention of secondary myocardial infarction by ASA in comparison with ohenprocoumon and placebo? Multicenter Controlled Trials, Ed. J.P. Boisset, C.R. Klimt, Inserm, 76:49.

Burley, D.M., Prout, B.J., Sutton, G.C., Taylor, S.H., Turner, J.R.B., Walker, W.C., 1979, Beta adrenergic receptor blockade in the treatment and prevention of myocardial infarction, VII. Asian-Pacific Congress of Cardiol. Abstr. 52.6.

Carleton, R.A., Sanders, C.A., Burack, W.R., 1960, Heparin administration after acute myocardial infarction, N. Engl. J. Med., 263:1002.

Carlson, L.A., Danielson, M., Ekberg, I., Klintemar, B., Rosenhamer, G., 1977, Reduction of myocardial reinfarction by the combined treatment with clofibrate and nicotinic acid, Atherosclerosis, 28:81.

Chapman, B.L., 1979, Effect of coronary care on myocardial infarct mortality, Br. Heart J., 42:386.

Cobb, L.A., Alvarez, H., Kopass, M.K., 1976, A rapid response system for out-of-hospital cardiac emergencies, Med. Clin. North Am., 60:283.

Conti, C.R., 1977, Unstable angina pectoris in Yu PN. Goodwin J.F. (eds) : Progress in Cardiology 6. Philadelphia Lea & Febiger p. 51.

Conti C.R., 1978, Current status of randomized prospective study on unstable angina, Adv. Cardiol., 22:130.

Coronary Drug Project Research Group, 1974, Factors influencing long-term prognosis after recovery from myocardial infarction - Three-year findings of the Coronary Drug Project, J. Chron. Dis., 27:267.

Coronary Drug Project Research Group, 1970, Initial findings leading to modifications of its research protocol, JAMA, 214:1303.

Coronary Drug Project Research Group, 1972, Findings leading to further modifications of its protocol with respect to dextrothyroxine, JAMA, 220:996.

Coronary Drug Project Research Group, 1973, Findings leading to discontinuation of the 2.5 mg/day estrogen group, JAMA, 226:652.

Coronary Drug Project Research Group, 1975, Clofibrate and niacin in coronary heart disease, JAMA, 231:360.

Coronary Drug Project Research Group, 1976, Aspirin in coronary heart disease, J. Chron. Dis., 29:625.

Coronary Drug Project Research Group, 1979, Cigarette smoking as a risk factor in men with a prior history of myocardial infarction, J. Chron. Dis., 32:415.

Craig, J.H., Byrne, E., Tiltman, R.C.B., 1978, Changing mortality from ischaemic heart disease and acute myocardial infarction, Med. J. Aust., 2:461.

Detre, K., Murphy, M.L., Hultgren, H., 1977, Effect of coronary bypass surgery on longevity in high and low risk patients, Lancet, ii:1243.

Drapkin, A., Merskey, C., 1972, Anticoagulant therapy after acute myocardial infarction : Relation of therapeutic benefit to patient's age, sex and severity of infarction, JAMA, 222:541.

Eisenberg, M., Bergner, L., Hallstrol, A., 1979, Paramedic programs and out-of-hospital cardiac arrest : II. Impact on community mortality, AJPH, 69:39.

Elwood, P.C., Cochrane, A.L., Burr., M.L., Sweetnam, P.M., Williams, G., Welsby, E., Hugues, S.J., Renton, R., 1974, A randomized controlled trial of acetylsalicylic acid in the secondary prevention of mortality from myocardial infarction, Br. Med. J., 1:436.

Elwood, P.C., Sweetnam, P.M., 1979, Aspirin and secondary mortality after myocardial infarction, Lancet, ii:1313.

European Coronary Surgery Study Group, 1979, Coronary-artery bypass surgery in stable angina pectoris : Survival at two years, Lancet, i:889.

Evemy, K.L., Pentecost, B.L., Intravenous and oral practolol in the acute stages of myocardial infarction, Europ. J. of Cardiol., 7:391.

Gazes, P.C., Mobley Jr., E.M., Faris Jr., H.M., Duncan, R.C., Humphries, G.B., 1973, Preinfarctional (unstable) angina A prospective study - Ten year follow-up. Prognostic significance of electrocardiographic changes, Circulation, 48:331.

Handley, A.J., Emerson, P.K.A., Fleming, P.R., 1972, Heparin in the prevention of deep vein thrombosis after myocardial infarction, Br. Med. J., 2:436.

Harpur, J.E., Kellett, R.J., Conner, W.T., Galbraith, H.-J.,B., Hamilton, M., Murray, J.J., Swallow, J.H., 1971, Controlled trial of early mobilisation and discharge from hospital in uncomplicated myocardial infarction, Lancet, ii:1331.

Hunt, D., Sloman, G., Christie, D., Penington, C., 1977, Changing patterns and mortality of acute myocardial infarction in a coronary care unit, Brit. Med. J., 1:795.

Jenkins, C.D., Zyzanski, S.J., Rosenman, R.H., 1976, Risk of new myocardial infarction in middle-aged men with manifest coronary heart disease, Circulation, 53:342.

Jennings, G., Model, D.G., Jones, M.B.S., Turner, P.P., Besterman, E.M.M., Kidner, P.H., 1976, Oral disopyramide in prophylaxis of arrhythmias following myocardial infarction, Lancet, i:51.

Kallio, V., Hämäläinen, H., Luurila, O., Hakkila, J., 1979, Multifactorial intervention programme on patients after myocardial infarction, Trans. of the Europ. Society of Cardiol., Vol. 1. No 2. Dublin.

Kloster, F.E., Kremkau, E.L., Ritzmann, L.W., Rahimtoola, S.H., Rösch, J., Kanarek, P.H., 1979, Coronary bypass for stable angina, N. Engl. J. Med., 300:149.

Leren, P. 1966, The effect of plasma cholesterol lowering diet in male survivors of myocardial infarction. A controlled trial, <u>Acta Med. Scand.</u>, suppl. 466.

Liberthson, R.R., Nagel, E.L., Hirschman, J.C., Nussenfeld, S.R., 1974, Prehospital ventricular defibrillation - Prognosis and follow-up course, <u>N. Engl. J. Med.</u>, 291:317.

Lie, K.I., Wellens, H.J., van Capelle, F.J., Durrer, D., 1974, Lidocaine in the prevention of primary ventricular fibrillation, <u>N. Engl. J. Med.</u>, 291:1324.

Lombardo, M., Selvin, A., Motolese, M., Belli, C., Pedroni, P., 1979, Beta-blocking treatment in 440 cases of acute myocardial infarction : A study with oxprenolol. Abstr. Florence Intern. Meeting M.I., 1979, No C145.

Marmorston, J., Moore, F.J., Hopkins, C.E., Kuzma, O.T., Weiner, J., 1962, Clinical studies of long-term estrogen therapy in men with myocardial infarction, <u>Proc. Soc. Exp. Biol. Med.</u>, 110:400.

Maroko, P.R., Hillis, L.D., Muller, J.E., Tavazzi, L., Heyndrickx, G.R., Ray, M., 1977, Favorable effects of hyaluronidase on electrocardiographics evidence or necrosis in patients with acute myocardial infarction, <u>N. Engl. J. Med.</u>, 296:898.

Mather, H.G., Pearson, N.G., Read, K.L.Q., Shaw, D.B., Steed, G.R., Thorne, M.G., Jones, S., Guerrier, C.J., Eraut, C.D., McHugh, P.M., Chowdury, N.R., Jafary, M.H., Wallace, T.J., 1971, Acute myocardial infarction : Home and hospital treatment, <u>Brit. Med. J.</u>, 3:334.

Mather, H.G., Morgan, D.C., Pearson, N.G., Read, K.L.Q., Shaw, D.B., Steed, G.R., Thorne, M.G., Lawrence, C.J., Riley, I.S., 1976, Myocardial infarction : A comparison between home and hospital care for patients, <u>Brit. Med. J.</u>, 1:925.

Morrison, L.M., 1960, Diet in coronary atherosclerosis, <u>JAMA</u>, 173:884.

Mulcahy, R., Hickey, N., Graham, I., McKenzie, G., 1975, Factors influencing longterm prognosis in male patients surviving a first coronary attack, <u>Brit. Heart J.</u>, 37.

Multicentre International Study, 1975, Improvement in prognosis of myocardial infarction by long-term beta-adrenoreceptor blockade using practolol : A multicentre international study, <u>Br. Med. J.</u>, 3:735.

National Exercice and Heart Disease Project, 1980, Effects of a prescribed supervised exercice program on mortality and cardiovascular morbidity in myocardial infarctions subjects : A randomized clinical trial, <u>CVD Epidem. Newsletter</u>, Council on Epidem. A.H.A. Ed. NO.O Barhani, No28:55.

Norris, R.M., Clarke, E.D., Sammel, N.L., Smith, W.M., Williams, B., 1978, Protective effect of propranolol in treatened myocardial infarction, <u>Lancet</u>, ii:907.

Norwegian Multicenter Study Group, 1981, Timolol-induced reduction in mortality and reinfarction in patients surviving acute myocardial infarction, <u>N. Engl. J. Med.</u>, 304:801.

Pantridge, J.F., 1974, Prehospital coronary care, Br. Heart J., 36:233.

Pantridge, J.F., Geddes, J.S., 1974, Primary ventricular fibrillation, Eur. J. Cardiol., 1/4:335.

Persantine-Aspirin Reinfarction Study (PARIS) Research Group, 1980, The Persantine-Aspirin Reinfarction Study, Circulation, 62:V-85.

Pitt, A., Lipp, H., Anderson, S.T., 1971, Lignocaine given prophylactically to patients with acute myocardial infarction, Lancet, i:612.

Physicians of the Newcastle upon tyne region, 1971, Trial of clofibrate in the treatment of ischaemic heart disease. Five-year study by a Group of Physicians ..., Brit. Med. J., 4:767.

Pohjola, S., Siltanen, P., Romo, M., Hwapakoski, J., 1979, Effect of quitting smoking on the longterm survival after myocardial infarction, Proc. 2nd Scient. Meeting Working Group on Epidem. and Prev. Europ. Society of Cardiol., No 033.

Rawles, J.M., Kenmure, A.C.F., 1976, Controlled trial of oxygen in uncomplicated myocardial infarction, Brit. Med. J., 1:1121.

Report of a Research Committee to the Medical Research Council, 1968, Controlled trial of soya-been oil in myocardial infarction, Lancet, ii:693.

Report by a Research Committee of the Scottish Society of Physicians, 1971, Ischaemic heart disease : A secondary prevention trial using clofibrate, Brit. Med. J., 4:775.

Report of the Sixty Plus Reinfarction Study Research Group, 1980, A double-blind trial to assess long-term oral anticoagulant therapy in elderly patients after myocardial infarction, Lancet, ii:889.

Research Committee, 1965, Low-fat diet in myocardial infarction. A controlled trial, Lancet, ii, 501.

Rose, G.A., Thomson, W.B., Williams, R.T.J., 1965, Corn oil in treatment of ischaemic heart disease, Brit. Med. J., 1:1531.

Rose, G., 1975, The contribution of intensive coronary care, Brit. J. Prev. Soc. Med., 29:147.

Rose, G., Hamilton, P.J.S., Keen, H., Reid, D.D., MacCartney, P., Jarrett, R.J., 1977, Myocardial ischaemia, risk factors and death from coronary heart disease, Lancet, i:105.

Rosenman, R.H., Friedman, M., Jenkins, C.D., Straus, R., Wurm, M., Kositchek, R., 1967, Recurring and fatal myocardial infarction in the Western Collaborative Group Study, Am. J. Cardiol., 19:771.

Scanlon, P.J., Nemickas, R., Moran, J.F., 1973, Accelerated angina pectoris. Clinical, hemodynamic, arteriographic and therapeutic experience in 85 patients, Circulation, 47:19.

Secondary prevention in myocardial infarction survivors, 1980, J. of the Int. Society & Fed. of Cardiol., Heart Beat No3.

Selzer, A., 1978, Use of anticoagulant agents in acute myocardial infarction : Statistics or Clinical judgment? Am. J. of Cardiol., 41:1315.

Sparrow, D., Dawber, T.R., Colton, T., 1978, The influence of cigarette smoking on prognosis after a first myocardial infarction, J. Chron. Dis., 31:425.

Stamler, J., Pick, R., Katz, L.N., Pick, A., Kaplan, B.M., Berkson, D.M., Century, D., 1963, Effectiveness of estrogens for therapy of myocardial infarction in middle-age men, JAMA, 183:632.

Telford, A.M., Wilson, C., 1981, Trial of heparin versus atenolol in prevention of myocardial infarction in intermediate coronary syndrome, Lancet, i:1225.

Valentine, P.A., Frew, J.L., Mashford, M.L., Sloman, J.G., 1974, Lidocaine in the prevention of sudden death in the prehospital phase of acute infarction, N. Engl. J. Med., 291:1327.

Veterans Administration Cooperative Urological Research Group (The), 1967, Treatment and survival of patients with cancer of the prostate, Surg. Gyn. & Obst., 1011.

Wasserman, A.J., Gutterman, L.A., Yoe, K.B., 1966, Anticoagulants in acute myocardial infarction : The failure of anticoagulants to alter mortality in randomized series, Am. Heart J., 71:43.

West, R.R., Henderson, A.H., 1979, Randomized multicentre trial of early mobilisation after uncomplicated myocardial infarction, Brit. Heart J., 42:381.

Wilhelmsson, C., Wilhelmsen, L., Vedin, J.A., Tibblin, G., Werkö, L., 1974, Reduction of sudden deaths after myocardial infarction by treatment with alprenolol, Lancet, i:1157.

Wilhelmsson, C., Elmfelt, D., Vedin, J.A., Tibblin, G., Wilhelmsen, L., 1975, Smoking and myocardial infarction, Lancet, i:415.

Yusuf, S., Ramsdale, D., Peto, R., Furse, L., Bennett, D., Bray, C., Sleight, P., 1980, Early intravenous atenolol treatment in suspected acute myocardial infarction, Lancet, ii:273.

Zainal, N., Carmichael, D.J.S., Griffiths, J.W., Besterman, E.M.M., Kidner, P.H., Gillham, A.D., Summers, G.D., 1977, Oral dispyramide for the prevention of arrhythmias in patients with acute myocardial infarction admitted to open wards, Lancet, ii:887.

THERAPEUTIC CONTROL OF ATHEROGENOUS PRIMARY HYPERLIPIDEMIAS

J.L. de Gennes

Service d'Endocrinologie Métabolisme
Hôpital de la Pitié, 83 Bd. de l'Hôpital
Prais 13ème - FRANCE

This report reexamines the objectives of medical treatment in primary (or idiopathic) hyperlipidemia. Secondary hyperlipidemias stemming from thyroid, cholestatic, diabetic, and renal etc. origins which require their own specific treatments have therefore been excluded from this discussion.

Therapeutic objectives must be precisely adjusted to the dangers incurred in each type, or more exactly, each class of primary hyperlipidemia; they must also take into account the place of these threats in the patient's own vital profile according to his age and sex. These dangers can be immediate as in the case of pancreatitis with massive hyperglyceridemia, or dangerously anticipated as, for example, in severely graded atherogenic hyperlipidemia. Conversely, they can be delayed to late term or even aleatory, particularly in females and when the grade of hyperlipidemia is minimal.

For this reason treatment of massive hyperglyceridemia, which is responsable for the often dramatic consequences of pancreatitis, must be differentiated from treatment of diverse atherogenic hyperlipidemias.

TREATMENT OF MASSIVE HYPERGLYCERIDEMIAS

Treatment of massive hyperglyceridemia aims to avoid all risks of acute or relapsing subacute pancreatitis which can occur in all classes of massive hyperglyceridemia when, as we have previously demonstrated, triglyceride levels exceed 1000 mg/dl or more (1).

In all of these forms the essential part of treatment is dietetic and not drug therapy. These diets however which aim to correct this hyperglyceridemia are varied and can be completely different according to the type of hyperglyceridemia involved.

1. Exogenous fat-dependent hyperglyceridemia

In exogenous type I fat-dependent hyperglyceridemia - which occasionally changes into type V - characterized by a positive decantation test at 4° and a heavy floating layer of chylomicrons alimentary restriction of long chain fatty-acid fats to no more than 5% of the total alimentary ration is an absolute necessity regardless of the difficult constraints imposed.

Consequently, in order to avoid the risk of an important imbalance in alimentary ration favoring carbohydrates which in turn would convert this type I hyperglyceridemia to type IV or type V as is often the case, it is desirable to readjust fat intake owing to the use of medium chain glycerides. These should not, however, exceed approximately 20% of caloric intake since above this amount they may reinforce an excess charge of prebetalipoproteins.

In most instances correction on a long term basis is only partial. Residual hyperglyceridemia remains after treatment. Triglyceride levels should subsequently be maintained below 1000 mg/dl. It is best to consider this disease as a hyperchylomicronemic (type I) form rather than a hyperlipomicronemic (type IV) form in order to avoid the probable, if not certain, atherogenic risk of the latter.

2. Mixed massive fat and carbohydrate-dependant hyperglyceridemia (real type V)

Only a diet regimen based upon a double restriction of fats and carbohydrates can totally correct mixed massive fat and carbohydrate-dependant hyperglyceridemia. Such a correction, often dramatic and complete, can be only time limited because this regimen leads to inevitable progressive weight loss in these patients. While this reduction is certainly desirable when an overweight preexists it can become undesirable and critical with normal or thin subjects - which is often the case in real type V hyperglyceridemia - and can lead to excessive weight loss and fatigue.

For long term treatment of these patients it is best to accept a partial dietary modification which preferentially limits long chain triglycerides and partially reduces carbohydrates so that a reasonable caloric ration is maintained

and allows for stabilized weight as a function of each patient's build and daily physical effort.

3. Endogenous hyperglyceridemia (type IV)

Endogenous type IV hyperglyceridemia which is characterized by increased prebetalipoproteins and a negative decantation
test (even after 48 hours), is the most frequently encountered
type of hyperglyceridemia. Tolerance to fats is excellent and
should be exploited when adjusting diet regimens. Because of
type IV's particular sensitivity to sugars and sugar derivatives (alcohol), dietary restrictions should first successively
center on eliminating alcohol, saccharose, fructose (honey,
sweets, fruits, fruit juices), and maltose (beer); only when
reduction of hyperglyceridemia is insufficient should other
glucide complexes found in the daily diet be limited. Carbohydrate intake should be reduced to 200-250 gms/24h which is
comparable to that of diabetic diet regimens.

If reduction is still incomplete in this type of endogenous hyperglyceridemia, residual hyperglyceridemia should be
treated with a complementary drug treatment analogous to that
which is usually employed in minor type IV hyperglyceridemia.
This in order to prevent an atherogenic risk which is sometimes
discussed and disputed, but which in our experience is not to
be neglected and can progres subclinically.

We have experienced that Clofibrate prescribed at the
usual 2 gm-day is perfectly adequate and completely corrects
these residual anomalies.

TREATMENT OF ATHEROGENIC HYPERLIPIDEMIAS

With the exception of certain minor excesses which can be
entirely controlled through dietary regimens and which shall be
reviewed later, treatment of atherogenic hyperlipidemia most
often combines dietetic measures and the use of hypolipidemic
drugs.

Three classes of atherogenic hyperlipidemia are at the
center of these therapeutic preoccupations :
- Familial hypercholesterolemia
- Mixed or Combined hyperlipidemia
- Minor type IV hyperglyceridemia

1. Familial hypercholesterolemia

Because of the atherogenic risk that has been demonstrated
for all increases in circulating cholesterol and more precisely LDL cholesterol when their respective critical thresholds

of 260 mg/dl and 190 mg/dl are exceeded familial hypercholesterolemia requires, if possible, absolutely perfect therapeutic
reduction to normal levels.

Dietary measures do not suffice as treatment except in
very minor forms which in fact do not necessarily belong
to the class of true familial hypercholesterolemia. Dietary
regimens should never be neglected however and always prescribed from the onset of treatment. If possible they should
preceed medication by several weeks in order to clearly assess
their contribution in lowering cholesterol levels which
except for certain rare cases (those which are quite sensitive
to the additon of exogenous cholesterol from eggs (2) for
example) rarely exceed -10% to -15%. A general reorientation
of regimen is preferable to a strictly calibrated diet which
soon becomes fastidious and is quickly abandoned. Exogenous
cholesterol should be limited to less than 300 mg per day and
fats rationed to 35 to 40% of total caloric intake. Vegetal
polyunsaturated fats should be substituted for animal saturated
fats (other than fish) in order to obtain a P/S ratio of
approximately 1.25. These measures usually amply suffice and
are generally well accepted by patients even on a long tern
basis.

In the heterozygotic form of this disease which is
clinically quasi-certain when the patient or his immediate
relatives present tendinous xanthomata, Clofibrate derivatives in association with an appropriate diet regimen can
lower not only cholesterol but also LDL cholesterol levels;
these reductions which are notably improved with the newer
Clofibrate derivatives (particularly fenofibrate) can decrease
these levels from 20-25% in the best of cases. Responses to
these drugs however are variable and have led to the classification of patients as good and poor responders : such classification becomes clear within the first six months of treatment.
Moreover responses are often limited and insufficient, thereby
requiring combined use of bile sequestrants such as Cholestyramine.

This drug appears to be more specific than the previous
medications in the correction of essential familial hypercholesterolemia of this type. It can be used alone and at the
onset of treatment. Final maintenance dose is one 4 gm packet
of Cholestyramine per gram/l of total circulating cholesterol
of the hypercholesterolemia to be treated. Maintenance doses
can be obtained only after very gradual and progressive incre-
ments of the original starting doses in order to palliate
digestive tract side effects.

In our experience however the combination of Cholestyramine and Clofibrate or its newer derivatives has proved to be the therapy of choice and enables the most thorough correction of these lipid anomalies. In addition the use of Cholesty-ramine alone often favors the appearance of hyperglyceridemia (3) which quickly disappears when Clofibrate or its derivatives are added to the treatment. We have found that nicotinic acid, as recommended by Carlson, is troublesome over long periods of time because of the intolerance reactions it provokes. However this drug should not be overlooked when other medical treat-ments fail to obtain positive results.

Finally, when confronted with objectives drug treatment resistance or poor treatment compliance ileal by-pass using Buchwald's techniques (4) may still be indicated although its indications are now limited because of recent improvements in medical treatment.

In the case of major grade Type II - which corresponds either to homozygotic familial hypercholesterolemia, characte-rized by the absence or deficiency of LDL receptors, or to double heterozygotic forms - the previous therapeutic measures often fail. Nevertheless Cholestyramine and Clofibrate should systematically be tried at the beginning of treatment followed by the adjunction of nicotinic acid when sufficiently tolera-ted prior to giving up drug treatment and turning toward therapeutic measures such as plasmaphoresis (5, 6, 7) or porto-caval shunts (8, 9) which remain 'heroic' and exceptional treatments.

In addition to the two previous grades, a large group of patients remains who are affected by a lesser grade of pure type IIa hyperchoelsterolemia which we have previously designa-ted as minor hypercholesterolemia (11), and which is found far more frequently in any population than the previous two forms. The lines of treatment in minor hypercholesterolemia are derived from those previously described for heterozygotic forms but they must take into account the relative ease of correction in this minor form. Consequently Cholestyramine is not syste-matically prescribed, as was previously detailed, and is reserved either for forms which are resistant or respond inadequately to Clofibrate or new Clofibrate derivatives. It is also reserved for treatment of young individuals needing long term therapy and thus, long term security, for whom physicians would hesitate to prescribe Clofibrate derivatives over prolonged periods lasting more than 15-20 years. With the exception of these difficulties the association of a diet regimen and Clofibrate derivatives can habitually totally correct lipid anomalies and achieve normal distribution of cholesterol; this reduction should be verified by dosing HDL cholesterol and subsequently calculating LDL cholesterol using the Friedwald and Fredrickson formula.

Only when cholesterol levels are very moderately elevated
- generally not in excess of 300 mg of total cholesterol
per 100 ml - can dietary treatment alone satisfactorily
correct these lipid anomalies on a long term basis. For
these cases real LDL cholesterol excess requiring treatment
should be verified by systematically checking HDL cholesterol.
Besided this common situation it is the hypercholesterolemia
found in children which initially requires dietary treatment
alone in order to delay, for general safety reasons, both the
age of onset, and the long term duration of drug treatment.

2. Mixed or Combined hyperlipidemia

Mixed or Combined hyperlipidemia strictly - identical and
exchangeable - according to J. Goldstein's or our own (10)
terminology are easier to treat and correct than essential
hypercholesterolemia regardless of the levels of lipid abnormalities.

Once again, even though dietary measures similar to those
prescribed in essential hypercholesterolemia are absolutely
necessary, with in addition restriction of sugar, sugar
derivatives, and glucides as in endogenous hyperglyceridemic
and diabetic regimens they must be accompanied by drug therapy.
For a large contingent of these cases medication can be
limited to Clofibrate derivatives : ordinary Clofibrate which
is active in these mixed forms should be tried initially.

This is notably the case in type III hyperlipidemia - a
perfect example of a major grade of mixed hyperlipidemia -
which is remarkably responsibe to ordinary Clofibrate, its
derivatives, and occasionally to estrogens in women, even when
synthetic and given per os. Type II + type IV, equally designated as IIb occurs more frequently than type III and is
present in both major and minor grades of mixed hyperlipidemia.

This form often responds quite well and completely to
Clofibrate derivatives. The hypercolesterolemic component
(type IIa) however may resist treatment longer than the
endogenous type IV hyperglyceridemic fraction. In this
case Cholestyramine should be added to the above treatment and
dosed as a function of residual hypercholesterolemia so that
total therapeutic correction can be achieved.

In addition to these mixed hyperlipidemias, we have
isolated a new subtype (12) with a slow prebetalipoprotein

which we have designated by analogy and commodity as type IVb (13). This subvariety is also distinctive because of its particular resistance to previous therapeutic measures even with respect to its endogenous hyperglyceridemic component. For this reason, it is radically different from type III hyperlipidemia with which it has often been abusively confounded. This new class of mixed hyperlipidemia which is fortunately less frequent than type IIb is particularly dangerous since it is highly resistant to the therapeutic arsenal and utilisation of all drug combinations in attempting to correct these anomalies may sometimes prove unsuccessfull. Probucol, a newly introduced therapeutic agent, may prove useful in surmounting this type of therapeutic resistance.

3. Minor type IV hyperglyceridemia

Minor type IV hyperglyceridemias are at the center of numerous controversies at present as to their atherogenic potential and the justification of their systematic therapeutic correction (14). From our standpoint, these hyperglyceridemias should be treated and corrected every time cholesterol levels are either globally increased or simply perturbed in their distribution with, as a result, decreased HDL cholesterol and a total cholesterol/HDL cholesterol ratio greater than 4.5. This is generally the case in these forms because of the inversed reciprocal relation that exists between the triglycerides of VLDL and HDL cholesterol (15).

Contrary to newly circulated opinions it is rare that the simple dietetic measures which were previously discussed in the treatment of massive endogenous hyperglyceridemia can, by themselves, maintain complete and permanent correction of residual lipidic anomalies. Most often, as a recent study has pointed out, complementary use of Clofibrate or its new derivatives is necessary if a normal level of HDL is to be reestablished (16).

CRITERIA FOR LONG TERM SECURITY IN DRUG TREATMENT OF HYPERLIPIDE-MIAS

If we are to avoid the pitfalls of hesitation and indecision, the search for criteria for long term security drug treatment of hyperlipidemia must be approached pragmatically and the benefits of treatment weighed against its risks. We should not forget (as, unfortunately, it is now often the case) the considerable threatening cardiovascular dangers that these patients – who have been duly identified as having atherogenic hyperlipidemia – risk because of their non-treatment and the non-correction of these lipid anomalies.
Such resigned and cowardly attitudes towards treatment are being

encountered more and more frequently as a result of ambiguous and
unsettling reports spread throughout the medical and lay communities following the recent studies undertaken by the Coronary Drug
Project (17) and particularly by the World Health Organization
whose prospective study analyzes the 5-year long term results of
Clofibrate on primary and secondary cardiovascular prevention
(18).

While these results should be taken into consideration and
exploited in order - as was the case in these two studies -
to avoid treating minor lipid anomalies with Clofibrate alone
when dietary measures should be the first and perhaps exclusively
treatment applied, these same results seem detrimental when they
encourage attitudes which ignore that the worst danger in true
atherogenic hyperlipidemia is the absence of effective corrective
treatment.

Neither of these studies is conclusive enough to force
abandoning the therapeutic resources of Clofibrate and its
derivatives at the present time as long as they are judiciously
prescribed; their success depends upon following the best therapeutic indications, associating an appropriate diet regiment, and
discerning good responders from poor ones for whom Clofibrate is
inadequate and requires replacement by other medications. Our own
experience with Clofibrate over the last fifteen years correlates
with many other studies and has shown that the most tangible
disadvantage of this drug resides in the increased risk of chole-
lithiasis (Fig. 1) which is most often confined to the gall
bladder and pure assymptomatic. In the future therefore this
risk must be reduced. This can be accomplished either by selecting new less lithogenic derivatives or through associations of
Clofibrate with drugs such as Cholestyramine or Ursolic acid, for
example, which prove to be advantageous.

As to the other tangible drawbacks of Clofibrate, its depressive effect on male sexual function, although highly variable,
merits serious consideration even if no precise explanation has
yet been proposed. This side effect is also found with many of
the other Clofibrate derivatives and may eventually compel
to abandon this drug.

Purely hepatic side effects due to Clofibrate or its derivatives are limited to an initial and temporary increase in SGPT
transaminase. In 20% of cases where Procetofen was utilized,
however, we have noted a larger and more durable increase in SGPT
levels which should therefore systematically be surveyed.

Potential carcinogenic dangers with Clofibrate and its
derivatives should certainly be studied most carefully by drawing
numerous long term animal toxicity trials using rodents and

other species as well as large-scale prospective and retrospective studies in humans. At present, however, it must be admitted that there has been no decisive or demonstrative proof of drug carcinogenicity in humans, and although this proof exists for women for oestroprogestative treatment the cases which have been duly proven as carcinogenic are still numerically small and have evidently not been sufficient to forbid this form of hormonal therapy.

Finally, the increase in total 'all-inclusive' non-cardiovascular mortality with Clofibrate which was significant in the WHO study (5, 18) and which has been largely responsible for the discredit and disaffection of this drug leading to its condemnation and premature abandonment in the treatment of atherogenic hyperlipidemia has not been demonstrated in any other study.

The unilateral informations do not allow to forget the more tangible imminent threats of the cardiovascular complications of this disease to the patient's lifespan which justify the use of this treatment.

The problem of drug safety should most certainly be attentively and extensively studied through animal experimentation. In addition, all advances in Clofibrate-derived molecules which can increase the margin of safety of these drugs without reducing their efficacy should be welcomed.

For the moment however no substances providing a better benefit to risk ratio have been found to replace the Clofibrate derivatives which are now available and must continue to be indispensable for treatment along wich Cholestyramine, nicotinic acid, and a few new rare products such as Probucol.

Indeed, with the correction of these lipid anomalies all of these drugs, often taken in association with one another, and accompanied by adequate diet regimens are beginning to manifest their effects of slowing, arresting, or reversing the cardiovascular complications of grave atherogenic hyperlipidemia whose forms have been described in this report. In addition to several favorable, although partial, indications coming out of the CDP as well as the WHO study*, much more promising reassurance is beginning to emerge from more contrasted studies where hyperlipidemia was more pronounced and better corrected. Such supportive findings were already indicated in our 1976 study comparing good

----
* It would indeed be advisable to repeat the entire WHO prospectivestudy with the combined use of an enhanced intake of polyunsaturated fats in order to obviate the decrease of P/S of circulating fat, which has been described after the use of Clofibrate alone without adequate diet.

and poor responders to treatment (20) as well as in Carlson's
study now in progress (3).

In a final analysis the effect of treatment on cardiovascular complications is the ultimate and only definitive criteria as to the efficacy of medical treatment. To obtain this
effectiveness, however, demands much effort, prudence, and discussion as to the final analysis of these results. We must be
particularly cautious of the skepticism and the temptation
to abandon these treatments as a result of the influence of
disputable interpretations of these studies which have been more
impressive with respect to the enormity of their numeric series
and their cost than their final significances. This is particularly true in view of the fact that with the therapeutic aids now
at our disposal, we perhaps already possess effective and safe
means to combat hyperlipidemia-induced atherosclerosis.

REFERENCES

1. J.L. de Gennes, G. Turpin, and J. Truffert, Les pancréatites
   des hyperlipidémies idiopathiques. Etude d'une série
   personnelle de 40 cas. Ann. Med. Interne, 125, 4:333
   (1974).
2. J. Davignon, N. Leboeuf, and S. Lussier-Cacan, Aspects nutri-
   tionnels du traitement des hyperlipidémies et de l'athéro-
   sclérose, Union Médicale, 109, 5:1 (1980).
3. G. Rosenhamer, and L.A. Carlson, Effect of combined clofibra-
   te-nicotinic acid treatment in ischemic heart disease,
   Atherosclerosis, 37, 129 (1980).
4. H. Buchwald, R.B. Moore, and R.L. Varco, Partial ileal bypass :
   a test of the lipid-atherosclerosis hypothesis in Atherosclerosis V, A.M. Gotto Jr, L.C. Smith and B. Allen,
   (eds.), Proceedings of the Fifth International Symposium on
   Atherosclerosis in Houston, novemver 6-9th 1979, 462.
5. J.L. de Gennes, R. Touraine, G. Maunand, and J. Truffert,
   Formes homozygotes cutanéo-tendineuses de xanthomatose
   hypercholestérolémique dans une observation familiale
   exemplaire. Essai de plasmaphérèse à titre de traitement
   héroïque, Soc. Med. des Hôp. de Paris, 118, 15:1377
   (1967).
6. J.L. de Gennes, S. Moorjani, M. Lou, D. Brun, and C. Gagne,
   Removal of cholesterol from blood by affinity binding to
   heparin-agarose : evaluation of treatment in homozygous
   familial hypercholesterolemia, Pediat. Res., 14:113 (1980).
7. G.R. Thompson, N.B. Myant, D. Kilpatrick, C.M. Oakly, M.J.
   Raphael, and R.E. Steiner, Assessment of long-term plasma
   exchange for familial hypercholesterolemia, Br. Heart. J.,
   43:680 (1980).

8. T.E. Starlz, H.P. Chose, C.W. Putnam, and K.A. Porter, Porto-caval shunt in hyperlipoproteinemia, Lancet, 2:940 (1973).

9. T.E. Starlz, L.J. Koep, and R. Weil, Portocaval shunt and hyperlipidemia, in Atherosclerosis V, A.M. Gotto Jr., L.C. Smith, and B. Allen (eds.), Proceeding of the Fifth International Symposium on Atherosclerosis in Houston, november 6-9th 1979, 450.

10. J.L. de Gennes, Les hyperlipidémies idiopathiques. Proposition d'une classification simplifiée, La Nouvelle Presse Médicale, 18:791 (1971).

11. J.L. de Gennes, F. Dairou, P. Hamon, and J. Truffert, Normalisation lipidique d'un dysbêtalipoprotéinémie de type III par l'éthinyl-oestradiol (50 ug par jour) chez une femme de 87 ans, Ann. Med. Interne, 131, 7:410 (1980).

12. J.L. de Gennes, F. Dairou, P. Hamon, and J. Truffert, Ultracentrifugal evidence of a special subtype of mixe hyperlipidemia, Atherosclerosis, 27:493 (1977).

13. J.L. de Gennes, F. Dairou, P. Hamon, and J. Truffert, L'hyperlipidémie mixte athérogène à surcharge principale en pré-bêtalipoprotéine lente (tyep IVb), La Nouvelle Presse Médicale, 10, 9:691 (1981).

14. S.B. Hulley, R.H. Rosenman, R.D. Bawol, and R.J. Brand, Epidemiology as a Guide to Clinical Decisions; the association between triglyceride and coronary heart disease, The New Engl. J. Med., 302, 25:1383 (1980).

15. A.R. Tall, and D.M. Small, Plasma high density lipoproteins, The New Engl. J. Med.,299:1232 (1978).

16. J.L. Witztum, M.A. Dillingham, W. Giese, J. Bateman, C. Diekman, E. Kammeyer, S. Weidman, and G. Schonfeld, Normalization of triglycerides in type IV hyperlipoproteinemia fails to correct low levels of high-density-lipoprotein cholesterol, The New Engl. J. Med., 16:907 (1980).

17. Coronary Drug Project Research Group : Clofibrate and niacin in coronary heart disease, JAMA, 231:360 (1980).

18. W.H.O. Cooperative trial on primary prevention of ischaemic heart disease using clofibrate to lower serum cholesterol : mortality follow-up, The Lancet, 8191:397 (1980).

19. J.L. de Gennes, J. Truffert, and P. Periac, Elévation des transaminases glutopyruviques sous traitement par Procétofène des hyperlipidémies idiopathiques. Fréquence et importance dans 443 cas traités, La Nouvelle Presse Médicale, 7, 27:2398 (1978).

20. J.L. de Gennes, Intervention trial for secondary CV prevention in primary atherogenous hyperlipidemias, in Atherosclerosis V, G. Schettler, Y. Toto, Y. Hata, and G. Klose (eds.), Proceedings of the Fourth International Symposium on Atherosclerosis in Tokyo, august 24-28th 1976, 686.

RADICAL THERAPY OF HYPERCHOLESTEROLAEMIA

AND ATHEROSCLEROSIS

G.R. Thompson

Medical Research Council Lipid Metabolism Unit
Hammersmith Hospital
London W12 OHS

INTRODUCTION

Before describing the various methods available for treating
severe hypercholesterolaemia and the accompanying atherosclerosis
it is first necessary to discuss the nature of the problem and define
the objectives to be achieved. It seems appropriate to start by
considering the pathology of fatal coronary heart disease (CHD), as
described by Roberts.[1] His autopsy findings can be summarised as
follows: Atherosclerotic lesions involve the entire coronary tree,
usually with 2 or 3 major branches critically stenosed, i.e.,
narrowed by more than 75%; the main stem of the left coronary artery
is critically stenosed in 25% of cases, this lesion always being
accompanied by severe triple vessel disease; critical stenoses are
always due to complicated plaques, of which fibrous tissue is the
major component but approximately 25% is lipid. These features
suggest that fatal CHD is usually associated with severe but not
necessarily irreversible atherosclerosis.

Relationship Between Hypercholesterolaemia and Atherosclerosis

The value of the major risk factors, namely serum cholesterol,
blood pressure and smoking, in predicting CHD is well known but it
is of interest that serum cholesterol was the only one which correlated with the extent of atherosclerosis at autopsy, as determined
during the Framingham Study.[2] This correlation was evident in males
with serum cholesterol values obtained as recently as 1 year before
death. This and other evidence of the predictive power of hypercholesterolaemia in individuals with clinically-evident CHD provides
hope that control of hypercholesterolaemia might improve prognosis,
even in the advanced stages of the disease.[3]

Additional evidence of the relationship between hypercholesterolaemia and the severity and extent of coronary atherosclerosis comes
from angiographic studies in patients with angina.[4-9]   Those with
hypercholesterolaemia tend to be younger than those without[10,11] and
more prone to multi-vessel involvement.[5]   Serial angiographic studies
show that coronary lesions more often progress in patients with hyperlipidaemia than in those with normal serum lipids.[12,13]   This association between hypercholesterolaemia and premature, severe and
progressive coronary atherosclerosis is especially evident in patients
with familial hypercholesterolaemia (FH).   The pathogenesis and
clinical features of this inherited disorder of low density lipoprotein (LDL) metabolism have been reviewed elsewhere[14] but can be
summarised briefly as follows: Increased LDL levels are present from
birth and are secondary to a partial (in heterozygotes) or near
complete (in homozygotes) deficiency of LDL receptors; the resultant
hypercholesterolaemia is extreme in homozygotes, in whom the early
development of atheromatous lesions of the aortic valve, supravalvular
region of the aorta and coronary ostia,[15] usually leads to death
before 30; heterozygotes have serum cholesterol levels intermediate
between normal subjects and homozygotes, associated with the onset in
early middle-age of severe and often fatal CHD.[16]

Hypercholesterolaemia and Coronary Artery Bypass Grafts

Angiographic studies have revealed a much higher incidence of
left main stem disease in FH patients than in subjects with other
risk factors such as hypertriglyceridaemia[17] or cigarette smoking.[18]
As mentioned earlier this lesion has an ominous association with
fatal CHD,[1] which is borne out by data on the influence of coronary
artery bypass grafting on prognosis.   In one series almost 40% of
medically treated patients with left main stem disease were dead
within a year compared with only 20% of those treated surgically,[19]
the corresponding figures for death within 4 years being 36% and 7%
in the larger Veterans Administration Study.[20]   There seems little
doubt that coronary artery bypass grafting improves the prognosis of
left main stem disease, and it seems reasonable to presume that this
procedure is being and will be performed relatively often in young
patients with FH or other forms of hypercholesterolaemia with which
that lesion is associated.[21]

There have been few studies of the anatomy and pathology of
coronary artery bypass grafts.   Barboriak et al.[22,23] have shown
that atheromatous changes can occur within 5 years, usually in the
grafts of patients who have remained hyperlipidaemic post-
operatively; one FH patient even developed such changes within 9
months.   Another larger autopsy series showed the occurrence of
atherosclerosis in 11% of grafts from normolipidaemic patients and

in 79% of those from hyperlipidaemic patients,[24] the mean time of onset being 29 months.   The authors concluded that saphenous vein grafts were more susceptible to hyperlipidaemia than native coronary arteries and that post-operative control of serum lipids was essential if graft atherosclerosis was to be prevented.

Objectives of Treatment

The main aim of treating hypercholesterolaemia is to arrest the progression or induce regression of the all too commonly associated and potentially fatal atherosclerotic lesions, or to prevent their development, as in the case of coronary artery bypass grafts;   the latter can be regarded as a form of primary prevention.   Because severe hypercholesterolaemia is commonly due to FH, most trials of radical therapy have been undertaken in patients with that disorder. The results, however, can probably be extrapolated to other less severe forms of hyperlipidaemia.

Studies in dogs, pigs and monkeys show that experimentally-induced atheroma will regress if hypercholesterolaemia is sufficiently well controlled,[25-28] but evidence of regression in man is largely anecdotal.   It has been suggested that regression of atherosclerosis in humans only occurs if the serum cholesterol is brought below 3.1 mmol/l (160 mg/dl).[28]   However, recent evidence shows that arrest or slowing of the rate of progression of lesions can be achieved, at least in FH patients, at somewhat higher levels of serum cholesterol, around 7 mmol/l (270 mg/dl), so long as the decrease in total cholesterol is accompanied by an increase in the HDL:LDL ratio.[29]   Thus ideally treatment should result in substantial reductions in plasma levels of LDL, and very low density lipoprotein (VLDL) where these are raised, whilst raising or leaving unchanged HDL levels.   In the light of these requirements let us now consider the various radical approaches which have been used to treat severe hypercholesterolaemia.

PORTACAVAL SHUNT

Portacaval shunt was first used to treat a patient with FH by Starzl et al. in 1973 on the rather empirical basis that this procedure relieved the secondary hyperlipidaemia of patients with glycogen-storage disease.[30]   Their patient, a homozygote, responded with a remarkable 60% fall in serum cholesterol and a 46 mm decrease in the gradient across her aortic valve,[31] but she died suddenly 18 months later, apparently from an arrhythmia.[32]   Since then Starzl et al. have carried out portacaval shunts in 4 more homozygotes and a severely affected heterozygote.[33]   All the homozygotes have shown some resolution of xanthomata but none have had quite such a striking reduction in serum cholesterol levels as the first case (Table 1). Mild abnormalities of liver function have been observed but there has

Table 1. Patients with Familial Hypercholesterolaemia Treated
with Portal Diversion at the University of Colorado
Health Sciences Center (adapted from Starzl et al.[33]).

No.	Age/Sex	Years post-op	Cholesterol mmol/l			Clinical State
			pre	post	Δ	
1	12 F	1.5	20.0	7.5	(-62%)	Homozygote. Died
2	7 F	6.5	26.0	10.4	(-60%)	"
3	8 M	5.5	26.0	13.2	(-49%)	"
4	5 M	2	20.8	13.4	(-36%)	"
5	14 M	0.5	22.9	15.6	(-32%)	"
6	52 M	0.25	14.9	10.1	(-32%)	Heterozygote

been no evidence of hepatic encephalopathy.   Stein et al.[34] undertook
this procedure on 4 homozygotes in South Africa with variable success
and have recently reviewed the results of these and the 30 other
portacaval shunts performed between 1973-1980, the majority of them
in homozygotes.[35]   Ages have ranged from 2-28 and the mean decrease
in serum cholesterol has been 40%.   In at least 3 instances thrombosis of the shunt has been held to be responsible for a failure of
the serum cholesterol to fall;   an increase in platelet aggregation
has been observed in 1 homozygote post-operatively,[36] which could be
relevant to the problem of shunt closure.

Mechanism of Effect of Portacaval Shunt

Investigation of the mechanism whereby portacaval shunt exerts
its effects have shown a progressive decrease in serum cholesterol
and triglyceride concentrations in normal dogs[37] accompanied by
atrophic changes in liver cells, including glycogen depletion and a
decrease in the rough endoplasmic reticulum.[38]   Similar histological
changes were observed in an FH homozygote.[30]   Studies in pigs have
shown a 50% decrease in cholesterol synthesis in liver biopsies[39] and
turnover studies suggest that this is accompanied by a decreased rate
of synthesis of LDL in vivo.[40]   It is difficult to account for these
changes simply in terms of a reduction in hepatic blood flow[41] and
other mechanisms have been proposed, including a reduction in the
amount of insulin reaching the liver.[38]

Kinetic studies by Bilheimer et al.[42] in a homozygote showed
marked decreases in the synthesis of both cholesterol and LDL protein
after a portacaval shunt but the only one of our patients to undergo
this procedure showed a less marked decrease in LDL synthesis.[43]
This particular patient showed a disappointingly slight decrease in

serum cholesterol which, together with an increasing aortic gradient, suggested that portacaval shunting alone was insufficient to prevent progression of her disease.[15]

Indications for Portacaval Shunt

One of the main drawbacks of undertaking a portacaval shunt is the variability of response and difficulty in predicting which patients are likely to do well. Furthermore, although the reduction in serum cholesterol averages 40%, this is usually insufficient to bring a homozygote's serum cholesterol down to anything approaching the normal range. However, the operation is relatively easy to perform and so far has been remarkably free from serious side-effects. Also it has the conceptual attraction of counteracting at least one of the metabolic abnormalities responsible for the hypercholesterolaemia of homozygotes, namely the increased synthesis of LDL. Although portacaval shunt alone may be insufficient to control hyper-cholesterolaemia adequately in most FH homozygotes, its effectiveness can be enhanced by other procedures such as plasma exchange or partial ileal bypass, as reviewed below. However, there seems little theoretical or practical justification for using it to treat patients with heterozygous FH.

PLASMA EXCHANGE

In 1967 De Gennes et al. undertook repetitive plasmapheresis in a patient with homozygous FH. This involved removing 800 ml blood several times a week over a period of 4 months.[44] The patient's hypercholesterolaemia was controlled effectively by this means but the inconvenience of manual plasmapheresis (described by the authors as 'traitment héroique') resulted in its eventual abandonment, and the patient subsequently died. The advent of the continuous-flow blood cell separator occurred at about the same time but was not exploited in the context of hypercholesterolaemia until 1972 when Turnberg et al.[45] used an IBM machine to treat successfully a patient with xanthomatous neuropathy due to primary biliary cirrhosis. These authors exchanged their patient's plasma with 1-2 litres of fresh frozen plasma (FFP) every 2-4 weeks for a period of 6 months. Three years later I and my colleagues[46] introduced the use of plasma exchange to treat FH, when we exchanged 2 homozygotes at monthly intervals using an Aminco centrifuge. Our approach was similar to that of Turnberg et al.[45] except that plasma protein fraction (PPF) was found to be a better replacement fluid than FFP. Since then we have undertaken plasma exchange in another 3 homozygotes and in 4 heterozygotes with CHD[47,48] and have recently reviewed our own experience and that of other authors.[49] To date plasma exchange has been reported in a total of 24 patients with severe hypercholesterol-aemia, as shown in Table 2. The commonest category of patient has

Table 2.   Published Reports of Hypercholesterolaemic Individuals
           Treated by Plasma Exchange, 1972-81 .

Source	Patients	Frequency & Duration	Other Measures
Turnberg et al.[45]	1 PBC	1/mth for 7 mth	
Thompson et al.[46]	2 FH hmz	1/mth for 4-8 mth	PCS in 1[15]
Berger et al.[50]	2 FH hmz	1-2/mth for 3-18 mth	PCS in 1
Simons et al.[51]	4 FH htz	1/mth for 13-18 mth	
Thompson et al.[47,48]	3 FH hmz)		
	4 FH htz)	2-4/mth for 5-38 mth	
King et al.[52]	2 FH hmz	2/mth for 21-30 mth	PIB in 1
Witzum et al.[53]	1 FH hmz	2/mth for 12 mth	
Berger et al.[54]	1 FH hmz	No details	
	1 FH htz	2/mth for 4 mth	
Stein et al.[55]	1 FH hmz)		
	1 FH htz)	2/mth for up to 16 mth	
	1 PBC)		

PBC, Primary biliary cirrhosis;   PCB, Portacaval shunt;
PIB, Partial ileal bypass

been homozygous FH (12) followed by heterozygous FH (11) and primary
biliary cirrhosis (2).

Plasma Exchange for Homozygous FH

Our 2 original patients were treated at monthly intervals with
relatively small volume (2-2.4 1) exchanges[46] but this combination
subsequently proved to be ineffective in preventing progression of
aorto-coronary disease, as judged by an increasing gradient across
their aortic valves.[47]   One of these patients died after an aortocoronary bypass, the other had a portacaval shunt which failed to
arrest her disease, and she too subsequently underwent coronary
artery bypass grafting, together with insertion of an aortic valve
prosthesis.[48]   She is now undergoing plasma exchange at 2-weekly
intervals which, together with her portacaval shunt, results in an
acceptably low mean serum cholesterol, as shown in Table 3.   The
Table also shows the 50-55% reduction in hypercholesterolaemia
achieved in 2 male homozygotes by approximately twice monthly,
large volume (3.2-4 1) plasma exchanges.   During the past 5 years
these 2 patients have each undergone well over 100 plasma exchanges
without mishap.   Their xanthomata have regressed and their aortocoronary atheromatous lesions have not progressed, as judged by

Table 3. Details of 3 Homozygotes Currently Undergoing Plasma Exchange at Hammersmith Hospital, London .

Patient	Current Age	Plasma Exchange			Serum Cholesterol mmol/l		
		No.	Duration[a]	PPF,1	Off PE	On PE[b]	Δ
1 Pre-PCS	30	9	10	2.0-2.4	16.1	11.4	-29%
Post-PCS		40	24	2.4	13.7	8.1	-41%
2	28	129	70	4.0	18.5	9.2	-50%
3	18	143	60	3.2-4.0	19.0	8.5	-55%

[a]Months   [b]Mean   PE, Plasma exchange;   PCS, Portacaval shunt

serial angiography and measurement of aortic gradients.[47]   The experiences of others who have treated homozygotes with twice monthly plasma exchange have been similarly favourable, including a 4-year-old child treated by Witzum et al.[53]   It is not clear whether the presence of a partial ileal bypass helped slow the rate of rise in plasma cholesterol after plasma exchange in the homozygote treated by King et al.[52] but the data of Berger et al.[54] show that the rate of rise in a homozygote who had had a portacaval shunt was much less than in another without a shunt, less even than a heterozygote.

Plasma Exchange for Heterozygous FH

Evidence that plasma exchange is beneficial to heterozygotes is more controversial than for homozygotes. We used it to treat 4 patients with CHD, 3 of whom achieved symptomatic benefit, with evidence of partial regression of coronary atheroma in one.[47]   In contrast, Simons et al.[51] and Stein et al.[55] considered that plasma exchange offered no advantage over conventional therapy.   However, the lack of improvement reported by Simons et al.[56] could have been due to their performing plasma exchange at only monthly intervals, as discussed elsewhere.[57]   Nevertheless the indications for plasma exchange in heterozygotes are less pressing than for homozygotes, chiefly because of the existence of effective therapeutic alternatives such as the combination of anion-exchange resins and nicotinic acid, or partial ileal bypass.   On the other hand, the better control of hypercholesterolaemia achievable by plasma exchange in heterozygotes make them potentially better candidates for testing the lipid hypothesis.[47]

Plasma Exchange for Primary Biliary Cirrhosis

Only 2 patients have been reported so far[45,55] but the response
has been good in both instances, with resolution of the painful
neuropathy caused by xanthomatous infiltration of peripheral nerves.
The main cause for hypercholesterolaemia in this condition is accumulation of an abnormal form of LDL called lipoprotein-X, which
consists largely of unesterified cholesterol and phospholipid which
have refluxed into plasma from obstructed biliary canaliculi.
Lipoprotein-X probably has a turnover rate similar to that of LDL in
FH, thus rendering it equally suitable for removal by plasma exchange
at 1-2 weekly intervals.

Parameters of Plasma Exchange

In effect plasma exchange achieves a short-term enhancement of
LDL catabolism by removing hypercholesterolaemic plasma and substituting lipoprotein-free PPF.   This action is particularly useful in
patients with FH, in whom defective catabolism is one of the main
reasons for high LDL levels, this defect being especially marked in
homozygotes.   Since LDL synthesis is increased to a greater extent
in homozygotes than in heterozygotes, this must also contribute to

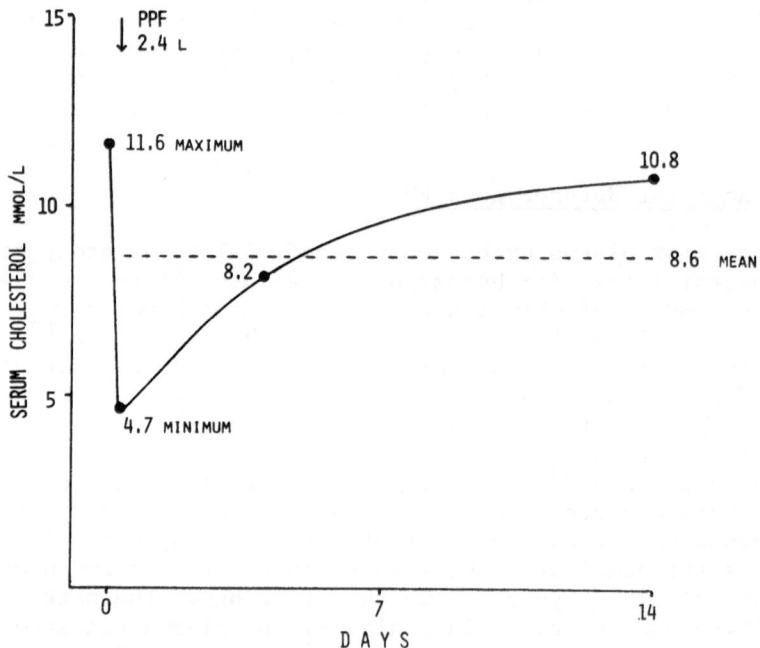

Fig. 1.   Changes in serum cholesterol after a single plasma
          exchange.   (From Thompson.[49])

the more rapid rebound in plasma cholesterol observed in homozygotes after plasma exchange.[58]

The changes in serum cholesterol which follow a single plasma exchange are illustrated in Fig. 1.   The immediate pre-exchange value is referred to as the maximum, the immediate post-exchange value as the minimum and the average during the period between exchanges as the mean.   The latter is calculated by integrating beneath the rebound curve and dividing the area by the duration between exchanges.   If all data were expressed in this manner this would enable results to be compared between different centres.

Various factors other than the state of the patient's LDL metabolism determine the cholesterol-lowering effect of plasma exchange, notably the ratio between plasma volume and the volume of PPF,[58] and the frequency with which the procedure is performed.   The rate of rebound after plasma exchange is also influenced by concomitant drug therapy, nicotinic acid being the most effective drug in homozygotes and cholestyramine in heterozygotes.[59]

The long-term effects of plasma exchange combined with drug therapy on serum cholesterol in an FH homozygote and a heterozygote are illustrated in Fig. 2.   Although mean serum cholesterol levels

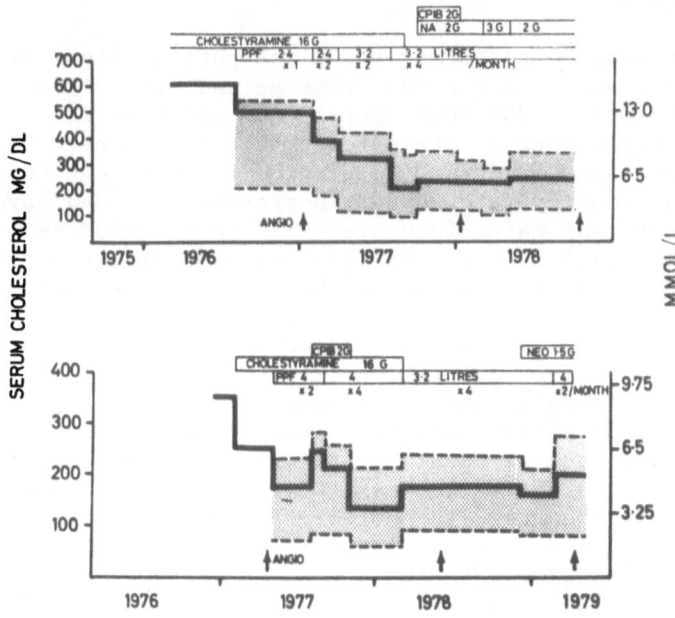

Fig. 2.   Long-term reduction of serum cholesterol level by combined drug therapy and plasma exchange in homozygous (top) and heterozygous (bottom) FH patients.   (From Thompson.[60])

within the normal range (<6.5 mmol/1) can be achieved by weekly
plasma exchange, in practice the procedure is usually performed every
2 weeks, for logistic reasons including the availability of PPF and
conservation of veins.

Future Developments

One drawback to plasma exchange is its non-specificity in that
both HDL and LDL get removed.   This can be overcome by selectively
removing LDL from plasma, as initially described by Lupien et al.[60]
who used heparin-agarose beads to remove VLDL and LDL from batches of
whole blood, which was then re-infused. A variation on this theme
has been described whereby plasma is collected and treated with
heparin-agarose and then kept and used as the exchange medium during
the subsequent plasma exchange.[62]   Recently, Stoffel and Demant[63]
described a method whereby LDL is removed continuously from plasma
during perfusion through a column containing anti-LDL antibodies
coupled to Sepharose.   This approach has considerable promise and
could eventually replace plasma exchange as the treatment of choice
for homozygous FH, especially where the expense or availability of
PPF are limiting factors.

PARTIAL ILEAL BYPASS

In 1964 Buchwald[64] performed the first partial ileal bypass for
hypercholesterolaemia.   Since that time he and his colleagues have
performed approximately 250 such operations, and have recently
reviewed their experience of its effects.[65]   They observed an
overall mean reduction in serum cholesterol of more than 40% in
patients with various types of hyperlipoproteinaemia and have shown
that this decrease was maintained over a 10 year period.[66]   The
procedure is relatively simple and involves bypassing the terminal
one-third or 200 cm of the ileum, whichever is the greater, by
sectioning the ileum and anastomosing its proximal cut-end to the
side of the caecum, the distal cut-end being closed.   This diverts
the intestinal contents away from the sites of absorption of both
vitamin B_{12} and bile salts and necessitates life-long injections of
vitamin B_{12}, 1000 μg every 3 months.   Post-operative diarrhoea can
be severe initially but is usually controllable with codeine phosphate
and gradually lessens during the next few months.   Exacerbations of
diarrhoea often respond well to cholestyramine.   Weight loss is
variable but averaged 5 kg at 3 months in Buchwald's series.[67]   No
serious side-effects have been reported; in particular the procedure
seems free from the hepatic dysfunction which accompanies the jejunal-
ileal bypass operation used to treat obesity.   However, occasionally
patients develop steatorrhoea and it is probably wise to monitor
appropriate indices of calcium metabolism and blood coagulation at
intervals.

Partial Ileal Bypass for Heterozygous FH

Buchwald et al.[68] described a 42% decrease in serum cholesterol after partial ileal bypass in a poorly-documented group of 24 patients, most of whom apparently had type II phenotypes. Some of these patients were said to have features compatible with FH, such as a positive family history and a poor response to dietary therapy. A more detailed study by Strisower et al.[69] demonstrated the LDL-lowering effects of partial ileal bypass in 2 FH heterozygotes whose hypercholesterolaemia had been resistant to lipid-lowering drugs. Subsequently, Miettinen and Lempinen[70] reported a mean decrease in serum cholesterol of 35% in 14 FH patients, together with an improvement in angina and regression of xanthomata. Subsequent studies by the same authors in 12 heterozygotes showed that partial ileal bypass lowered serum cholesterol to a two-fold greater extent than even 32 g daily of cholestyramine.[71] Russell et al.[72] reported a very similar reduction in serum cholesterol (34%) 1 year after partial ileal bypass in 10 heterozygotes, all of whom had failed to respond to or had become intolerant of drug therapy. Recently, we have studied 8 heterozygotes, in whom the serum cholesterol fell by 25% on 16 g daily of cholestyramine and by 38% 2 months after partial ileal bypass, as compared with the levels achieved on diet alone.[73] LDL cholesterol fell by 36% post-operatively but HDL cholesterol did not change.

These various results, summarised in Table 4, clearly show that partial ileal bypass provides a highly effective and permanent means of reducing serum cholesterol which is mainly achieved by a decrease in LDL levels. HDL cholesterol and plasma triglyceride concentrations remained unchanged.[72,73] Interestingly, the 2 patients

Table 4. Results of Partial Ileal Bypass in Patients with Heterozygous Familial Hypercholesterolaemia

Source	No. of Patients	Time post-op	Serum Cholesterol mmol/l		
			pre	post	Δ
Buchwald et al.[65,66,68]	24[a]	1 year	9.7	5.8	-40%
Miettinen & Lempinen[71]	12	3 weeks	12.7	8.3	-35%
Miettinen[81]	27[b]	9 years	15.0	9.3	-38%
Russell et al.[72]	10	4 months	11.6	7.5	-35%
" " "		1 year		7.6	-34%
Spengel et al.[73]	8	2 months	12.2	7.6	-38%

[a]Type II, presumed FH
[b]Data probably include 2 homozygotes

studied by Strisower et al.[69] showed a post-operative rise in HDL,
with an increase in the ratio of $HDL_2:HDL_3$.   This effect and the
marked increase in the ratio of HDL:LDL cholesterol which occurs
after partial ileal bypass should theoretically result in a substantial reduction in the risk of developing CHD.[65]   Whether or not this
will occur is the subject of a current trial, albeit in patients with
existing CHD.[74]

        Information on the effects of partial ileal bypass on the
arterial wall is scanty but 2 radiographic surveys have been reported.
In the first, 22 patients underwent coronary angiography before and
$3\frac{1}{2}$ years after the operation;   lesions progressed in 23%, regressed
in 14% and did not change or were unclassifiable in the remainder.[75]
The second series involved 7 patients studied before and 2 years after
the operation, 5 of whom showed angiographic progression over this
period despite a 48% reduction in serum cholesterol.[76]   Thus although
partial ileal bypass is undoubtedly a potent means of controlling
hypercholesterolaemia, evidence that this exerts a major impact on
established CHD is, at best, equivocal.

Partial Ileal Bypass for Homozygous FH

        In contrast to heterozygotes partial ileal bypass has proved
disappointing in homozygotes.   In 3 instances serum cholesterol
levels actually rose[77,78] whereas in 2 others decreases of only 16%[79]
and 23%[71] were observed.   The best results were reported in 2 children in Honolulu, whose serum cholesterol levels decreased by 38%.[80]
Although it would seem inadvisable to use partial ileal bypass as the
sole means of treating homozygotes, the combination of partial ileal
bypass followed by portacaval shunt or vice versa has been shown to
decrease the serum cholesterol by around 50%.[81]   Possibly this
synergistic effect is due to suppression by the portacaval shunt of
the compensatory increase in hepatic cholesterol synthesis which
accompanies partial ileal bypass, as discussed below.

Mechanism of Hypocholesterolaemic Effect of Partial Ileal Bypass

        The rationale for partial ileal bypass was originally based on
the mistaken hypothesis that cholesterol is absorbed preferentially
in the ileum whereas it is actually absorbed mainly in the jejunum,
as discussed elsewhere.[82]   It is probable that the reduction in
cholesterol absorption which has been reported[83] is due partly to
rapid intestinal transit and partly to the impaired bile acid absorption which is the primary result of bypassing the ileum.   Bile acid
excretion is increased four-fold, with[84] or without[71] an accompanying
increase in neutral sterol excretion.   The increased excretion of
bile acids leads to an increased rate of turnover of cholesterol to
bile acids and a compensatory increase in cholesterol synthesis,[85]

the net effect in most patients being a decrease in the amount of cholesterol present in plasma and elsewhere in the body.[84]

Studies of LDL turnover in heterozygotes show that LDL catabolism is stimulated to a greater extent by partial ileal bypass than by cholestyramine,[83] possibly because the former increases bile acid excretion to a greater extent.[71] Interestingly the increase in LDL catabolism after both procedures is almost entirely due to an increase in receptor-mediated LDL catabolism.[83,86] This suggests that increases in bile acid synthesis lead to an increased demand for cholesterol by the liver which is met to some extent by an increased rate of LDL uptake via hepatic LDL receptors. If so, lack of these putative receptors in homozygotes might explain the failure of partial ileal bypass to influence their hypercholesterolaemia.

CONCLUSIONS

Repeated plasma exchange with PPF at 2-weekly intervals is currently the most effective method of controlling hypercholesterol-aemia in homozygous FH and has proved to be safe over periods exceeding 5 years. The post-exchange rise in serum cholesterol can be slowed by concomitant therapy with nicotinic acid or by a portacaval shunt. The latter is usually less efficient than plasma exchange in controlling hypercholesterolaemia in homozygotes but its effects can be augmented by combining it with a partial ileal bypass. Partial ileal bypass is the treatment of choice for patients with hetero-zygous FH in whom drug therapy has proved difficult or ineffective, although plasma exchange provides a non-invasive alternative. Whether these measures will prevent or reverse atherosclerosis in FH remains to be shown but there is some evidence that they arrest the progression of the disease.

Efforts should be made in every instance in which radical therapy is employed to monitor its effects. Apart from measuring serum cholesterol, photographic records should be made of changes in size of xanthomata and changes in cardiac diameter should be assessed by X-ray and ECG. The latter also provides an index of myocardial ischaemia. Echocardiography provides a non-invasive means of assessing narrowing of the aortic root[15] but at the present time the most accurate assessment of coronary and aortic involvement is provided by serial angiographic studies, including measurement of the gradient across the aortic valve. These various investigations provide objective evidence as to whether hypercholesterolaemia and atherosclerosis are being controlled effectively, and enable the need for additional measures, such as cardiac surgery, to be assessed.

REFERENCES

1. W. C. Roberts, The status of the coronary arteries in fatal
    ischemic heart disease, Cardiovasc. Clinics 7:1 (1975).
2. M. Feinleib, W. B. Kannel, C. G. Tedeschi, T. K. Landau, and
    R. J. Garrison, The relation of antemortem characteristics
    to cardiovascular findings at necropsy, Atherosclerosis
    34:145 (1979).
3. G. Rose, Detection of high coronary risk, Postgrad. Med. J.
    52:452 (1976).
4. W. L. Proudfit, E. K. Shirey, and F. M. Sones, Selective cine
    coronary arteriography. Correlation with clinical findings
    in 1000 patients, Circulation 33:901 (1966).
5. R. G. Murray, A. Tweddel, J. L. H. C. Third, I. Hutton, W. S.
    Hillis, A. R. Lorimer, and T. D. V. Lawrie, Relation between
    extent of coronary artery disease and severity of hyperlipo-
    proteinaemia, Brit. Heart J. 37:1205 (1975).
6. D. C. Banks, E. B. Raftery, and S. Oram, Clinical significance
    of the coronary arteriogram, Brit. Heart J. 33:863 (1971).
7. A. M. Gotto, G. A. Gorry, J. R. Thompson, J. S. Cole, R. Trost,
    D. Yeshuron, and M. E. Debakey, Relationship between plasma
    lipid concentrations and coronary artery disease in 496
    patients, Circulation 56:875 (1977).
8. M. H. Frick, D. Dahlen, K. Berg, M. Valle, and P. Hekali, Serum
    lipids in angiographically assessed coronary atherosclerosis,
    Chest 73:62 (1978).
9. P. J. Jenkins, R. W. Harper, and P. J. Nestel, Severity of
    coronary atherosclerosis related to lipoprotein concentration,
    Brit. Med. J. 2:388 (1978).
10. V. Fuster, R. L. Frye, D. C. Connolly, M. A. Danielson, L. R.
    Elveback, and L. T. Kurland, Arteriographic patterns early in
    the onset of the coronary syndromes, Brit. Heart J. 37:1250
    (1975).
11. R. A. Heinle, R. I. Levy, D. S. Frederickson, and R. Gorlin,
    Lipid and carbohydrate abnormalities in patients with angio-
    graphically documented coronary artery disease, Amer. J.
    Cardiol. 24:178 (1969).
12. C. E. Bemis, R. Gorlin, H. G. Kemp, and M. V. Herman,
    Progression of coronary artery disease, Circulation 47:455
    (1973).
13. D. T. Nash, G. Gensini, H. Simon, T. Arno, and S. D. Nash, The
    Erysicthon Syndrome. Progression of coronary atherosclerosis
    and dietary hyperlipidemia, Circulation 56:363 (1977).
14. G. R. Thompson, Familial hypercholesterolaemia, in:"The Lipo-
    protein Molecule," H. Peeters, ed., Plenum Press, New York
    (1978).
15. J. M. Allen, G. R. Thompson, N. B. Myant, R. Steiner, and C.M.
    Oakley, Cardiovascular complications of homozygous familial
    hypercholesterolaemia, Brit. Heart J. 44:361 (1980).

16. J. Slack, Risk of ischaemic heart disease in familial hyperlipo-proteinaemic states, Lancet 2:1380 (1969).

17. A. Bloch, R. E. Dinsmore, and R. S. Lees, Coronary arteriographic findings in type-II and type-IV hyperlipoproteinaemia, Lancet 1:928 (1976).

18. D. D. Sugrue, G. R. Thompson, C. M. Oakley, I. M. Trayner, and R. E. Steiner, Contrasting patterns of coronary atherosclero-sis in normocholesterolaemic smokers and patients with famil-ial hypercholesterolaemia, Brit. Med. J. in press (1981).

19. J. V. Talano, P. J. Scanlon, W. R. Meadows, M. Kahn, R. Pifarre, and R. M. Gunnar, Influence of surgery on survival in 145 patients with left main coronary artery disease, Circulation 52(Suppl.1):105 (1975).

20. K. Detre, M. L. Murphy, and H. Hultgren, Effect of coronary by-pass surgery on longevity in high and low risk patients, Lancet 2:1243 (1977).

21. J. Crittin, D. D. Waters, P. Theroux, and H. F. Mizgala, Left main coronary artery stenosis in young patients, Chest 76:508 (1979).

22. J. J. Barboriak, K. Pintar, and M.E. Korns, Atherosclerosis in aortocoronary vein grafts, Lancet 2:621 (1974).

23. J. J. Barboriak, G. E. Batayias, K. Pintar, and M. E. Korns, Pathological changes in surgically removed aortocoronary vein grafts, Ann. Thor. Surg. 21:524 (1976).

24. J. T. Lie, G. M. Lawrie, and G. C. Morris, Aortocoronary bypass saphenous vein graft atherosclerosis. Anatomic study of 99 vein grafts from normal and hyperlipoproteinemic patients up to 75 months post-operatively, Amer. J. Cardiol. 40:906 (1977).

25. M. L. Armstrong, E. D. Warner, and W. E. Connor, Regression of coronary atheromatosis in Rhesus monkeys, Circulation Res. 27:59 (1970).

26. M. L. Armstrong, and M. B. Megan, Lipid depletion in athero-matous coronary arteries in Rhesus monkeys after regression diets, Circulation Res. 30:675 (1972).

27. A. Daoud, J. Jarmolych, J. M. Augustyn, K. E. Fritz, J. K. Singh, and K. T. Lee, Regression of advanced atherosclerosis in swine, Arch. Pathol. Lab. Med. 100:372 (1976).

28. R. G. Depalma, S. Koletsky, E. M. Bellon, and W. Insull, Failure of regression of atherosclerosis in dogs with moderate cholesterolemia, Atherosclerosis 27:297 (1977).

29. P. T. Kuo, K. Hayase, J. B. Kostis, and A. E. Moreyra, Use of combined diet and colestipol in long-term (7-7½ years) treat-ment of patients with type II hyperlipoproteinemia, Circulation 59:199 (1979).

30. T. E. Starzl, H. P. Chase, C. W. Putnam, and K. A. Porter, Portacaval shunt in hyperlipoproteinaemia, Lancet 2:940 (1973).

31. T. E. Starzl, H. P. Chase, C. W. Putnam, and J. J. Nora, Follow-up of patient with portacaval shunt for the treatment of hyperlipidaemia, Lancet 2:714 (1974).

32. T. E. Starzl, H. P. Chase, C. W. Putnam, J. J. Nora, R. H. Fennell, and K. A. Porter, Portacaval shunt in hyperlipid-aemia, Lancet 2:1263 (1974).

33. T. E. Starzl, L. Koep, and R. Weil, Portacaval shunt for type II hyperlipidemia, in"Atherosclerosis V," A. M. Gotto, L. C. Smith, and B. Allen, ed., Springer-Verlag, New York (1980).

34. E. A. Stein, J. Pettifor, C. Mieny, K. W. Heimann, I. Spitz, I. Bersohn, I. Saaron, and M. Dinner, Portacaval shunt in four patients with homozygous hypercholesterolaemia, Lancet 1:832 (1975).

35. E. A. Stein, and C. J. Glueck, Homozygous hypercholesterolaemia: treatment by portacaval shunt, in:"Atherosclerosis V," A. M. Gotto, L. C. Smith, and B. Allen, ed., Springer-Verlag, New York (1980).

36. O. Faergeman, J. Gormsen, and H. Meinertz, Anti-platelet drugs and portacaval anastomosis for homozygous hypercholesterol-aemia, Lancet 2:1416 (1976).

37. J. T. Coyle, M. Z. Schwartz, A. T. Marubbio, R. L. Varco, and H. Buchwald, The effect of portacaval shunt on plasma lipids and tissue cholesterol synthesis in the dog, Surgery 80:54 (1976).

38. T. E. Starzl, K. Watanabe, K. A. Porter, and C. W. Putnam, Effects of insulin, glucagon and insulin/glucagon infusions on liver morphology and cell division after complete porta-caval shunt in dogs, Lancet 1:821 (1976).

39. H. P. Chase, and T. Morris, Cholesterol metabolism following portacaval shunt in the pig, Atherosclerosis 24:141 (1976).

40. T. E. Carew, R. P. Saik, K. H. Johansen, C. A. Dennis, and D. Steinberg, Low density and high density lipoprotein turnover following portacaval shunting in swine, J. Lipid Res. 17:441 (1976).

41. A. C. Nestruck, S. Lussier-Cacan, M. Bergseth, M. Bidallier, J. Davignon, and Y. L. Marcel, The effect of portacaval shunt on plasma lipids and lipoproteins in swine, Biochim. Biophys. Acta 488:43 (1977).

42. D. W. Bilheimer, J. L. Goldstein, S. M. Grundy, and M. S. Brown, Reduction in cholesterol and low density lipoprotein synthesis after portacaval shunt surgery in patient with homozygous familial hypercholesterolemia, J. Clin. Invest. 56:1420 (1975).

43. A. K. Soutar, N. B. Myant, and G. R. Thompson, Simultaneous measurement of apolipoprotein B turnover in very-low- and low-density lipoproteins in familial hypercholesterolaemia, Atherosclerosis 28:247 (1977).

44. J.-L. DeGennes, R. Touraine, B. Maunand, J. Truffert, and P. Laudat, Formes homozygotes cutaneo-tendineuses de xanthomatose hypercholestérolémique dans une observation familiale exem-

plaire. Essai de plasmaphérèse à titre de traitment héroique. Bull. Mem. Soc. Hôp. Paris 118:1377 (1967).

45. L. A. Turnberg, M. P. Mahoney, M. H. Gleeson, C. B. Freeman, and A. H. Gowenlock, Plasmaphoresis and plasma exchange in the treatment of hyperlipaemia and xanthomatous neuropathy in patients with primary biliary cirrhosis, Gut 13:976 (1972).

46. G. R. Thompson, R. Lowenthal, and N. B. Myant, Plasma exchange in the management of homozygous familial hypercholesterol-aemia, Lancet 1:1208 (1975).

47. G. R. Thompson, N. B. Myant, D. Kilpatrick, C. M. Oakley, M. J. Raphael, and R. E. Steiner, Assessment of long-term plasma exchange for familial hypercholesterolaemia, Brit. Heart J. 43:680 (1980).

48. G. Thompson, N. Myant, C. Oakley, R. Steiner, and R. Sapsford, Combined medico-surgical strategy for severe familial hyper-cholesterolaemia, in:"Atherosclerosis V," A. M. Gotto, L. C. Smith, and B. Allen, ed., Springer-Verlag, New York (1980).

49. G. R. Thompson, Plasma exchange for hypercholesterolaemia, Lancet 1:1246 (1981).

50. G. M. B. Berger, J. L. Miller, F. Bonnici, H. S. Joffe, and D. W. Dubovsky, Continuous flow plasma exchange in the treat-ment of homozygous familial hypercholesterolemia, Amer. J. Med. 65:243 (1978).

51. L. A. Simons, J. C. Gibson, J. P. Isbister, and J. C. Biggs, The effects of plasma exchange on cholesterol metabolism, Atherosclerosis 31:195 (1978).

52. M. E. E. King, J. L. Breslow, and R. S. Lees, Plasma-exchange therapy of homozygous familial hypercholesterolemia, New Engl. J. Med. 301:1457 (1980).

53. J. L. Witzum, J. C. Williams, R. Ostlund, L. Sherman, G. Siccard, and G. Schonfeld, Successful plasmapheresis in a 4 year old child with homozygous familial hypercholesterolemia, J. Pediat. 97:615 (1980).

54. G. M. B. Berger, F. Bonnici, H. S. Joffe, and D. W. Dubovsky, Plasma exchange in the treatment of familial hypercholesterol-emia, in:"Atherosclerosis V," A. M. Gotto, L. C. Smith, and B. Allen, ed., Springer-Verlag, New York (1980).

55. E. A. Stein, C. J. Glueck, A. Wesselman, E. R. Owens, S. Nichols, and P. Vink, Repetitive intermittnet flow plasma exchange in patients with severe hypercholesterolemia, Atherosclerosis 38:149 (1981).

56. L. A. Simons, J. J. Morgan, J.C. Gibson, J. P. Isbister, and J. C. Biggs, Regression of atherosclerosis, Atherosclerosis 35:345 (1980).

57. G. R. Thompson, and N. B. Myant, Regression of atherosclerosis, Atherosclerosis 35:347 (1980).

58. G. R. Thompson, Plasma exchange for hypercholesterolaemia: a therapeutic mode and investigative tool, Plasma Ther. 1:5 (1980).

59. G. R. Thompson, Long-term plasma exchange in severe familial hypercholesterolaemia, in:"Proceedings of the Workshop on

Therapeutic Plasma and Cytapheresis," in press (198-).

60. G. R. Thompson, Plasma exchange in hyperlipidemia, in: "Therapeutic Plasma Exchange," H. Gurland, V. Heinze, and H. A. Lee, ed., Springer-Verlag, Berlin Heidelberg (1981).

61. P-J. Lupien, S. Moorjani, and J. Awad, A new approach to the management of familial hypercholesterolaemia: removal of plasma cholesterol based on the principle of affinity chromatography, Lancet 1:1261 (1976).

62. B. Graisely, M. Cloarec, S. Salmon, J. Polonovski, C. Polonovski, J. M. Delacotte, J. Gardent, J. Cavalier, D. Vergoz, and C. Salmon, Extracorporeal plasma therapy for homozygous familial hypercholesterolaemia, Lancet 2:1147 (1980).

63. W. Stoffel, and T. Demant, Selective removal of apolipoprotein B-containing serum lipoproteins from blood plasma, Proc. Nat. Acad. Sci. USA 78:611 (1981).

64. H. Buchwald, Lowering of cholesterol absorption and blood levels by ileal exclusion, Circulation 29:713 (1964).

65. H. Buchwald, R. B. Moore, and R. L. Varco, Partial ileal bypass: a test of the lipid-atherosclerosis hypothesis, in:"Athero-sclerosis V," A. M. Gotto, L. C. Smith, and B. Allen, ed., Springer-Verlag, New York (1980).

66. H. Buchwald, R. B. Moore, and R. L. Varco, Ten years clinical experience with partial ileal bypass in management of the hyperlipidaemias, Ann. Surg. 180:384 (1974).

67. R. B. Moore, H. Buchwald, R. L. Varco, et al., The effect of partial ileal bypass on plasma lipoproteins, Circulation 62:469 (1980).

68. H. Buchwald, R. B. Moore, G. B. Lee, I. D. Frantz, and R. L. Varco, Treatment of hypercholesterolemia.Combined dietary, surgical, and bile-salt binding resin therapy, Arch. Surg. 97:275 (1968).

69. E. H. Strisower, R. M. Kradjian, A. V. Nichols, E. Coggiola, and J. Tsai, Effect of ileal bypass on serum lipoproteins in essential hypercholesterolemia, J. Atheroscl. Res. 8:525 (1968).

70. T. A. Miettinen, and M. Lempinen, Ileal bypass operation in familial hypercholesterolemia, Scand. J. Clin. Lab. Invest. Suppl. 113:55 (1970).

71. T. A. Miettinen, and M. Lempinen, Cholestyramine and ileal by-pass in the treatment of familial hypercholesterolaemia, Eur. J. Clin. Invest. 7:509 (1977).

72. D. Russell, V. Fritz, C. Mieny, D. Mendelsohn, B. I. Joffe, and H. C. Seftel, Treatment of familial hypercholesterolaemia by partial ileal bypass, S. A. Med. J. 55:237 (1979).

73. F. A. Spengel, A. Jadhav, R. G. M. Duffield, C. B. Wood, and G. R. Thompson, Cholesterol reduction in familial hyper-cholesterolaemia: superiority of partial ileal bypass over cholestyramine, Lancet in press (1981).

74. R. B. Moore, J. M. Long, J. P. Matts, K. Amplatz, R. L. Varco, H. Buchwald, and The Posch Group, Plasma lipoproteins and

coronary arteriography in subjects in the program on the surgical control of the hyperlipidemias. Preliminary report, Atherosclerosis 32:101 (1979).

75. L. Knight, R. Scheibel, K. Amplatz, R. L. Varco, and H. Buchwald, Radiographic appraisal of the Minnesota partial ileal bypass study, Surg. Forum 23:141 (1972).

76. R. R. Henderson, and G. G. Rowe, The progression of coronary atherosclerotic disease as assessed by cine-coronary angiography, Amer. Heart J. 86:165 (1973).

77. J. A. Davis, I. D. A. Johnston, C. D. Moutafis, and N. B. Myant, Ileal bypass in hypercholesterolaemia, Lancet 2:971 (1966).

78. S. M. Grundy, E. H. Ahrens, and G. Salen, Interruption of the enterohepatic circulation of bile acids in man: comparative effects of cholestyramine and ileal exclusion on cholesterol metabolism, J. Lab. Clin. Med. 78:94 (1971).

79. H. Buchwald, R. B. Moore, I. D. Frantz, and R. L. Varco, Cholesterol reduction by partial ileal bypass in a paediatric population, Surgery 68:1101 (1970).

80. J. F. Balfour, and R. Kim, Homozygous type II hyperlipoprotein-emia treatment. Partial ileal bypass in two children, J. Amer. Med. Ass. 227:1145 (1974).

81. T. A. Miettinen, Comparison of cholestyramine, ileal by-pass and portocaval shunt in the treatment of familial hypercholest-erolemia, in:"Atherosclerosis V," A. M. Gotto, L. C. Smith, and B. Allen, ed., Springer-Verlag, New York (1980).

82. G. R. Thompson, and A. M. Gotto, Ileal bypass in the treatment of hyperlipoproteinaemia, Lancet 2:35 (1973).

83. H. Buchwald, and R. L. Varco, Partial ileal bypass for hyper-cholesterolemia and atherosclerosis, Surg. Gynaecol. Obstet. 124:1231 (1967).

84. R. B. Moore, I. D. Frantz, and H. Buchwald, Changes in chole-sterol pool size, turnover rate, and fecal bile acid and sterol excretion after partial ileal bypass in hypercholest-eremic patients, Surgery 65:98 (1969).

85. C. D. Moutafis, N. B. Myant, and S. Tabaqchali, The metabolism of cholesterol after resection or by-pass of the lower small intestine, Clin. Sci. 35:537 (1968).

86. J. Shepherd, C. J. Packard, S. Bicker, T. D. V. Lawrie, and H. G. Morgan, Cholestyramine promotes receptor-mediated low-density-lipoprotein catabolism, New Engl. J. Med. 302:1219 (1980).

DRUG CONTROL OF HYPERCHOLESTEREMIA AND PLATELET FUNCTION

E. Tremoli, P. Maderna, S. Colli and R. Paoletti

Institute of Pharmacology and Pharmacognosy
University of Milan, Milan
Italy

Atherosclerosis is a major disease which involves the response of different cell systems to vascular injury (1, 2). Normal endothelium possesses thromboresistant capacities, due to the synthesis of several factors, including heparin-like proteoglycans, a plasminogen activator and prostacyclin (3, 4, 5).

Endothelial injury results in the alteration of the endothelial cell monolayer with a concomitant smooth muscle cell proliferation (6, 7). The protein synthesis and deposition, such as collagen, and lipid accumulation within proliferating smooth muscle cells and macrophages initiate and contribute to the development of the atherosclerotic lesions (8, 9). Circulating platelets adhere to the damaged endothelium (10), and trigger a sequence of reactions leading to the accumulation of aggregated platelets on the injured areas (11, 12).

Platelets then produce mitogenic factors inducing smooth muscle cell proliferation (13, 14). Although the role of the platelet derived growth factor in plasma is not yet established, it may be hypothesized that the platelet interaction and the consequent release reaction at the site of vascular injury can establish favourable conditions for the smooth muscle cell proliferation and for the organization of the atherosclerotic plaque (15). Therefore the role of platelet function in the development of atherosclerosis, particularly under conditions associated with the presence of the major risk factors for the disease (smoking, high blood pressure, dislipidemias) appears of specific interest.

PLATELET FUNCTION IN HYPERCHOLESTEREMIA

Since Carvalho et al (16) have shown that platelets from type
IIa hypercholesterolemic patients are more sensitive to the in
vitro aggregation induced by several aggregating agents, as
compared with those of normal subjects, the interest on the
relationship between abnormal plasma lipid composition and platelet function and biochemistry has been raised (17, 18).

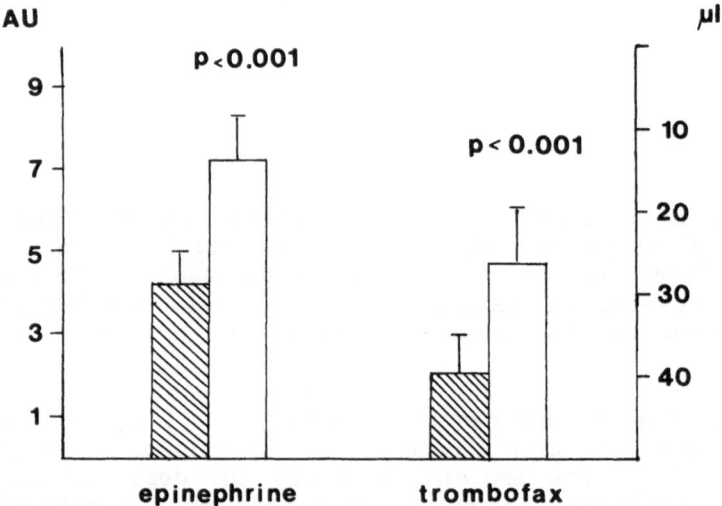

Fig. 1. Threshold platelet aggregatory concentrations of epi-
       nephrine and thrombofax in type IIa hypercholesterolemic
       patients. AU (aggregation units) define serial 1/2
       dilutions of a stock solution (1 mg/ml for epinephrine).
       1 µl of the final solution was added to 0.25 ml of
       PRP.

In our laboratory it has been demonstrated in a large group
of type IIa hypercholesterolemic subjects that not only the
platelet response to aggregating agents (fig. 1 and 2) is altered
but also the synthesis of arachidonic acid metabolites by platelets, such as malondialhehyde (a mesure of lipid peroxidation) and
thromboxane B_2 is increased (table 1) (19, 20, 21).

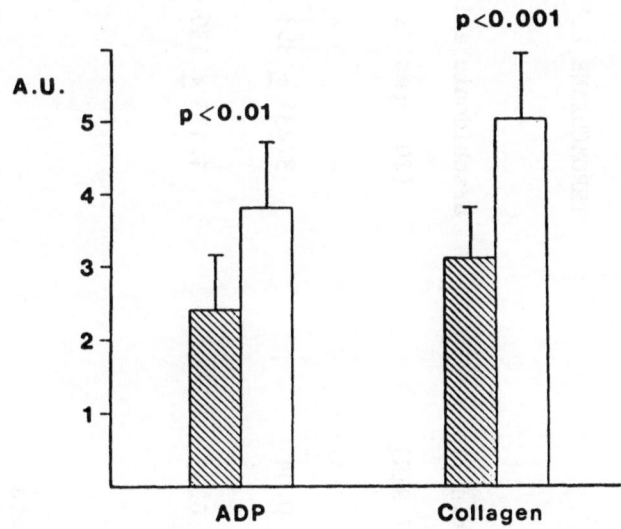

Fig. 2. Threshold aggregatory concentrations of ADP and collagen.
AU defined in Fig. 1. Stock solution for ADP : 1mM, for
collagen : 1 mg/ml.

The platelet hypersentivity appears to be related to the
modification of the cell membrane composition, possible due
to the altered cholesterol and phospholipid content of the
cells (21).

The incubation of normal platelets with cholesterol rich
liposomes results, in fact, in increased amounts of released
arachidonic acid by thrombin stimulated platelets and in a
significantly higher thromboxane B_2 synthesis, comparing with
platelets incubated with cholesterol poor liposomes (22).

In addition the incubation of platelets from type IIa patients with plasma from normal subjects, does not reestablish the
normal platelet response to aggregating agents (21). These
findings have been confirmed also in experimental animals (26).
Platelets from rabbits fed one month with a high cholesterol diet

Table 1. Malondialdehyde and Thromboxane B_2 formation by platelets form type IIa and controls.

	MALONDIALDEHYDE*		THROMBOXANE B_2**
	collagen	thrombin	arachidonic acid
	(30 μg/ml)	(25 U/ml NIH)	(20 μmol/l)
TYPE IIa (25)	0.91 ± 0.05°	0.82 ± 0.04°	3.231 ± 353°
CONTROLS (31)	0.58 ± 0.04	0.52 ± 0.03	1.175 ± 130

* = nmoles/3x10^8 platelets; ** = ng/10^9 washed platelets

°p < 0.001

Values represent the mean ± S.E.M.

(2%), show increased sensitivity to the in vitro aggregation induced by collagen and arachidonic acid (23). Plasma exchange experiments indicate that the normal plasma lipid environment, at least in relatively short time experiments, does not correct platelet hypersensitivity (23). The phospholipid/cholesterol ratio, however, in the same group of rabbits, is signficantly lowered, whereas data from hypercholesterolemic platelets indicate that both phospholipid and cholesterol content are increased, with a resulting unaltered ratio (24).

The difference between the human and the animal model may be due to the acute induction of hypercholesteremia in rabbits, or to the relatively short dietary period, resulting in lipid abnormalities different from those which occur in human type IIa hypercholesteremia (25).

Other investigators have shown that also beta-thromboglobulin levels in plasma from type IIa patients are increased (26). Beta-thromboglobulin is considered a predictable index of in vivo platelet activation and release reaction (27, 28). Therefore treatments aimed to the reduction of platelet aggregation and the release reaction appear to be indicated in these patients.

ANTIAGGREGATING THERAPY IN TYPE IIA HYPERCHOLESTEREMIC SUBJECTS

The effect of Indobufen, a new inhibitor of platelet aggregation (29), has been evaluated in a group of type IIa hypercholesteremic patients and compared with the effect on normocholesteremic subjects matched for sex and age, in order to verify if the activity of the drug was similar in the two groups. Indobufen (200 mg twice a day) or placebo were administered according to a cross over design for three days with four days interval. Blood samples were taken before, 3 hours after the administration and 12 from the last administration.

Indobufen treatment completely suppressed the epinephrine second wave and arachidonic acid sodium salt (AASS) induced aggregation, when the tests were performed using threshold concentrations of both aggregating agents (table 2). In addition malondialdehyde production by platelets incubated with increasing concentrations of thrombin was completely inhibited both in patients as in controls, up to twelve hours from the last administration of the drug with all thrombin concentrations (table 3). The concentrations of either epinephrine or arachidonic acid reversing the inhibitory effect exerted by the drug were also determined after the Indobufen adminstration to evaluate the potency of the drug. These concentrations of aggregating agents are defined as the overcoming concentrations (OC).

After Indobufen treatment the OCs for arachidonic acid

Table 2. Platelet responses (normal and abnormal) before and during Indobufen treatment.

	Controls (n=8)			Patients (n=8)		
	Number of tests	Normal tracings	Abnormal tracings	Number of tests	Normal tracings	Abnormal tracings
Before and during placebo	64	64	0	64	64	0
During drug therapy	64	0	64	64	0	64

Platelet responses from controls and type IIa patients to the aggregation induced by thres-hold concentrations of epinephrine and AASS are considered.

E. Tremoli et al., Pharmacol. Res. Comm. 13:847 (1981).

Table 3. Malondialdehyde (nM/3.10^8 platelets) production by platelets from controls and type IIa patients before and during Indobufen and/or placebo treatment. Values during placebo treatment x ± SEM of four separate determinations for each subject according to protocol; +p < 0.001, ++p < 0.05 vs corresponding controls.

	Thrombin	Before treatment	Placebo	Indobufen treatment 1st day 3h	3rd day 3h	4th day 12h
Controls	2.5	0.10 ± 0.03	0.17 ± 0.02	n.d.°	n.d.°	n.d.°
	5	0.33 ± 0.04	0.28 ± 0.02	"	"	"
	7.5	0.39 ± 0.07	0.32 ± 0.02	"	"	"
	10	0.40 ± 0.07	0.38 ± 0.02	"	"	"
	15	0.55 ± 0.06	0.45 ± 0.03	"	"	"
	20	0.56 ± 0.06	0.51 ± 0.01	"	"	"
	25	0.59 ± 0.05	0.57 ± 0.02	"	"	"
Patients	2.5	0.22 ± 0.04	0.21 ± 0.02	"	"	"
	5	0.44 ± 0.05	0.41 ± 0.01++	"	"	"
	7.5	0.48 ± 0.05	0.50 ± 0.02++	"	"	"
	10	0.52 ± 0.04	0.57 ± 0.03++	"	"	"
	15	0.64 ± 0.07+	0.66 ± 0.02++	"	"	"
	20	0.67 ± 0.07+	0.67 ± 0.02++	"	"	"
	25	0.68 ± 0.07+	0.74 ± 0.02++	"	"	"

° n.d. = not detectable

E. Tremoli et al., Pharmacol. Res. Comm. 13:847 (1981)

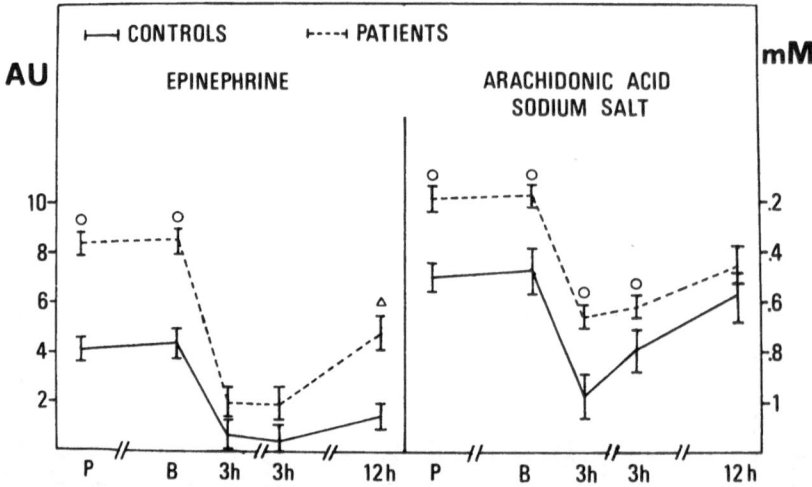

Fig. 3. OCs for epinephrine and AA sodium salt in patients and
controls after Indobufen therapy (see text).
° p < 0.001   Δ p < 0.05
P = placebo
B = baseline

were significantly lower in the patient group after three and
twelve hours from the administration of the drug (fig. 3).

    The same results were obtained when epinephrine was used to
stimulate platelets. Significantly lower epinephrine concentrations were necessary to overcome the inhibitory effect of the
drug.   The most impressive finding was that after Indobufen
therapy, platelets from type IIa patients, challenged with very
high epinephrine concentrations (0.5 - 8 μg/ml PRP) showed a
double wave of aggregation (fig. 4), indicating the complete
aggregation independent from the arachidonic acid pathway.   No
malondialdehyde production in fact by platelets stimulated with
increasing thrombin concentrations could be detected under the
same experimental conditions. Rao et al. have shown that exposure

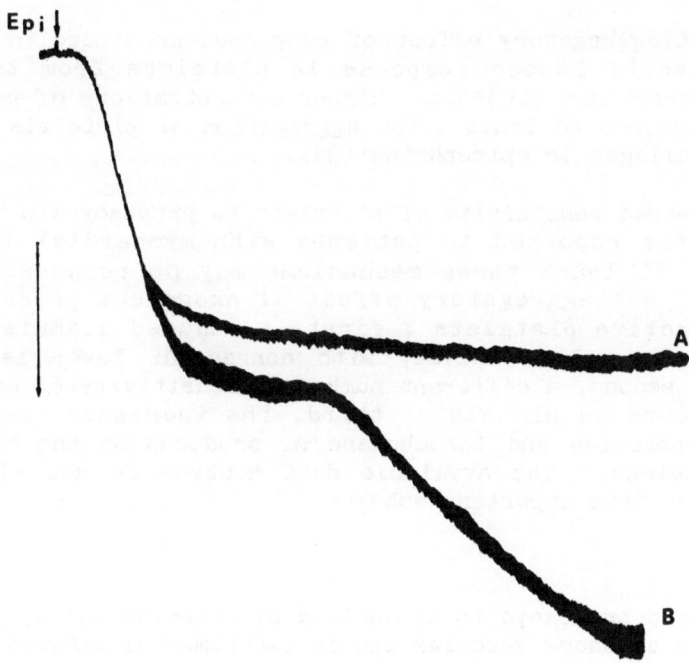

Fig. 4. Aggregatory response to 2 μ g/ml epinephrine in control
(A) and type IIa patient (B) after Indobufen treatment (12
hours).

of aspirin treated platelets to epinephrine results in a second
aggregatory wave, following ADP or thrombin, in the absence of
prostaglandin synthesis and/or release reaction (30). Another
tempting explanation may consider the possibility of an increased
percentage of newly formed cells, with different biochemical and
functional reactivity.

These differences may not be as important in an in vivo
situation, considering the relatively high amounts of inducer
employed to stimulate in vitro platelets. It is however of
interest to note that the potency of antiaggregating agents

needs to be checked also under pathological conditions to define the most suitable treatment schedule.

PROSTACYCLIN AND HYPERCHOLESTEREMIA

The antiaggregatory effect of exogenous prostacyclin elicits a significantly lesser response in platelets from type IIa hypercholesterolemic subjects. Higher concentrations of prostacyclin are required to inhibit the aggregation of platelets induced either by collagen or epinephrine (31).

A decreased sensitivity of platelets to prostacyclin has also been recently reported in patients with myocardial ischemia (32, 33). At least three mechanisms may be responsible for the reduced antiaggregatory effect of exogenous prostacyclin in hyperreactive platelets : first, a reduced stimulation of the adenylate cyclase enzyme, with consequent lower levels of cyclic AMP; second, a different number or sensitivity of prostacyclin receptors on platelets; third, the increased amounts of cyclic endoperoxide and thromboxane A_2 produced by the hypersensitive platelets. The available data however do not allow any conclusion on this important subject.

CONCLUSIONS

A reduced prostacyclin production by arterial walls, particularly by the coronary vascular bed in experimental atherosclerosis has been observed (34). In addition no prostacyclin has been measured in atherosclerotic plaques (35). Thus it could be conceivable to hypothesize that during the atherosclerotic process the platelet and vascular cyclooxygenase can be differently affected.

Gryglewski et al. (36) suggest that the presence of lipid peroxides in atherosclerotic aortas (37, 38) results in a reduced or absent prostacyclin production, due to the selective inhibition by lipid peroxides on the prostacyclin synthetase, with no effect on the platelet cyclooxygenase. Thus the natural antioxidants, such as alpha-tocopherol would exert beneficial effects reducing or eliminating the lipid peroxidation (39).

In addition increased lipid peroxidation has been reported in low density lipoprotein fractions from patients with coronary heart disease and hyperlipidemia, compared to those of normal subjects (40). If this peroxidation is present in vivo in blood or it is an in vitro artefact, due to the lipoprotein isolation, remains to be established. No informations are yet available on the prostacyclin formation in patients with type IIa hypercholesteremia, also because of the well known inconsistency of the blood measurement of the prostacyclin metabolites. Nordoy et al. have reported that increasing LDL concentrations inhibit

PGI$_2$ production by human cultured endothelial cells (41), thus contributing to the hypothesis of a selective inhibitory effect in dislipidemias on vascular protocyclin. Other studies, however, will provide more informations on this important subject.

REFERENCES

1. R. Ross, Atherosclerosis : a problem of the biology of arterial wall cells and their interactions with blood components, Arteriosclerosis, 1:293 (1981).
2. J.E. French, Atherosclerosis in relation to the structure and function of the arterial intima, with special reference to the endothelium, Int. Rev. Exp. Pathol., 5:253 (1966).
3. E.A. Jaffe, C.R. Minick, B. Adelman, C.G. Becker, and R. Nachman, Synthesis of basement membrane collagen by cultured human endothelial cells, J. Exp. Med., 144:209 (1976).
4. F.B. Klynstra, E. Boelsma-van Houte, and C.J.F. Boh, Acid mucopolysaccharides and atherosclerosis, Lancet, 2:1150 (1967).
5. D.J. Loskutoff, and T.S. Edgington, Synthesis of a fibrinolytic activator and inhibitor by endothelial cells, Proc. Natl. Acad. Sci. USA, 74:3903 (1977).
6. R. Ross, and J. Glomset, Atherosclerosis and the arterial smooth muscle cell, Science, 180:1332 (1973).
7. R. Ross, and J. Glomset, The pathogenesis of atherosclerosis, N. Engl. J. Med., 295:369, 420 (1976).
8. M.B. Stemerman, and R. Ross, Experimental atherosclerosis? Fibrous plaque formation in primates, an electron microscopy study, J. Exp. Med., 136:769 (1972).
9. M.A. Gimbrone, Endothelial dysfunction and the pathogenesis of atherosclerosis, in : 'Atherosclerosis V', A.M. Gotto, L.C. Smith, B. Allen (eds.) Proc. 5th International Symposium Atherosclerosis, New York, Springer Verlag, 415 (1980).
10. J.F. Mustard, M.A. Packham, The role of blood and platelets in atherosclerosis and the complications of atherosclerosis, Thromb. Diath. Haemorrh., 33:444 (1975).
11. H. Holmsen, Biochemistry of the platelet release reaction, 'Biochemistry and Pharmacology of platelets', Ciba Foundation Symposium, Elsevier Norht Holland Biomedical Press, Amsterdam, 175 (1975).
12. H. Holmsen, The platelet, its membrane physiology and biochemistry, 'Clinics in Hematology', WB. Sanders Co. London, 2:235 (1972).
13. R. Ross, J. Glomset, B. Kariya, and L. Harker, A platelet-dependent serum factor that stimulates the proliferation of arterial smooth muscle cells in vitro, Proc. Natl. Acad. Sci. USA, 75:4001 (1975).
14. H.N. Antoniades, C.D. Scher, and C.D. Stiles, Purification of human platelet derived growth factor, Proc. Natl. Acad. Sci. USA, 76:1809 (1979).

15. R. Ross, and A. Vogel, The platelet derived growth factor, Cell, 14:203 (1978).

16. A.C.A. Carvalho, R.W. Colman, and R.S. Lees, Platelet function in hyperlipoproteinemia, N. Engl. J. Med., 290:434 (1974).

17. A. Nordoy, and J.M. Rodset, Platelet function and platelet phospholipids in patients with hyperbetalipoproteinemia : effect of nicotinic acid and clofibrate, Circulation, 50:570 (1974).

18. R. Fabrizewski, and K. Worowski, Enhancement of platelet aggregation and adhesiveness by lipoproteins, J. Ather. Res., 8:988 (1968).

19. E. Tremoli, P. Maderna, M. Sirtori, and C.R. Sirtori, Platelet aggregation and malondialdehyde formation in type IIa hypercholesterolemic patients, Haemostasis, 8:47 (1979).

20. E. Tremoli, G.C. Folco, E. Agradi, and C. Galli, Platelet thromboxanes and serum cholesterol, Lancet, 1:107 (1979).

21. A.C.A Carvalho, and R.S. lees, Platelets intravascular coagulation and fibrinolysis in hyperlipidemias : relationship to thromboembolic complications, Acta Med. Scand., suppl. 642:101 (1980).

22. M.J. Stuart, J.M. Gerrard, and J.G. White, Effect of cholesterol on production of thromboxane B_2 by platelets in vitro, N. Engl. J. Med., 302:6 (1980).

23. E. Tremoli, G.C. Ghiselli, P. Maderna, S. Colli, and C.R. Sirtori, Metformin reduces platelet hypersensitivity in hypercholesterolemic rabbits, Atherosclerosis, 41:53 (1982).

24. K.M. Shastri, A.C.A. Carvalho, and R.S. Lees, Platelet function and platelet lipid composition in dyslipoproteinemias, J. Lipid Res., 21:467 (1980).

25. J.L. Rodriguez, G.C. Ghiselli, D. Torreggiani, and C.R. Sirtori, Very low density lipoproteins in normal and cholesterol-fed rabbits : lipid and protein composition and metabolism, Atherosclerosis, 23:73 (1976).

26. J. Zahavi, J.D. Betteridge, N.A.G. Jones, D.J. Galton, and V.V. Kakkar, Enhanced in vivo platelet release reaction and malondialdehyde formation in patients with hyperlipidemia, The Amer. J. Med., 70:59 (1981).

27. C.A. Ludlam, Evidence for the platelet specificity of Beta-thromboglobulin and studies on its concentrations in healthy individuals, Br. J. Haematol., 41:271 (1979).

28. J. Dawes, R.C. Smith, D.S. Pepper, The release distribution and clearance of human Beta-thromboglobulin and platelet factor 4, Thromb. Res., 12:851 (1978).

29. V. Tamassia, G. Corvi, L.M. Fuccella, E. Moro, G. Tosolini, and E. Tremoli, Indobufen (K 3920), a new inhibitor of platelet aggregation : effect of food on bioavailability, pharmocokinetic and pharmacodynamic study during repeated oral administration to man, Europ. J. Clin. Pharmacol., 15:329 (1979).

30. G.H.R. Rao, G.J. Johnson, and J.G. White, Influence of epi-
    nephrine on the aggregation response of aspirin-treated
    platelets, Prostaglandins and Medicine, 5:45 (1980).
31. E. Tremoli, P. Maderna, S. Colli, in preparation.
32. J. Mehta, P. Mehta, and P. Couli, Platelet function studies in
    coronary heart disease. IX. Increased platelet prosta-
    glandin generation and abnormal platelet sensitivity to
    prostacyclin and endoperoxide analog in angina pectoris,
    Am. J. Cardiol., 46:943 (1980).
33. H. Sinzinger, G. Schernthaner, and J. Kaliman, Sensitivity of
    platelets to prostaglandins in coronary heart disease and
    angina pectoris, Prostaglandins, 22:773 (1981).
34. A. Dembinska-Kiec, T. Gryglewska, A. Zmuda, and R.J. Gryglews-
    ki, The generation of prostacyclin by arteries and by
    coronary vascular bed is reduced in experimental athero-
    sclerosis in rabbits, Prostaglandins, 14:1025 (1977).
35. V. D'Angelo, S. Villa, M. Mysliwiec, M.B. Donati, and G. de
    Gaetano, Defective fibrinolytic and prostacyclin-like
    activity in human atheromatous plaques, Thromb. Haemost.,
    38:535 (1978).
36. R.J. Gryglewski, Prostaglandins, Platelets and Atherosclero-
    sis, CRC Reviews, 290 (1980).
37. K. Fukuzumi, Lipids in atherosclerotic artery. The cause of
    atherosclerosis from the vieuw point of fat chemistry,
    Fette, Seifen, Anstrichm. 11:953 (1969).
38. J. Filipovic, and M. Rutemoller, Comparative studies on fatty
    acid synthesis in atherosclerotic and hypoxic human aorta,
    Atherosclerosis, 24:457 (1976).
39. M. Steiner, and J. Anastasi, Vitamin E, an inhibitor of the
    platelet release reaction, J. Clin. Invest., 57:732 (1976).
40. A. Szczeklik, R.J. Gryglewski, B. Domagala, A. Zmuda, J.
    Hartwich, E. Wozny, M. Grzywacz, J. Madej, and T. Gryglews-
    ka, Serum lipoproteins, lipid peroxides and prostacyclin
    biosynthesis in patients with coronary heart disease,
    Prostaglandins, 22:795 (1981).
41. A. Nordoy, B. Svensson, D. Wiebe, and J.C. Hoak, Lipoproteins
    and the inhibitory effect of human endothelial cells on
    platelet function, Circulation Res., 43:527 (1978).

INDEX

405